ADVANCES IN EXTRA-CORPOREAL PERFUSION THERAPIES

Edited by **Michael S. Firstenberg**

Advances in Extra-corporeal Perfusion Therapies
http://dx.doi.org/10.5772/intechopen.72562
Edited by Michael S. Firstenberg

Contributors

Pedro José Curi-Curi, Umberto Borrelli, Vladimir Ganyukov, Roman Sergeevich Tarasov, Dmitry Shukevich, Ivan Vereshchagin, Cristiano Amarelli, Jaime Hernandez-Montfort, Pia Wintermark, Asim Al Balushi, Samara Zavalkoff, Luiz Fernando Caneo, Vitor Barzilai, Zhongjun Wu, Robert Conway, Douglas Tran, Bartley Griffith, Antonio Loforte, Giuditta Coppola, Carlo Mariani, Francesco Grigioni, Giuseppe Marinelli, Gregorio Gliozzi, Takashi Murashita, Fevzi Sarper Türker, Faruk Ozalp, Stephan Schueler, Koen De Decker, Carmen Silvia Valente Barbas, Roberta Palazo, Gustavo Matos, Wai Ching , Simon Sin, Pauline Yeung Ng, Chun Wai Wallace Ngai, Chi Keung Peter Lai, Wai Kit Ricky Chan, Yuen Tin Andy Mok, Michael S. Firstenberg

First published in London, United Kingdom, 2019 by IntechOpen
IntechOpen is the global imprint of INTECHOPEN LIMITED, registered in England and Wales, registration number: 11086078, The Shard, 25th floor, 32 London Bridge Street
London, SE19SG – United Kingdom
Printed in Croatia

British Library Cataloguing-in-Publication Data
A catalogue record for this book is available from the British Library

Additional hard copies can be obtained from orders@intechopen.com

Advances in Extra-corporeal Perfusion Therapies, Edited by Michael S. Firstenberg
p. cm.
Print ISBN 978-1-78984-913-4
Online ISBN 978-1-78984-914-1

For EU product safety concerns:
IN TECH d.o.o., Prolaz Marije Krucifikse Kozulić 3, 51000 Rijeka, Croatia,
info@intechopen.com or visit our website at intechopen.com.

Meet the editor

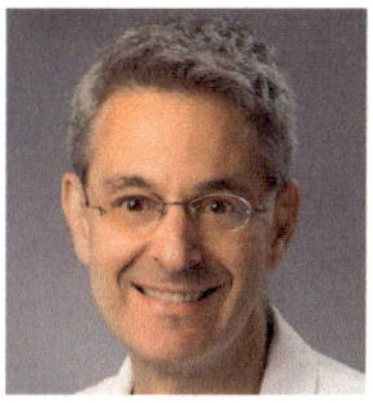

Dr. Michael S. Firstenberg is a board-certified thoracic surgeon practicing adult cardiac surgery at The Medical Center of Aurora (Colorado, USA) where he serves as the Chief of Cardiothoracic and Cardiovascular Surgery. He currently holds adjunct appointments in the Colleges of Medicine and Graduate Studies at Northeast Ohio Medical University. He also has a faculty appointment at Rocky Vista University. He attended Case Western Reserve University Medical School, received his general surgery training at University Hospitals in Cleveland, and completed a Fellowship in Thoracic Surgery at Ohio State University. He also obtained advanced training in heart failure surgical therapies at the Cleveland Clinic. He has lectured worldwide and written more than 100 peer-reviewed articles, numerous textbook chapters, and edited several books. In addition, he is active in numerous professional societies, clinical research projects, and multidisciplinary leadership committees.

Contents

Preface

Extracorporeal membrane oxygenation (ECMO), also known as extracorporeal life support (ECLS), has evolved to be a mainstream therapy for those requiring cardiac and/or pulmonary support for acute heart, lung, or heart and lung failure and who are failing convention medical therapies. With now thousands of cases being performed each year worldwide, it is rapidly evolving into a valuable tool in the management of critically ill patients. However, there is still much to be learned from a technology that is controversial, invasive, often costly, and limited by a lack of convincing randomized trials. As experiences continue to grow, the hope is that outcomes will improve with better patient selection, better technologies, better guidelines and protocols for management, and a general understanding of the importance of a team-based approach to managing extremely complex and sick patients. Critical to the success of ECMO therapy is the recognition that therapy must be initiated early before the onset of multiorgan dysfunction, neurologic complications, and the pathophysiologic consequences of irreversible shock. While veno-venous ECMO is often considered for pulmonary support and venoarterial for cardiac or cardiopulmonary support, the overlap in the management of acute heart and lung injuries can complicate decision making regarding the specific details of initiating therapy. Hopefully, the goal of this text—the second edition on the topic—is to lend further insights into some of the challenges that face providers, at all levels, who are interested in ECMO or use it routinely

This text is separated into several different areas—each focused on different aspects—of the management of patients who require extracorporeal support. While there are several chapters on general indications for ECMO—such as for respiratory failure, cardiogenic shock, and postcardiotomy shock—there are several chapters that focus on specific applications. These specific indications include, for example, the use of ECMO for high-risk catheter-based interventions, complications following heart transplant, and unusual applications in the neonate/newborn. Several chapters also focus on challenging topics regarding the use of ECMO and include advanced concepts such as flow optimization, pump circuit design, and the relationship to ventricular assist devices. An important topic that is also addressed is the role of simulation training as a critical component to the development and maintenance of competency of a high-quality ECMO program.

A theme common to many of the chapters is the importance of team communication with the focus on optimizing timely care for critically ill patients. Without doubt, the importance of early initiation of therapy prior to the sequelae of shock, hypoxemia, and hypotension resulting in end-organ damage and neurologic dysfunction cannot be overemphasized. Furthermore, once the decision is made to support a patient on ECMO, a primary goal is to allow the heart and/or lungs to rest and recover. Prevention of complications while on ECMO is also paramount to good outcomes and is discussed in many of the chapters that focus on specific applications of ECMO.

Undoubtedly, ECMO is rapidly expanding throughout the world as it evolves into a valuable tool for the management of critically ill patients in cardiogenic shock or acute respiratory failure (or often a combination of both) regardless of the etiology. Hopefully, as the technology expands, and providers become more experienced with the specific indications, patient selection, pump circuit technology and interactions with human physiology, and the foundations for effect team functioning will be outcomes that will continue to be important. This text serves only as an update, and is by no means comprehensive, to the rapidly expanding literature on the topic of extracorporeal support.

Michael S. Firstenberg, MD FACC FAIM
Chief, Cardiothoracic and Vascular Surgery
Director, Adult ECMO Program
Associate Professor of Surgery and Integrative Medicine (Adjunct)
Graduate Adjunct Faculty, College of Graduate Studies
Northeast Ohio Medical Universities
Rootstown, Ohio, USA

Teaching Faculty
The Rocky Vista University
Parker, Colorado, USA

The Medical Center of Aurora and Rose Hospitals
Aurora, Colorado, USA

Chapter 1

Introductory Chapter: ECMO - Growing Indications, Applications, and Understanding of a Complex Supportive Therapy

Michael S. Firstenberg and Jennifer M. Hanna

Additional information is available at the end of the chapter

http://dx.doi.org/10.5772/intechopen.81777

1. Introduction

This volume represents the second in a series of texts focused on extra-corporeal membrane oxygenation (ECMO), also known as extra-corporeal life support (ECLS) [1]. Over the years, there has been a continuous evolution of this therapy from a salvage form employed only in extreme cases in which all other treatment options have failed to a technology which is now considered a critical component in the toolbox of therapies and technologies used for acute cardiopulmonary failure. While initial experiences reported few survivors, these poor outcomes clearly had multifactorial etiologies [2]. Difficulties with primitive pump and circuit designs and technologies, a poor understanding of which patients derive the greatest benefit from this therapy, little understanding of the long-term physiologic implications of patient-circuit biologic interactions, a lack of management guidelines, and a generally limited understanding of managing patients and therapy-related complications while on "longer" term cardiopulmonary bypass have all contributed to the complexities of successful implementation of ECMO into mainstream medical and surgical practices. Nevertheless, over the past three decades, there has been continued refinement in all aspects of ECMO therapies, with a growing understanding of the role of ECMO as a life-saving therapy and potential bridge to transplantation while awaiting organ availability. ECMO has evolved into a treatment option that allows for an acutely injured heart and or lungs to heal, either allowing for recovery or serving as a "bridge" to a more definitive long-term end-organ replacement option such as ventricular assist devices or cardiopulmonary transplantation [3]. Many of these complex topics are addressed in this contemporary volume. However, there remains, without a doubt, much more to learn and understand. The successes of the ECMO technology reflect the tremendous efforts, dedication, and commitment by providers and researchers at all levels who recognize the enormous potential for ECMO to save lives and present options to those who would otherwise have none [4].

This volume reflects the substantial work of those, worldwide, who have dedicated a tremendous amount of time and energy into better understanding of how to achieve better outcomes with this complex technology. The common theme of this work has been the recognition that teamwork is the most important variable that contributes to clinical success.

Developing a comprehensive "ECMO team" is one of the first steps in building a successful program. This team must be prepared to initiate therapy at any time and in any setting, from those as controlled as an operating room to those as chaotic as an emergency room. While the specific members of the team might vary from program to program, there are several key features that must be established in advance. It is well recognized that effective teams must communicate and work well together—there must be uniform trust and a collective value attached to the expertise that each member brings to the bedside. It likewise needs to be recognized that traditional medical and professional hierarchies might be considered "old-fashioned" and potentially ineffective, if not dangerous. Additionally, there must be a willingness to embrace the concepts of crew resource management (CRM). The foundation of CRM is that every member of the team has a voice and that each voice is valued and respected. All members of the team must be encouraged, if not empowered, to speak up, particularly when there are safety concerns. In the context of an ECMO team, membership must include all of the following related disciplines, including, but not limited to (and in no particular order of importance, as all are important):

- Surgeons (cardiothoracic, general, trauma, emergency medicine)
- Critical care intensivists (pulmonary, surgical)
- Medical specialists (infectious disease, neurology, cardiology)
- Perfusionists
- Pharmacists
- Nursing (bedside, advanced practice providers)
- Respiratory therapists
- Palliative care
- Hospital leadership and administration
- … and, most importantly, a Champion for the program to lead the team

As a function of the tremendous dedication of resources needed to establish a successful ECMO program, there must be a well-established network of support and encouragement from hospital administration and leadership (**Figure 1**) [5].

Increasingly, in medicine there is a recognition that optimal outcomes, especially with complex and high-risk interventions, can be achieved using simulation training to help prepare

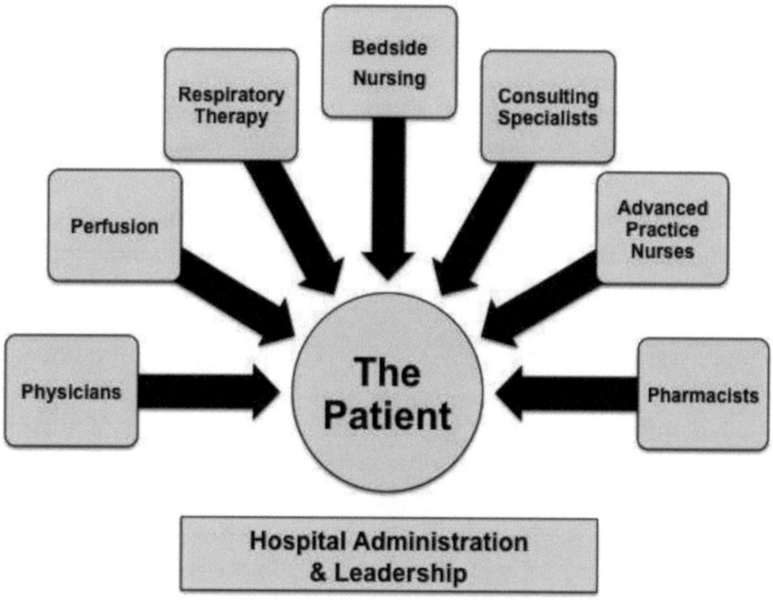

Figure 1. ECMO "team." Adopted from Reference intro chapter in Vol 1 (Ref [1]).

the team to respond in an effective and efficient manner. Especially in the case of time-sensitive therapies such as ECMO, in which minutes sometimes can determine an outcome, simulation training must be a component of every program and practiced regularly. In addition, the equipment and team must be prepared to implement this therapy at any time with established protocols, guidelines, and goals of therapy [6]. The chapter by Dr. Sin Wai Ching emphasizes and outlines these topics.

While patient selection is a critical aspect of ECMO therapy, determining the type of therapy to initiate and how is likewise paramount. In the previous text, some of the topics related to cannulation techniques [7] and pump/circuit design and development were addressed [8]. The chapter by Borrelli further elaborates on these technical aspects of pump/circuit design by outlining their 23-year experience with pump positioning and holder systems.

Regarding the specifics of patient selection and implementing ECMO therapy, it is important to understand how ECMO can (or should) be applied in specific clinical circumstances. Particularly, with regard to understanding the fundamental differences in veno-veno ECMO (VV-ECMO) for pulmonary support and veno-arterial ECMO (VA-ECMO) for cardiac or cardiopulmonary support, several chapters discuss general clinical topics related to the specifics of therapy. These include chapters in cardiogenic shock, severe acute respiratory distress syndrome, and generalized applications for longer-term support. More focused topics include:

- Primary graft failure after heart transplantation (Caneo)
- Post-cardiotomy cardiogenic shock (Murashita)
- Unusual applications in the newborn (Wintermark)
- Applications and support in high-risk percutaneous cardiac interventions (Ganyukov)

It cannot be emphasized enough that a key component to a successful program is appropriate patient selection. Despite all of the advances in ECMO therapies over the years, even successful programs have outcomes that range from 60 to 70% survival for veno-veno pulmonary support and 25–35% for veno-arterial cardiopulmonary and emergent cardiopulmonary resuscitation applications (E-CPR) [9, 10]. Lower success rates that improve over time and with experience, improvements in institutional protocols, and better (and more-timely) patient selection can be expected during the early phases of program development. Alternatively, as is seen with other areas of innovative clinical therapies, programmatic successes and improving outcomes spur attempts at treating higher-risk patients, resulting in a paradoxical loss in these successes. Programs with inordinately high success rates may be depriving salvageable patients the opportunity for survival because their indications are slightly out of the boundaries of the traditional indications for therapy. Programmatic attempts to support lower-risk patients on ECMO are not uncommon and are typically based on institutional (and personal) biases and outcomes. A series of successes with low-risk patients then rationalizes attempts to salvage the higher-risk patient. Conversely, lower than desired outcomes in higher-risk patients might then limit selection back to patients with low-risk characteristics. Regardless, institutional checks and balances as well as systems for reviewing metrics (clinical and financial) and outcomes should be established. Team engagement at all levels—from bedside nursing to top administrative leadership—is critical and cannot be emphasized enough. Membership and participation in the Extra-Corporeal Life Support Organization (ELSO: https://www.elso.org) should be encouraged, as it can provide data to help benchmark institutional success. Membership can also provide a community in which to partner with colleagues, exchange ideas, and as a resource for timely and important developments in the field.

Unusual patient populations represent one of the most rapidly expanding populations for ECMO. For example, early experiences with ECMO to support overwhelming septic shock in the setting of necrotizing soft tissues infections and the long-term, albeit anecdotal, good outcomes in this clinical scenario have prompted greater enthusiasm for otherwise potentially "hopeless" cases [11, 12]. There is also growing evidence supporting the role of ECMO to support high-risk catheter-based interventions, as discussed in the chapter by Dr. Ganyukov and colleagues [13]. However, such applications are limited to high-risk procedures in the catheterization laboratory, defined as those with impaired ventricular function and complex anatomy, or to reduce the risk of inherently high-risk or complex interventions, such as percutaneous aortic valve procedures (i.e., transcatheter aortic valve replacement), coronary or cardiac structural interventions, or electrophysiologic ablative procedures for complex arrhythmias. The key goal of providing ECMO support during these procedures is to reduce the risks of end-organ dysfunction. Hemodynamic instability (or even acute failure) during such procedures could be reduced by using ECMO to provide support for brief periods of time until the pathology is corrected (i.e., the coronary artery is stented or valve dilated) [14].

Managing patients on ECMO represents one of the greatest clinical challenges in all of medicine. Management on ECMO can be divided into several areas, and management decisions must be made in the context of the complex limitations of caring for patients on ECMO. For example, in many areas, there are little, if any, randomized evidence, established protocols, or even well-developed guidelines. Even simple interventions, like transporting patients on ECMO, require team-based decision-making regarding the potential risks and benefits [15].

Nevertheless, there are growing data to support some of the challenging aspects of caring for ECMO patients. Some of these topics, while discussed in the first volume [1], are expounded upon in this text. Such examples include chapters on flow optimization and reduction of ventricular distention by Dr. Amarelli and the application and role of modified ultrafiltration in pediatric patients by Curi-Curi and colleagues.

As with any intervention on complex and high-risk patients, transparent, frequent, and honest updates and communications with the family are critical to managing expectations. It is always important to emphasize that all communications should focus on the reality that even in ideal circumstances, morbidity and mortality in patients needing ECMO continue to be high. However, despite potentially long post-ECMO hospitalizations and recoveries, survivors can potentially return to productive lives [6].

2. Conclusions

The goal of this text is to demonstrate further that ECMO continues to evolve as a mainstream therapy for patients experiencing acute, severe, medically refractory cardiac and/or pulmonary

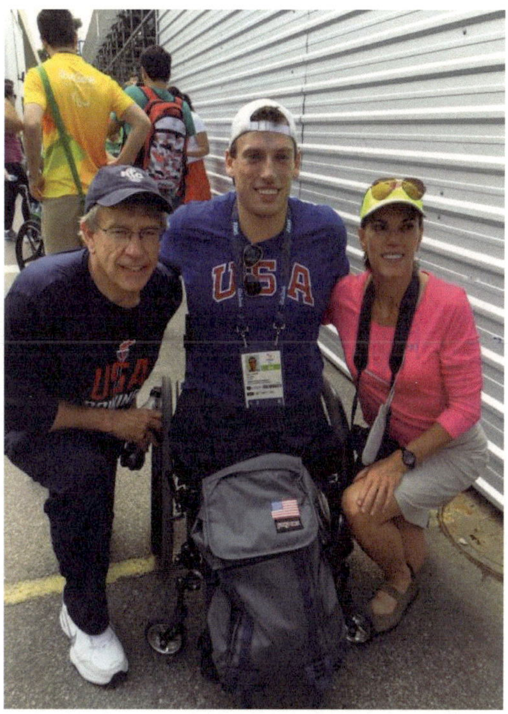

Figure 2. BH (center in wheelchair) with his parents after qualifying for the finals in the single-scull, arms and shoulder only, rowing competition in the 2016 Paralympics in Rio de Janeiro. BH, a five-time USA national champion in the event, represented the USA in Rio as a member of the Olympic team. In 2016 he was elected US Rowing "Rower of the Year". Several years prior, BH lost both legs to complications of a necrotizing soft tissue infection and required cardiopulmonary support with veno-arterial ECMO due to overwhelming septic shock. Picture used by permission by all represented [11, 12].

failure. Contemporary trials continue to define the role of ECMO as the search for better outcomes evolve [16]. However, as technology improves, guidelines get developed, protocols get refined, and experience grows, without a doubt, outcomes will improve [17]. ECMO, as a function of its invasiveness, need for substantial resources, and high-risk/high-reward, and novel technologies (i.e., the pump and oxygenators) often generates much institutional interest and intrigue. Unfortunately, many patients, despite such heroic efforts, die on ECMO—even when everything appears to have been done "right." As important as it is to learn from all outcomes, it is critical that everyone cherishes all victories. Victories can inspire, give hope, and motivate a team even when further treatments appear futile (**Figure 2**). Even though there is still much to learn on the topic of ECMO, the goal of this text is to continue to build on the growing foundation of experiences and the current literature. If nothing else, the hope is to help inspire those intrigued by and who believe in the potential benefits of ECMO [18].

Author details

Michael S. Firstenberg[1,2*] and Jennifer M. Hanna[1]

*Address all correspondence to: msfirst@gmail.com

1 Teaching Faculty, Rocky Vista University College of Osteopathic Medicine, Parker, Colorado, USA

2 Adjunct Faculty, College of Graduate Studies, Northeast Ohio Medical University, Rootstown, Ohio, USA

References

[1] Firstenberg MS. Introductory chapter: Evolution of ECMO from salvage to mainstream supportive and resuscitative therapy, extracorporeal membrane oxygenation. In: Firstenberg MS, editor. IntechOpen; 2016;**1**:3-10. Chapter 1. DOI: 10.5772/64345. Available from: https://www.intechopen.com/books/extracorporeal-membrane-oxygenation-advances-in-therapy/introductory-chapter-evolution-of-ecmo-from-salvage-to-mainstream-supportive-and-resuscitative-thera

[2] Zapol WM, Snider MT, Hill JD, Fallat RJ, Bartlett RH, Edmunds LH, et al. Extracorporeal membrane oxygenation in severe acute respiratory failure. A randomized prospective study. Journal of the American Medical Association. 1979;**242**(20):2193-2196

[3] Bartlett RH, Roloff DW, Custer JR, Younger JG, Hirschl RB. Extracorporeal life support: The University of Michigan experience. Journal of the American Medical Association. 2000;**283**(7):904-908

[4] Australia and New Zealand Extracorporeal Membrane Oxygenation (ANZ ECMO) Influenza Investigators, Davies A, Jones D, Bailey M, Beca J, Bellomo R, Blackwell N,

Forrest P, Gattas D, Granger E, Herkes R, Jackson A, McGuinness S, Nair P, Pellegrino V, Pettilä V, Plunkett B, Pye R, Torzillo P, Webb S, Wilson M, Ziegenfuss M. Extracorporeal membrane oxygenation for 2009 influenza A(H1N1) acute respiratory distress syndrome. Journal of the American Medical Association. 2009;**302**(17):1888-1895. Epub 2009 Oct 12

[5] Firstenberg MS, Swaminath D. Left ventricular failure—Extra-corporeal membrane oxygenation: An update. World Society of Cardiothoracic Surgeons Journal. 2016;**1**(1):12-14

[6] Firstenberg MS, Espinal EA, Abel EE, Tripathi RS, Papadimos TJ. Extracorporeal Membrane Oxygenation for Acute Cardiopulmonary Failure. Revista Argentina de Cirugia Cardiovascular. 2013;**9**:16-36. http://www.caccv.org.ar/raccv/V11-N01-06.pdf

[7] Chand Ramaiah, Ashok Babu . ECMO cannulation techniques, extracorporeal membrane oxygenation. Michael S. Firstenberg. IntechOpen; 2016;**1**:65-77. Chapter 4. DOI: 10.5772/64338. Available from: https://www.intechopen.com/books/extracorporeal-membrane-oxygenation-advances-in-therapy/ecmo-cannulation-techniques

[8] Khodeli N, Chkhaidze Z, Partsakhashvili J, Pilishvili O, Kordzaia D. Practical and theoretical considerations for ECMO system development, extracorporeal membrane oxygenation. Firstenberg MS, editor. IntechOpen; 2016. DOI: 10.5772/64267. Available from: https://www.intechopen.com/books/extracorporeal-membrane-oxygenation-advances-in-therapy/practical-and-theoretical-considerations-for-ecmo-system-development

[9] Rastan AJ, Dege A, Mohr M, Doll N, Falk V, Walther T, et al. Early and late outcomes of 517 consecutive adult patients treated with extracorporeal membrane oxygenation for refractory postcardiotomy cardiogenic shock. The Journal of Thoracic and Cardiovascular Surgery. 2010;**139**(2):302-311, 311.e1

[10] Peek GJ, Mugford M, Tiruvoipati R, Wilson A, Allen E, Thalanany MM, et al. CESAR trial collaboration. Efficacy and economic assessment of conventional ventilatory support versus extracorporeal membrane oxygenation for severe adult respiratory failure (CESAR): A multicentre randomised controlled trial. Lancet. 2009;**374**(9698):1351-1363

[11] Firstenberg MS, Abel E, Blais D, Louis LB, Steinberg S, Sai-Sudhakar C, et al. The use of extracorporeal membrane oxygenation in severe necrotizing soft tissue infections complicated by septic shock. The American Surgeon. 2010;**76**(11):1287-1289

[12] Pastoressa M, Haxton B, Firstenberg MS. Complex necrotizing soft-tissue infections managed with extra-corporeal membrane oxygenation: 10 year follow-up. International Journal of Academic Medicine. In press

[13] Spina R, Forrest AP, Adams MR, Wilson MK, Ng MK, Vallely MP. Veno-arterial extracorporeal membrane oxygenation for high-risk cardiac catheterisation procedures. Heart, Lung & Circulation. 2010;**19**(12):736-741. Epub 2010 Sep 24. Review

[14] Rihal CS, Naidu SS, Givertz MM, Szeto WY, Burke JA, Kapur NK, Kern M, Garratt KN, Goldstein JA, Dimas V, Tu T. 2015 SCAI/ACC/HFSA/STS clinical expert consensus statement on the use of percutaneous mechanical circulatory support devices in cardiovascular care: Endorsed by the American Heart Assocation, the Cardiological Society of India, and Sociedad Latino Americana de Cardiologia Intervencion; affirmation of value by the

Canadian Association of Interventional Cardiology-Association Canadienne de Cardiologie d'intervention. Journal of the American College of Cardiology. 2015;**65**(19):e7-26

[15] Hill S, Hejal R, Bowling SM, Firstenberg MS. Neurologic complications in patients receiving extracorporeal membrane oxygenation for influenza H1N1: Morbid but not futile. International Journal of Academic Medicine. 2016;**2**(1):22

[16] Combes A, Hajage D, Capellier G, Demoule A, Lavoué S, Guervilly C, et al. Extracorporeal membrane oxygenation for severe acute respiratory distress syndrome. New England Journal of Medicine. 2018;**378**(21):1965-1975

[17] Schmid C, Philipp A, Hilker M, Rupprecht L, Arlt M, Keyser A, et al. Venovenous extracorporeal membrane oxygenation for acute lung failure in adults. The Journal of Heart and Lung Transplantation. 2012;**31**(1):9-15

[18] Tulman DB, Stawicki SPA, Whitson BA, Gupta SC, Tripathi RS, Firstenberg MS, et al. Veno-venous ECMO: A synopsis of nine key potential challenges, considerations, and controversies. BMC Anesthesiology. 2014;**14**:65

Section 1

Applications

Chapter 2

Cardiogenic Shock

Fevzi Sarper Türker

Additional information is available at the end of the chapter

http://dx.doi.org/10.5772/intechopen.76688

Abstract

Cardiogenic shock (CS) is an end-organ hypoperfusion associated with heart failure. Any reason impairing acute left ventricular (LV) or right ventricular (RV) function may cause CS. The only way to avoid CS is to provide early reperfusion in myocardial infarction (MI) patients. CS is characterized by permanent or transient rearrangement of the entire circulatory system. According to the current IABP-SHOCK II trial, 74% of the patients with CSMI are treated with norepinephrine, 53% of them with dobutamine, 26% of them with epinephrine, 4% of them with levosimendan, and 4% of them with dopamine. Percutaneous circulatory support devices such as intra-aortic balloon pump (IABP), LV assist device (LVAD), or extracorporeal life support (ECLS) create treatment options for selected patients such as CS, cardiopulmonary resuscitation, or high-risk pPCI and CABG. Extracorporeal Life Support Organization (ELSO, 2017) evaluated that the use of ECLS/VA-ECMO should be considered when the mortality risk exceeds 50% despite optimal conventional treatment in case of acute severe heart or pulmonary failure, whereas it should be assessed as a primary indication when it exceeds 80%. Early and effective revascularization is the best treatment option for CS. Thus, the organizations on the national and global basis will play the most effective role for the short- and long-term survival of patients.

Keywords: cardiogenic shock, multiple organ failure, inotropes, left ventricular assist devices

1. Introduction

Cardiogenic shock (CS) is one of the most important issues dealt by cardiologists today and still needs solutions. Prevention, accurate diagnosis, urgent intervention, effective support for heart failure, and multi-organ failure (MOF) are what this endeavor involves [1]. More than 90% of patients arriving at the hospital with acute myocardial infarction (MI) are likely to survive [2]. CS occurs in approximately 5–8% of inpatients with ST-elevation myocardial infarctions (STEMI) and has a mortality rate of more than 30% [1]. CS is caused by end-organ hypoperfusion due to impaired cardiac pump function. Although CS-related mortality has declined significantly over the past decade, it continues to remain high, especially in cases of its coexistence with ischemic heart disease. Acute coronary syndrome (ACS) is still the most common cause of CS despite significant advances that have been made in its diagnosis and treatment. The most successful form of treatment is primary percutaneous coronary intervention (pPCI), which is carried out as rapidly as possible [3]. The recent research has suggested that the peripheral vasculature and neurohormonal and cytokine systems also play a role in the pathogenesis and persistence of CS.

In cases where CS complicates MI (CSMI), only one in two patients survives after 1 year [4, 5]. In a large study including 5782 patients, CSMI had developed in 2.5% of the patients with STEMI before admission to hospital, in 4.3% of them on the first day of hospitalization, and in 2.3% of them afterward [6]. For non-STEMI (NSTEMI) patients, these ratios were 1.2% for each condition [6]. Mortality rates were 45.7% before the hospitalization, 32.8% in the early period, and 54.1% in the late period [7]. Of 1422 CSMI patients, in the SHOCK Trial Registry, a shock is developed following left ventricular failure in 78.5% of them, acute mitral insufficiency in 6.9% of them, acute ventricular septal defect in 3.9% of them, right ventricular failure in 2.8% of them, cardiac tamponade in 1.4% of them, and other reasons in 6.7% of them [8].

2. Diagnosis and causes

2.1. Definition

CS is an end-organ hypoperfusion associated with heart failure. In terms of the hemodynamic parameters used in the definition of CS, it is characterized by a systolic blood pressure of 80–90 mmHg, a cardiac index below 1.8 L min^{-1} m^{-2} without support and below 2.0–2.2 L min^{-1} m^{-2} with support, a mean arterial baseline under 30 mmHg, and a pulmonary capillary wedge pressure of 15 or >18 mmHg [9].

2.2. Diagnosis

However, it is not necessary to measure these parameters in order to make the diagnosis of CS. Hypotension is not observed at the start in one-fourth of the patients diagnosed with CSMI. In this case, the diagnosis is made according to the clinical findings of organ hypoperfusion including extremity coldness, oliguria, and changes in mental condition such as agitation. It is imperative to distinguish MI-related complications, from primarily mechanical complications. The main complications are ventricular septal defect, free wall, and papillary muscle rupture developing after MI. Usually, if it is the first MI event and there is no anterior involvement, it should be considered that mechanical complications may have occurred. First of all, diagnosing CSMI should begin by quickly obtaining a 12-lead ECG (STEMI) and examining the clinical findings with respect to CS. In rare instances, the diagnosis of NSTEMI can be made based on the clinical criteria and troponin levels. Performing a rapid echocardiography (ECHO) before PCI may discount these complications, and, at the same time, the detection of any pre-angiographic valve disease may alter the revascularization approach. Bleeding, infection, and/or intestinal ischemia may also cause shock in cases of MI. In these situations, patient survivability depends on being skeptical and makes a rapid diagnosis along with correct intervention.

2.3. Causes

Anything that impairs acute left ventricular (LV) or right ventricular (RV) function may cause CS. In cases of acute myopericarditis, tako-tsubo, and hypertrophic cardiomyopathy, shock may present with ST elevation in which cardiac markers are released without coronary artery disease. Stress-induced cardiomyopathy, also known as apical ballooning or tako-tsubo cardiomyopathy, is a syndrome of acute LV dysfunction after emotional or respiratory distress leading to CS in 4.2% of cases [10]. Chordal rupture caused by degenerative diseases and trauma and acute valvular insufficiency caused by endocarditis may also cause CS. Severe aortic insufficiency (regurgitation) or coronary involvement developing as a result of aortic dissection may cause CS. Stress occurring in cases of severe aortic or mitral stenosis can cause shock. Cardiac tamponade and massive pulmonary embolism may cause shock without pulmonary congestion.

2.4. Risk identification

The only way to avoid CS is to provide early reperfusion in MI patients. In a randomized trial, CS occurred less frequently compared to PCI in STEMI patients treated with thrombolytic therapy within the first 2 hours of symptom onset before hospitalization (1.3 vs. 5.3%, $p = 0.032$) [11]. Low blood pressure and accelerated heart rhythm in patients admitted to hospital suggest shock. Advanced age, anterior MI, hypertension, diabetes mellitus, multivessel coronary artery disease, previous MI or angina, or being diagnosed with heart failure, STEMI, and left bundle branch block are risk factors for the development of CS [12].

3. Physiopathology

CS is characterized by permanent or transient rearrangement of the entire circulatory system. The primary cause of many CS instances is the failure of LV pump function, but other components of the circulatory system, inadequate compensation, or additional defects can also contribute to this condition. The fact that surviving patients demonstrate improved functionality explains that all or some of these changes are completely reversible.

3.1. Left ventricle

The degree of LV myocardial dysfunction usually initiates CS. In most cases, it is not severe. Left ventricular dysfunction reflects newly onset irreversible damage, reversible ischemia, and previous infarct-related injury in CS. Myocardial injury causes systolic and diastolic dysfunction. Low blood pressure helps by reducing afterload due to the unique position of the heart even though it causes damage at the same time by impairing the coronary blood flow. It can lead to an increase in ischemia and cell death at the border and remote zone of the infarct area. Reduction in coronary perfusion causes deterioration in perfusion of the heart and other vital organs by causing a decline in cardiac output (CO). Metabolic impairments occur inside and outside of the infarct region. Hypoperfusion leads to catecholamine discharge, resulting in an increase in contractility and peripheral blood flow, while, at the same time, increased contractility causes increased oxygen demand on the part of the myocardium, as well as arrhythmia and myocardial toxic effects [13]. Systemic inflammation may play a limiting role in peripheral vascular compensatory response or may only be considered as an epiphenomenon. Revascularization makes the ischemia disappear, but increased CO or LV ejection fraction (LVEF) could not be shown as a benefit of revascularization. Revascularization significantly increases the quality of life as well as survival rates [14, 15].

Vasoconstrictors and inotropic agents are able to correct CO and peripheral circulation temporarily, but they do not break this vicious cycle. Although rapid intra-aortic balloon pump (IABP) application improves ischemia transiently and supports the circulation, it is not the final solution. Correcting coronary occlusion through surgery or PCI will break the vicious cycle and increase survival.

In the light of CS's complex pathophysiology, the cause of shock in many cases is a severe impairment in contractility and moderate disruption in the LVEF [16]. LVEF was found approximately 30% in the SHOCK trial [17]. In terms of LVEF value, the SHOCK trial obscures many post-MI studies in which LVEF decreases with or without heart failure. The LVEF in this study generally does not indicate that the magnitude of myocardial damage causes CS, although it is measured in patients with inotropic and/or IABP support. LVEF is the same in the acute phase of CS, and 2 weeks later, its functional status is different [18]. Even when there are conditions in which there is no serious mitral regurgitation and the LV is preserved, CS still develops in some patients [19]. LVEF is a prognostic indicator in patients who end up with shock. The size of the LV is small or normal in about half of patients with CS [19]. LV dilatation is an adaptive mechanism of failure in order to provide stroke volume in the early phase. LV dilatation in the chronic phase may be maladaptive. The LV end-diastolic volume was shown to increase slightly to 15 mL as a result of the serially performed echo within the first 2 weeks in the survivors of CS [18].

3.2. Right ventricle

The RV may cause or contribute to CS. Shock based on the dominance of the RV occurs in 5% of CSMI cases. RV insufficiency may limit CO, ventricular interdependence, or both of them by decreasing LV filling. The treatment of patients with RV dysfunction and shock focuses not on reducing CO and on maintaining adequate right heart filling pressure in order to provide adequate LV preload in the conventional sense. However, in these patients, there is usually a very high RV end-diastolic pressure above 20 mmHg due to RV dysfunction [20]. The increase in RV end-diastolic pressure shifts the interventricular septum to the left via mechanical pressure, thus impairing the functions by reducing the filling [21]. This means that aggressive fluid resuscitation in RV dysfunction is actually the incorrect method. Inotropic therapy should be initiated if it persists despite optimization of RV end-diastolic pressure in the CS secondary to the RV. Maintaining RV end-diastolic pressures between 10 and 15 mmHg provides the best CO [22]. Inhaled nitric oxide (NO) may be useful in reducing pulmonary vascular resistance and promoting forward flow. Shock secondary to RV dysfunction has a mortality rate as high as that of shock secondary to LV dysfunction. The benefit of revascularization was similar in the SHOCK registry for patients with primarily RV dysfunction and those with primarily LV dysfunction [20].

Hypoperfusion of the extremities and vital organs is a sign of CS. MI-induced CO reduction and persistence of ischemia both result in the release of catecholamines leading to constriction of the peripheral arteries and, thus, affecting the maintenance of perfusion to the vital organs. Attempts to improve peripheral and coronary circulation at the expense of elevation in afterload by increasing the levels of vasopressin and angiotensin II at the beginning of MI and shock will subsequently lead to impairment in myocardial functions. The continuation of neurohormonal cascade activation will also increase acute pulmonary edema while attempting to improve perfusion by causing water and salt retention. The reflex increase of systemic vascular resistance (SVR) mechanism is not fully effective. The SHOCK trial showed that SVR was at mean levels during CS despite vasopressor treatment and that in some cases it was even as low as in a septic shock [23]. Sepsis was suspected in 18% of the cohort of the SHOCK trial, 74% of which developed positive bacterial cultures. SVR was lower in these patients, and low SVR preceded the clinical diagnosis of infection and culture positivity by days [23].

Findings and observations of MI may cause systemic inflammatory response syndrome (SIRS). Inappropriate vasodilation as part of SIRS results in impaired perfusion of the intestinal tract leading to the transmigration of bacteria and sepsis. As the duration of shock increases, so the possibility of SIRS increases [24].

Sometimes, the medications given can contribute to the development of CS. Numerous medications such as beta-blockers, angiotensin-converting enzyme inhibitors, and morphine were associated with the development of shock. The early use of these treatments contributes in a small way to increase the risk of CS. However, given the large patient population receiving this treatment, the number of incidents it causes significant [25, 26]. The timing of CS (early after medication initiation) in the placebo-controlled, randomized trials of β-blockage and angiotensin-converting enzyme inhibition combined with their mechanisms of action indicates that they may contribute to the development of CS in those at high risk.

Diuretics may also contribute to the development of post-MI shock [14]. The earliest effect of ischemia is usually a reduction in LV compliance. MI may cause pulmonary edema before a drop occurs in CO. The redistribution of intravascular volume to the lungs causes a clear decline in the volume of circulating plasma before heart failure. High-dose diuretics administered subsequently further reduce plasma volume. Low diuretic dose coupled with low-dose nitrates and positional measures to decrease preload (e.g., seated position with legs down) should be attempted in patients with MI and pulmonary edema to avoid precipitating shock. Excessive volume loading in patients with RV infarction may also cause or contribute to shock.

4. Treatment

4.1. Supportive treatment

For MI, giving aspirin and heparin routinely along with antithrombotic treatment is recommended. Since emergency coronary artery bypass grafting (CABG) therapy can be required depending on the results of coronary angiography, clopidogrel therapy may be delayed to the period after emergency angiography. There are indications of clopidogrel in all patients who are to undergo PCI, and this will be useful in MI patients with shock depending on the information obtained from non-shock MI patients. The use of vasodilators including negative inotropes and nitroglycerin should be avoided. The arterial oxygen and pH levels should be kept within normal limits in order to minimize the ischemia. Intensive insulin therapy improves survival in critically ill patients with hyperglycemia and is a recommended course of action in complicated MI [27]. An easy indication should be established in order to initiate mechanical ventilation with mask or endotracheal intubation. Positive end-expiratory pressure reduces preload and afterload. Mechanical ventilation also reduces respiratory workload.

4.2. Hemodynamic management

Pulmonary artery (PA) (Swan-Ganz) catheterization is frequently recommended in order to confirm the diagnosis of CS. There has been a decline in the use of PA catheters following the controversy caused by a prospective observational study suggesting that PA catheters are associated with poor outcome [28]. The use of PA catheters in severely hypotensive patients with MI can be performed according to patient [27]. At present, many clinics do not prefer PA catheter for CS treatment anymore. Clinical assessment with ECHO is a reasonable alternative: Both PA systolic pressure and wedge pressure can be accurately estimated with Doppler ECHO. In particular, finding a short mitral deceleration time (≤140 ms) is highly predictive of pulmonary capillary wedge pressure ≥20 mmHg in CS [19].

4.3. Pharmacological treatment

According to the German-Austrian CSMI guideline, dobutamine should be preferred as an inotrope option, norepinephrine as a vasopressor option, and levosimendan over phosphodiesterase III inhibitors in case of refractiveness to catecholamines [29]. In the current IABP-SHOCK II trial, 74% of the patients with CSMI were treated with norepinephrine, 53% of them with dobutamine, 26% of them with epinephrine, 4% of them with levosimendan, and 4% of them with dopamine [5, 30].

Since the survival outcomes of high-dose vasopressor use are poor, pharmacological support including these agents should be kept to a minimum [31]. This indicates the underlying serious hemodynamic derangement and toxic effects. Inotropic agents play a central role in the treatment because the event initiating the shock is contractile dysfunction. Unfortunately, inotropes increase myocardial ATP consumption, so when the heart fails and supply is already limited, short-term hemodynamic healing occurs at the expense of increased oxygen demand. In order to provide coronary and systemic perfusion, the use of inotropic and vasopressor agents is required until IABP is placed or shock recovers. Norepinephrine is recommended in cardiac hypotension due to its high potential [27]. Both dopamine and norepinephrine have inotropic properties, but dobutamine is often required in addition.

4.3.1. Norepinephrine

The mean arterial pressure is effectively increased by intravenous infusions of norepinephrine at 0.1–1 μg/kg/min. According to the SOAP II study conducted using 1679 patients who developed shock due to various etiologies, norepinephrine with a rate of 45.9% showed a 50.2% lower mortality rate compared to dopamine in the total population and produced significantly lower arrhythmia particularly atrial fibrillation (12.4 vs. 24.1%). Norepinephrine showed significantly better survival rates than dopamine treatment in the prospectively defined subgroup of CS patients [32].

4.3.2. *Dobutamine*

The inotropic dose range of dobutamine is between 2 and 20 μg/kg/min [33]. Based on the results of a multicenter cohort observational study on 1058 shock patients, following the German-Austrian guideline recommendations, the use of dopamine is an independent risk factor for mortality (p = 003), while this is not the case for dobutamine and norepinephrine [34]. Based on prospectively collected real-life data, epinephrine should be used only for resuscitation because it produces advanced organ damage and it is associated with higher mortality compared to dobutamine, levosimendan, and norepinephrine [35]. The European Association of Cardiology guidelines recommended the combination of levosimendan with a vasopressor agent in CSMI patients refractory to catecholamines or using it with a phosphodiesterase III inhibitor such as enoximone or milrinone, with or without dobutamine in intractable CS (ICS) patients [33]. The use of levosimendan or phosphodiesterase III inhibitors in shock patients who previously used chronic beta-blockers provides a better stabilization than dobutamine, and the results are similar to those with acute decompensated heart failure [36]. The German-Austrian CSMI guidelines recommend levosimendan, not PDE III inhibitors [29]. More importantly, PDE III inhibitors are not recommended at all in STEMI patients according to the guidelines of the European Society of Cardiology (ESC) [37].

4.3.3. *Phosphodiesterase III inhibitors*

Enoximone (Perfan™) and milrinone are selective PDE III inhibitors that increase inotropy and decrease systemic vascular resistance. They do not cause changes in myocardial oxygen consumption.

At the same time, they can be combined with dobutamine, because their combined inotropic effect is greater than that of dobutamine and PDE III inhibitor alone [38]. When "bridge to transplantation" was evaluated according to a prospective randomized trial, it did not prove superior to dobutamine, and it also caused high treatment costs [27].

4.3.4. *Levosimendan (Simdax™)*

Levosimendan, which has been used for the treatment of decompensated heart failure, is a calcium-sensitizing drug with inotropic agents. It increases the myocardial contractility with vasodilatory properties; meanwhile, diastolic relaxation is not impaired. It increased the cardiac contractility mediated by calcium sensation of troponin C, vasodilation through the opening of potassium channels on the sarcolemma of smooth muscle cells in the vasculature, and cardioprotection through the opening of mitochondrial potassium channels in the cardiomyocytes.

A single-center prospective randomized study comparing levosimendan and a PDE III inhibitor enoximone examined 88 patients with CSMI refractory to catecholamines. The endpoint was identified as the resolution of shock, but the study was prematurely terminated by the ethics committee due to the significant superiority of levosimendan in the transient analyses. Only 32 CSMI patients could be evaluated. The primary endpoint of 30-day survival was found to be significantly higher in the levosimendan group than in the enoximone group (69% 11/16 vs. 37%, 6/16) [38]. According to nonrandomized trials, levosimendan has positive effects such as increasing CO, LV stroke work index, and systemic vascular resistance [39, 40]. It has also been documented to improve right ventricular function by increasing the RV cardiac power index (rVCPI) and decreasing pulmonary vascular resistance [39]. A small-scale study with 22 CSMI patients comparing levosimendan therapy with dobutamine treatment did not reveal any difference in 1-year mortality [41].

4.4. Percutaneous assist devices

Percutaneous circulatory support devices such as IABP, LV assist device (LVAD), or extracorporeal life support (ECLS) create treatment options for selected patients such as CS, cardiopulmonary resuscitation, or high-risk pPCI and CABG.

Percutaneous mechanical cardiac support (pMCS) devices, venoarterial extracorporeal membrane oxygenation (VA-ECMO), and ECLS applications are quite appealing for patients with CSMI because these therapeutic approaches offer an option that can improve cardiac output by avoiding the cardiotoxic effects of catecholamine therapy. IABP as passive pMCS and many active pMCS and VA-ECMO/ECLS are used [42–46]. However, in a review of an IABP-SHOCK II trial conducted on 600 patients with CSMI, it was observed that no benefit was provided in postinfarction CS treated with IABP and without mechanical complications compared to conventional treatment. This condition was downgraded from Class I (level of evidence C) to Class IIIA in the European guidelines [5, 47]. The use of active pMCS and VA-ECMO, and the advantages that they can create, should be respected. However, there are no high-quality RCTs supporting the general use of active pMCS in patients with refractory CSMI [48, 49]. As a result, ESC guidelines do not suggest the routine use of IABP in CS [33, 37, 50, 51]. It can be used simultaneously in refractory CS for a short term as a bridge leading to the implantation of a durable left ventricular assist device depending on the age, comorbid factors, and neurological status of the patient [52]. ECLS/VA-ECMO may provide a respiratory support in patients with the coexistence of severe cardiac and pulmonary insufficiency. Although there are no randomized trials that can assess ECLS/VA-ECMO in CS, observational studies have shown that it is useful in CS occurring during acute and chronic heart failure and cardiac arrest patients [53, 54]. Current ESC guidelines for heart failure suggest the use of ECLS/VA-ECMO or other support devices for the treatment of acute heart failure until cardiac and organ functions are improved in CS.

Extracorporeal Life Support Organization (ELSO) 2017 suggested that the use of ECLS/VA-ECMO should be considered when the mortality risk exceeds 50% despite optimal conventional treatment in case of acute severe heart or pulmonary failure, whereas it was suggested as a primary indication when the rate exceeds 80%. The main goal of the ECLS/VA-ECMO is to provide rapid circulatory and respiratory stabilization until an adequate improvement in cardiac loading is obtained in refractory CS. Although there are no controlled randomized

http://dx.doi.org/10.5772/intechopen.76688

trials on the efficacy of ECLS/VA-ECMO, it was established as an indication of Class IIb in European guidelines and indication of Class IIa in American guidelines after observational studies demonstrated its beneficial effects on survival compared to conventional treatment [51, 54, 55]. Early application of ECLS/VA-ECMO was recommended to prevent imminent multi-organ failure since it maximizes cardiac recovery potential [46]. The ECLS VA-ECMO is also used in postcardiotomy CS occurring in the range 0.2–6% after cardiac operation [56].

There is a relative contraindication in patients that have recovered from life-incompatible conditions, in situations where preexisting conditions adversely affect the quality of life (the state of the central nervous system, end-stage malignancy, high-risk systemic bleeding complications), and in conditions that would not cause any benefit such as extreme old age or dependency; anatomical obstructions, if the treatment would take too long; or the existence of a fatal disease.

4.4.1. IABP

This has been the mainstay of mechanical CS treatment for a long period of time. IABP has become the most commonly used pMCS in the last decade. Some 10,000 IABPs were implanted in Germany alone in 2009 [57]. IABP, which is made of a polyurethane membrane mounted on a vascular 7.0–8.0 Fr catheter, is positioned in the descending thoracic aorta just distal to the left subclavian artery. This device matches its inflation and deflation times according to the cardiac cycle. The use of IABP improves coronary and peripheral circulation by increasing LV performance with diastolic balloon inflation and reduces afterload with systolic balloon deflation. IABP enables an increase in diastolic blood pressure and decrease in end-systolic pressure without affecting the mean blood pressure, cardiac output, cardiac power index, serum lactate levels, or by changing the doses of catecholamines. Accurate timing of inflation and deflation provides optimal support. Not all patients benefit from the support of IABP. It is a good prognostic indicator if it provides hemodynamic benefit [58]. If the procedure can be performed quickly, it should be applied as soon as possible before revascularization or transfer and in the presence of experienced operators. In the large National Registry of Myocardial Infarction, the use of IABP was independently associated with survival at centers with higher rates of IABP use [59], whether or not PCI, fibrinolytic therapy, or no reperfusion was used [43]. Some of the many nonrandomized trials on the use of IABP in CSMI are positive, but those with neutral outcomes have also been seen [46]. Sjauw et al. summarized the available data in a systematic review and meta-analysis on IABP in STEMI patients with and without CS including nine cohorts of patients with CSMI (n = 10,259). The use of IABP in patients treated with thrombolysis showed a significant decrease in 30-day mortality by 18% when compared to unsupported needs of highly revascularization rates. In contrast, the use of IABP in patients treated with pPCI showed a significant increase in 30-day mortality by 6% [60].

A randomized IABP-SHOCK trial conducted with 45 PCMI-treated patients with CSMI proved that the simultaneous administration of IABP did not correct multi-organ dysfunction syndrome (MODS) and hemodynamics [61]. When an IABP-SHOCK II trial that had been performed afterward was examined, it was seen that the administration of IABP along with early revascularization on 600 patients with CSMI had no effect on 30-day, 6-month, and

12-month mortality [5, 47]. In a review made by the Cochrane group, the treatment of IABP was compared with the standard treatment (n = 384) and three LVAD treatments (n = 45) in four randomized clinical trials covering a total of 790 patients with CSMI in which the majority of whom had been treated with the pPCI. No difference was noted in terms of 30-day mortality in the group treated with IABP compared to the group in which IABP was not used. It is thought that it can theoretically cause fewer complications and better support due to the improvement in the current technology coupled with improvements in automation, flexibility in treatment algorithms, and advances in placement speed and sheathless insertion thanks to its smaller catheter body, but there is no information to support these considerations.

IABP has rare but serious complications such as major bleeding, stroke, and local and systemic infections. When compared with LVAD and ECLS, it has the lowest complication rate. Limb ischemia is the most commonly occurring vascular complication, but their rates have been reduced due to its small-diameter catheter and sheathless insertion. Aortic dissection, retroperitoneal hemorrhage, femoral hematomas, arteriovenous fistulas, and femoral pseudoaneurysms, which may be seen in any femoral artery procedure, may also occur in IABP. Ischemia and necrosis in certain areas may occur with the embolization of aortic atherosclerotic components to the peripheral vascular bed. Visceral organs may be affected adversely as a result of inappropriate balloon catheter diameter and placement. In contrast to all of these clinical observations, randomized IABP-SHOCK II trial revealed that high complication rates secondary to IABP were not observed in patients treated with IABP.

4.4.2. LVADs

LV assist devices (LVADs) are theoretically appealing since they break the vicious ischemia cycle by providing temporary circulatory support, breaking hypotension and myocardial dysfunction, enabling recovery from the stunned and hibernating myocardium, and allowing the reversal of neurohumoral change. Active pMCS is hemodynamically more potent than IABP [42, 43, 46, 48]. However, device-related complications and permanent organ damage are the most important limiting factors. LVADs support the return of the oxygenated blood drained from the left side of the heart into the systemic arteries with pulsed circulation or continuous flow by circulating it through a device. Surgically implanted LVADs pump the blood taken from the apex of the left ventricle via a cannula.

4.4.2.1. The TandemHeart (CardiacAssist Inc., Pittsburgh, PA)

The TandemHeart is a left atrial-to-femoral arterial LVAD device. It drains the blood through a cannula placed in the left atrium entering from the femoral vein transseptally. The blood returns to a systemic artery, the femoral artery, and perfuses into the thoracic and abdominal aorta in a retrograde manner. The system is capable of delivering flow up to 4.0 L/min at 7500 rpm. The patients with CSMI treated with TandemHeart and Impella® family placed by passing through the aortic valve and pPCI were evaluated in small randomized clinical trials [48]. In the meta-analysis of four trials randomizing 148 patients treated with TandemHeart, Impella®, or Impella CP®, the results were compared with the patient group treated with IABP [48, 62–65]. Although hemodynamics were better in patients treated with pMCS, no

http://dx.doi.org/10.5772/intechopen.76688

significant difference was detected in terms of mortality, but complications such as bleeding and leg ischemia were higher in that group.

4.4.2.2. The Impella® (Abiomed)

The Impella® pump is a nonpulsatile axial flow pump consisting of a suction cannula with a turbine positioned in the LV in order to push the blood into the ascending aorta. It has three versions 2.5, 5, and CP. Impella® is inserted through the femoral artery by 2.5 and CP standard catheterization procedures into the ascending aorta and then placed in the left ventricle by passing it through the aortic valve. The inlet area, located at the distal tip of the cannula, has four openings that allow the blood to be drained into the inlet and channeled through the cannula. The placement of Impella 5.0® is the same except that it requires surgical cutdown. The axial flow pump system reduces the left ventricular load and causes a reduction in the LV wall stress.

The Impella 2.5®, Impella CP®, Impella 5.0®, and Impella LD® catheters, in conjunction with the Automated Impella® Controller (collectively, "Impella® System Therapy"), are temporary ventricular support devices intended for short-term use (≤4 days for the Impella 2.5® and Impella CP® and ≤6 days for the Impella 5.0® and Impella LD®) and indicated for the treatment of ongoing cardiogenic shock that occurs immediately (<48 h) following acute myocardial infarction or open heart surgery or in the setting of cardiomyopathy, including peripartum cardiomyopathy, or myocarditis as a result of isolated left ventricular failure that is not responsive to optimal medical management and conventional treatment measures (including volume loading and use of pressors and inotropes, with or without IABP). The intent of Impella® System Therapy is to reduce ventricular work and to provide the circulatory support necessary to allow heart recovery and early assessment of residual myocardial function (http://www.abiomed.com/impella/impella-25) (**Figure 1**).

4.4.2.3. HeartMate PHP (Thoratec Corporation)

This axial device system is composed of a percutaneously inserted, Nitinol-covered cannula through the femoral artery, integrated with a tribune (impeller) having a diameter of 13 Fr. Its major design feature is a collapsible elastomeric impeller and Nitinol cannula giving this device the lowest profile insertion cannula with the highest flow. When it is placed by passing through the aortic valve once, it may create a continuous flow of more than 4 L/min at reasonable operating speeds, resulting in reduced LV end-diastolic pressure and volume. When it has to be replaced again, the system collapsed by 13 Fr. The information is limited to a small registry trial made up of 46 patients, and the results of which have not been published yet.

4.4.2.4. The iVAC 2L (Terumo Interventional Systems)

The iVAC 2L system is introduced percutaneously through the femoral artery and can provide a pulsatile support of approximately 2 L/min using an extracorporeal membrane pump via a 17 Fr cannula. In the systolic phase of the heart, the blood is aspirated from the LV through the catheter lumen into the membrane pump. During the diastolic phase, the pump

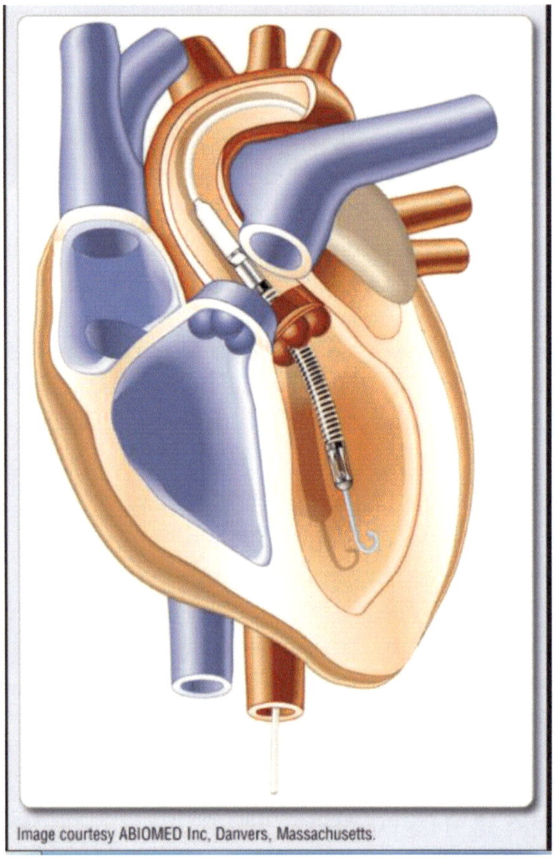

Figure 1. Installation of Impella®.

ejects the blood back through the catheter, then reopens the catheter valve, and delivers the blood to the ascending aorta through the side outflow port, thereby creating an "extra heart beat." Data are limited to a small case series, and the clinical impact of this device needs to be investigated further (**Figure 2**).

4.4.3. VA-ECMO

Advances made since the introduction of the first cardiopulmonary bypass system in 1953 have enabled the development of percutaneous devices. In fact, today's VA-ECLS devices consist of venous and arterial cannulas, tubing, a membrane oxygenator with gas blender, a continuous flow centrifugal pump, and a heat exchanger compensating for heat loss originating from extracorporeal circulation. Generally, a 16–19 Fr arterial cannula is placed in the ascending aorta, and an 18–21 Fr venous cannula is placed in the right atrium. The blood drained from the right atrium is pumped into the heat exchanger and membrane oxygenator and eventually returns to the femoral artery. The blood is drained from the main points separated from cardiopulmonary bypass (CPB) devices into an open reservoir passively, whereas there is a closed circuit in the VA-ECLS devices, and negative pressure is applied for venous blood

http://dx.doi.org/10.5772/intechopen.76688

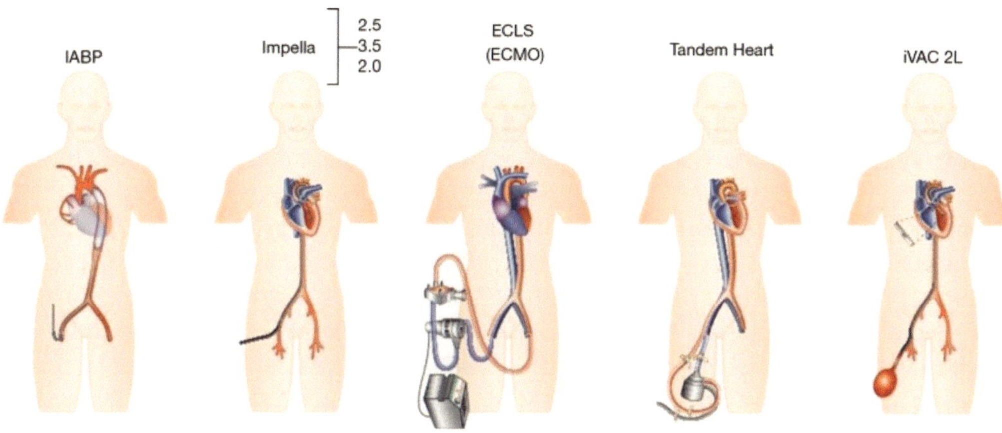

Figure 2. Mechanical cardiac support devices.

return [66]. The pump continues to provide pulsatile arterial blood pressure with the continuous flow until the circulation is fully supported by a cardiopulmonary bypass device. ECLS is used in LV, RV, and biventricular insufficiency with the flow exceeding 5 L/min.

Venoarterial extracorporeal oxygenation or its synonym extracorporeal life support (ECLS) and LVAD were commonly used as a bridge for heart transplantation in CS patients [67]. ECLS takes the blood circulation out of the body into a membrane oxygenator and takes some of the workload of the right and left heart and lungs. While anticoagulation is required for ECLS and percutaneous LVAD, it may be optional for surgically implanted LVADs. In reports concerning the large LVAD series, 74% of 49 surviving patients underwent transplantation, and 87% of the transplant patients in whom LVAD was placed surgically also survived and were discharged [68, 51]. Although early LVAD and extracorporeal life support and subsequently transplantation have been recommended as an alternative approach to emergency revascularization, these non-systematic direct comparative and observational studies have yielded contradictory results. In a study conducted with surgical LVAD with and without CABG, the mortality was found to be higher in patients with CABG in whom LVAD was inserted in the early period after MI [69].

While VA-ECMO may support pulmonary functions along with cardiac functions, they also have the advantage of being implanted in distant centers [46, 70]. After the publication of the neutral results of the IABP-SHOCK trial, the number of VA-ECMO applications increased dramatically [57]. The application number was 500 in Germany in 2012 increasing to 3000 in 2014 [57]. This worrisome increase in the use of VA-ECMO in CSMI patients is a very serious issue that needs to be assessed in more detail since it does not rely on concrete evidence but rather on conventional wisdom based on pathophysiology and the positive results published in observational studies [49, 71]. An increase of 3–6 L/min in the flow, which is provided by VA-ECMO and which is necessary, cannot ensure the survival of CSMI patients. There are drawbacks involved in using these devices as a result of the high rates of complications such as the large cannula sizes, major bleeding, lower extremity ischemia, compartment syndrome, amputation, stroke, severe infections, difficult weaning, lack of direct left ventricular unloading, and increase in afterload [72, 73]. Attempts to counteract the problem of left ventricular loading and increase in afterload with VA-ECMO are being made with the combination of an unloading device such as IABP or the use of Impella® [74, 75]. Better weaning and lower in-hospital and 28-day mortality were reported with Impella® of VA-ECMO along with IABP in a propensity-matched national registry [74]. Considering the lack of RCTs, systematic reviews should be taken into account as well as two small nonrandomized registries (n = 95) comparing VA-ECMO with IABP and Impella® and two other studies (n = 140) conducted with Impella RD® and TandemHeart [54, 75]. Considering the 30-day survival rate of VA-ECMO, in this meta-analysis, it is obviously superior to IABP with 33% absolute survival rate. No benefit was observed when compared with ECLS and pMCS (Impella®, TandemHeart). In conclusion, the total meta-analysis did not indicate any significant benefits. When addressed as a whole, the meta-analysis data of VA-ECMOs/ECLS and pMCS are inconsistent: on the one hand, pMCSs are not better than IABP, whereas, on the other, VA-ECMOs/ECLS are better than IABP while they are not better than pMCSs. Of course, there is a need for higher-quality RCTs to be able to answer the questions about the routine use of VA-ECMO/ECLS in treatment-resistant CS patients [44, 49]. It is seen that 75% of the survivors after ECLS are able to go about their daily life, 25% of them return to work or school, and 57% of them are not limited in their usual activities. However, when compared to a normative age-matched population, significantly lower quality-of-life indices are reported [76].

4.5. Reperfusion

Coronary revascularization probably with pPCI should be planned as soon as possible in STEMI/NSTEMI patients with impaired pump function. In the IABP-SHOCK II trial conducted with 600 patients between 2009 and 2012, emergency coronary revascularizations were performed with pPCI in 95.8% of them and with CABG in 3.5% usually after unsuccessful pPCI, and revascularization was not performed only in 3.2% of them [5]. Early coronary revascularization is the key recommendation for treatment of CSMI patients [29, 32, 33, 37, 50, 51]. The SHOCK trial conducted with 302 CSMI patients between 1993 and 1998 revealed a tendency for early revascularization compared to conservative treatment whether with pPCI (64%) or CABG (36%) in terms of 30-day mortality (56.0 vs. 47.6%; $p = 0.11$) [77]. However, the 6-month (49.7 vs. 36.9%; $p = 0.027$), 12-month (46.7 vs. 33.6%; $p < 0.04$), and even 6-year (32.8 vs. 19.6%; $p = 0.03$) survival rates, for early revascularization, are significantly high [77–79]. SMASH (Swiss Multicenter Trial of Angioplasty for SHOCK) trial, which is the second study suitable for early coronary revascularization, was prematurely terminated due to low participation after only 55 CSMI patients were included. This study seemed neutral regarding 30-day mortality [5]. The low mortality rates of CSMI patients in the data registry reports of numerous countries such as France, Italy, Switzerland, Sweden, and the United States in the past 30 years were attributed to the increased rates of pPCI [3]. The "real-world" situation in Germany is reflected by the registry data addressing 2.818 CSMI-treated patients, of whom 85% were treated with pPCI, 4.2% with CABG, and 8.9% with noninterventional treatment. Hospital mortality rates were 42% for pPCI, 21.7% for CABG, and 47.8% for noninterventional treatment [80].

4.5.1. Types of revascularization

The preferred approach is primary percutaneous coronary intervention (pPCI). The decision to carry out revascularization in CSMI patients with multivessel disease or left main coronary artery should be made depending on the patient's medical information, coronary anatomy, procedural risks, potential delays in treatment, and patient preferences in cooperation with a "heart team" composed of cardiologists and surgeons [32, 81, 82]. Registry data indicated similar mortality rates between pPCI and CABG, while they sometimes suggested that CABG was better [80, 81]. Chest pain units and shock centers in the network generated for MI patients should allow to rapid transfer of CSMI patients to those centers where cardiac catheterization and pPCI are performed [33, 37, 83]. Only in cases in which emergency cardiac catheterization cannot be performed in a reasonable time period, systemic fibrinolysis should be preferred as the second best option, and cardiac catheterization should be performed because systemic fibrinolysis is not as effective as catheter revascularization [84].

The standard concept for pPCI in CSMI patients is reopening only the culprit coronary lesion. Even though 70–80% of CSMI patients in fact have multivessel disease, the mortality rate of opening multiple vessels in the same session is high. According to the registry data of the IABP-SHOCKII trial, a significant difference could not be demonstrated between multivessel pPCI and the culprit lesion only pPCI in terms of 12-month mortality [85]. The European Society of Cardiology guidelines recommend the implantation of a drug-eluting stent (DES) over bare metal stents (BMS) in patients with STEMI and also in NSTEMI patients with acute coronary syndrome [29, 37]. However, the roles of DES and BMS are still indefinite. All the long-term causes of mortality were better in those who underwent DES implantation, while the other two were neutral in a retrospective analysis [86, 87]. Still, even though using DES instead of BMS does not have any adverse effect, the use of DES is still recommended in CSMI patients.

5. Conclusion

Examining the patients with CS, we can see that we have many problems to deal with and solve. Due to ever-increasing risk factors for MI, particularly due to rapidly increasing world population, aging populations, and tobacco use, the number of CS patients is increasing day by day despite the serious advances and solutions in ACS. Although pMCS devices manufactured specifically with advancing technology are considered to be good solutions, they do pose new and serious problems. They are not suitable for every country or society due to their high application and device costs and particularly due to the fact that they cannot guarantee life. We need to allocate more resources to the abovementioned problems for the sake of public health through the world, and we need to produce pMCS devices that are suitable for each population, easy to apply, inexpensive, transportable, permanent, and effective so that the patient can be transferred to a cardiac center no matter where the patient is. One clear fact revealed by this study is the lack of clarity with respect to pMCS indications due to a low number of controlled randomized clinical trials. Early and effective revascularization is the best treatment option for CS. To this end, those organizations operating on both national and global bases are going to play the most active role for the short-term and long-term survival of patients.

Conflict of interest

None declared.

Fund

This chapter is funded by İpek Medikal in Turkey.

Author details

Fevzi Sarper Türker

Address all correspondence to: sarperturker@gmail.com

Cardiovascular Clinic, Elazığ Education and Research Hospital, University of Health Sciences, Elazığ, Turkey

References

[1] Reynolds HR, Hochman JS. Cardiogenic shock. Current concepts and improving outcomes. Circulation. 2008;**117**:686-697

[2] Nabel EG, Braunwald E. A tale of coronary artery disease and myocardial infarction. The New England Journal of Medicine. 2012;**366**:54-63

[3] Nuding S, Werdan K, Prondzinsky R. Optimal course of treatment in acute cardiogenic shock complicating myocardial infarction. Expert Review of Cardiovascular Therapy. 2018 Feb;**16**(2):99-112

[4] Schurtz G, Laine M, Delmas C, Kerbaul F, Puymirat E, Lemesle G, Bonello L. Mechanical support in cardiogenic shock complicating acute coronary syndrome: Ready for prime time? Current Vascular Pharmacology. 2018 Jan 16. DOI: 10.2174/157016111666618011616 5544. [Epub ahead of print]

[5] Thiele H, Zeymer U, Neumann FJ, et al. Intra-aortic balloon counterpulsation in acute myocardial infarction complicated by cardiogenic shock (IABP-SHOCK II): Final 12 month results of a randomised, open-label trial. Lancet. 2013;**382**:1638-1645

[6] Nguyen HL, Yarzebski J, Lessard D, et al. Ten-year (2001-2011) trends in the incidence rates and short-term outcomes of early versus late onset cardiogenic shock after hospitalization for acute myocardial infarction. Journal of the American Heart Association. 2017 Jun 7;**6**(6):pii: e005566. DOI: 10.1161/JAHA.117.005566

[7] Bangalore S, Gupta N, Guo Y, et al. Outcomes with invasive vs conservative management of cardiogenic shock complicating acute myocardial infarction. The American Journal of Medicine. 2015;**128**:601-608

[8] Hochman JS, Buller CE, Sleeper LA, et al. Cardiogenic shock complicating acute myocardial infarction—Etiologies, management and outcome: A report from the SHOCK trial registry. SHould we emergently revascularize occluded coronaries for cardiogenic shocK. Journal of the American College of Cardiology. 2000;**36**:1063-1070

[9] Giannuzzi P, Imparato A, Temporelli PL, de Vito F, Silva PL, Scapellato F, Giordano A. Doppler-derived mitral deceleration time of early filling as a strong predictor of pulmonary capillary wedge pressure in postinfarction patients with left ventricular systolic dysfunction. Journal of the American College of Cardiology. 1994;**23**:1630-1637

[10] Gianni M, Dentali F, Grandi AM, Sumner G, Hiralal R, Lonn E. Apical ballooning syndrome or takotsubo cardiomyopathy: A systematic review. European Heart Journal. 2006;**27**:1523-1529

[11] Steg PG, Bonnefoy E, Chabaud S, Lapostolle F, Dubien PY, Cristofini P, Leizorovicz A, Touboul P. Impact of time to treatment on mortality after prehospital fibrinolysis or primary angioplasty: Data from the CAPTIM randomized clinical trial. Circulation. 2003;**108**:2851-2856

[12] Lindholm MG, Kober L, Boesgaard S, Torp-Pedersen C, Aldershvile J. Cardiogenic shock complicating acute myocardial infarction: Prognostic impact of early and late shock development. European Heart Journal. 2003;**24**:258-265

[13] Beyersdorf F, Buckberg GD, Acar C, Okamoto F, Sjostrand F, Young H, Bugyi HI, Allen BS. Cardiogenic shock after acute coronary occlusion: Pathogenesis, early diagnosis, and treatment. The Thoracic and Cardiovascular Surgeon. 1989;**37**:28-36

[14] Hochman JS. Cardiogenic shock complicating acute myocardial infarction: Expanding the paradigm. Circulation. 2003;**107**:2998-3002

[15] Hollenberg SM, Kavinsky CJ, Parrillo JE. Cardiogenic shock. Annals of Internal Medicine. 1999;**131**:47-59

[16] Ramanathan K, Harkness SM, Nayar AC, Cosmi JE, Sleeper LS, White HD, Davidoff R, Hochman JS. Cardiogenic shock in patients with preserved left ventricular systolic function: Characteristics and insight into mechanisms. Journal of the American College of Cardiology. 2004;**241A**:43

[17] Stevenson LW, Miller LW, Desvigne-Nickens P, Ascheim DD, Parides MK, Renlund DG, Oren RM, Krueger SK, Costanzo MR, Wann LS, Levitan RG, Mancini D. Left ventricular assist device as destination for patients undergoing intravenous inotropic therapy: A subset analysis from REMATCH (Randomized Evaluation of Mechanical Assistance in Treatment of Chronic Heart Failure). Circulation. 2004;**110**:975-981

[18] Yehudai L, Reynolds HR, Schwarz SA, Hrkness SM, Picard MH, Davidoff R, Hochman JS. Serial echocardiograms in patients with cardiogenic shock: Analysis of the SHOCK trial. Journal of the American College of Cardiology. 2006;**47**(suppl A):111A

[19] Reynolds HR, Anand SK, Fox JM, Harkness S, Dzavik V, White HD, Webb JG, Gin K, Hochman JS, Picard MH. Restrictive physiology in cardiogenic shock: Observations from echocardiography. American Heart Journal. 2006;**151**(890):e9-e15

[20] Jacobs AK, Leopold JA, Bates E, Mendes LA, Sleeper LA, White H, Davidoff R, Boland J, Modur S, Forman R, Hochman JS. Cardiogenic shock caused by right ventricular infarction: A report from the SHOCK registry. Journal of the American College of Cardiology. 2003;**41**:1273-1279

[21] Brookes C, Ravn H, White P, Moeldrup U, Oldershaw P, Redington A. Acute right ventricular dilatation in response to ischemia significantly impairs left ventricular systolic performance. Circulation. 1999;**100**:761-767

[22] Zhang C, Xu X, Potter BJ, Wang W, Kuo L, Michael L, Bagby GJ, Chilian WM. TNF-alpha contributes to endothelial dysfunction in ischemia/reperfusion injury. Arteriosclerosis, Thrombosis, and Vascular Biology. 2006;**26**:475-480

[23] Kohsaka S, Menon V, Lowe AM, Lange M, Dzavik V, Sleeper LA, Hochman JS. Systemic inflammatory response syndrome after acute myocardial infarction complicated by cardiogenic shock. Archives of Internal Medicine. 2005;**165**:1643-1650

[24] Brunkhorst FM, Clark AL, Forycki ZF, Anker SD. Pyrexia, procalcitonin, immune activation and survival in cardiogenic shock: The potential importance of bacterial translocation. International Journal of Cardiology. 1999;**72**:3-10

[25] Meine TJ, Roe MT, Chen AY, Patel MR, Washam JB, Ohman EM, Peacock WF, Pollack CV Jr, Gibler WB, Peterson ED. Association of intravenous morphine use and outcomes in acute coronary syndromes: Results from the CRUSADE Quality Improvement Initiative. American Heart Journal. 2005;**149**:1043-1049

[26] ACE Inhibitor Myocardial Infarction Collaborative Group. Indications for ACE inhibitors in the early treatment of acute myocardial infarction: Systematic overview of individual data from 100,000 patients in randomized trials. Circulation. 1998;**97**:2202-2212

[27] Antman EM, Anbe DT, Armstrong PW, Bates ER, Green LA, Hand M, Hochman JS, Krumholz HM, Kushner FG, Lamas GA, Mullany CJ, Ornato JP, Pearle DL, Sloan MA, Smith SC Jr, Alpert JS, Anderson JL, Faxon DP, Fuster V, Gibbons RJ, Gregoratos G, Halperin JL, Hiratzka LF, Hunt SA, Jacobs AK. ACC/AHA guidelines for the management of patients with ST-elevation myocardial infarction: Executive summary: A report of the American College of Cardiology/American Heart Association Task Force on Practice Guidelines (Writing Committee to Revise the 1999 Guidelines for the Management of Patients With Acute Myocardial Infarction). Circulation. 2004;**110**:588-636

[28] Connors AF Jr, Speroff T, Dawson NV, Thomas C, Harrell FE Jr, Wagner D, Desbiens N, Goldman L, Wu AW, Califf RM, Fulkerson WJ Jr, Vidaillet H, Broste S, Bellamy P, Lynn J, Knaus WA, SUPPORT Investigators. The effectiveness of right heart catheterization in the initial care of critically ill patients. Journal of the American Medical Association. 1996;**276**:889-897

[29] Werdan K, Russ M, Buerke M, et al. Cardiogenic shock due to myocardial infarction: Diagnosis, monitoring and treatment: A German-Austrian S3 Guideline. Deutsches Ärzteblatt International. 2012;**109**:343-351

[30] Orban M, Limbourg T, Neumann FJ, et al. ADP receptor antagonists in patients with acute myocardial infarction complicated by cardiogenic shock: A post hoc IABP-SHOCK II trial subgroup analysis. EuroIntervention. 2016;**12**:e1395-e1403

[31] Valente S, Lazzeri C, Vecchio S, Giglioli C, Margheri M, Bernardo P, Comeglio M, Chiocchini S, Gensini GF. Predictors of in-hospital mortality after percutaneous coronary intervention for cardiogenic shock. International Journal of Cardiology. 2007;**114**:176-182

[32] van Diepen S, Katz JN, Albert NM et al. Contemporary management of cardiogenic shock: A scientific statement from the American Heart Association. Circulation. 2017 Oct 17;**136**(16):e232-e268

[33] Ponikowski P, Voors AA, Anker SD, et al. 2016 ESC Guidelines for the diagnosis and treatment of acute and chronic heart failure: The Task Force for the diagnosis and treatment of acute and chronic heart failure of the European Society of Cardiology (ESC) Developed with the special Downloaded by [University of Pennsylvania] at 03:10 10 January 2018 Accepted Manuscript 22 contribution of the Heart Failure Association (HFA) of the ESC. European Heart Journal. 2013;**37**:2129-2200

[34] Sakr Y, Reinhart K, Vincent JL, et al. Does dopamine administration in shock influence outcome? Results of the Sepsis Occurrence in Acutely Ill Patients (SOAP) Study. Critical Care Medicine. 2006;**34**:589-597

[35] Tarvasmäki T, Lassus J, Varpula M, et al. Current real-life use of vasopressors and inotropes in cardiogenic shock—Adrenaline use is associated with excess organ injury and mortality. Critical Care. 2016;**20**:208

[36] Mebazaa A, Nieminen MS, Filippatos GS, et al. Levosimendan vs. dobutamine: Outcomes for acute heart failure patients on beta-blockers in SURVIVE. European Journal of Heart Failure. 2009;**11**:304-311

[37] Ibanez B, James S, Agewall S, et al. 2017 ESC Guidelines for the management of acute myocardial infarction in patients presenting with ST-segment elevation: The Task Force for the management of acute myocardial infarction in patients presenting with ST-segment elevation of the European Society of Cardiology (ESC). European Heart Journal. 2017

[38] Gilbert EM, Hershberger RE, Wiechmann RJ, et al. Pharmacologic and hemodynamic effects of combined beta-agonist stimulation and phosphodiesterase inhibition in the failing human heart. Chest. 1995;**108**:1524-1532

[39] Russ MA, Prondzinsky R, Carter JM, et al. Right ventricular function in myocardial infarction complicated by cardiogenic shock: Improvement with levosimendan. Critical Care Medicine. 2009;**37**:3017-3023

[40] Christoph A, Prondzinsky R, Russ M, et al. Early and sustained haemodynamic improvement with levosimendan compared to intraaortic balloon counterpulsation (IABP) in cardiogenic shock complicating acute myocardial infarction. Acute Cardiac Care. 2008; **10**:49-57

[41] Samimi-Fard S, García-González MJ, Domínguez-Rodríguez A, et al. Effects of levosimendan versus dobutamine on long-term survival of patients with cardiogenic shock after primary coronary angioplasty. International Journal of Cardiology. 2008;**127**:284-287

[42] Thiele H, Ohman EM, Desch S, et al. Management of cardiogenic shock. European Heart Journal. 2015;**36**:1223-1230

[43] Blumenstein J, de Waha S, Thiele H. Percutaneous ventricular assist devices and extracorporeal life support: Current applications. EuroIntervention. 2016;**12**(Suppl X):X61-X67

[44] Combes A, Brodie D, Chen YS, et al. The ICM research agenda on extracorporeal life support. Intensive Care Medicine. 2017;**43**:1306-1318

[45] Sandhu A, McCoy LA, Negi SI, et al. Use of mechanical circulatory support in patients undergoing percutaneous coronary intervention: Insights from the National Cardiovascular Data Registry. Circulation. 2015;**132**:1243-1251

[46] Werdan K, Gielen S, Ebelt H, et al. Mechanical circulatory support in cardiogenic shock. European Heart Journal. 2014;**35**:156-167

[47] Thiele H, Zeymer U, Neumann FJ, et al. Intraaortic balloon support for myocardial infarction with cardiogenic shock. New England Journal of Medicine. 2012;**367**:1287-1296

[48] Thiele H, Jobs A, Ouweneel DM, et al. Percutaneous short-term active mechanical support devices in cardiogenic shock: A systematic review and collaborative meta-analysis of randomized trials. European Heart Journal. 2017 Dec 14;**38**(47):3523-3531. DOI: 10.1093/eurheartj/ehx363. in press

[49] Prondzinsky R, Werdan K. Extracorporeal life support during cardiac arrest and cardiogenic shock-how good is the evidence really. Annals of Translational Medicine. 2017;**5**:58

[50] Roffi M, Patrono C, Collet JP, et al. 2015 ESC Guidelines for the management of acute coronary syndromes in patients presenting without persistent ST-segment elevation: Task Force for the Management of Acute Coronary Syndromes in Patients Presenting without Persistent STSegment Elevation of the European Society of Cardiology (ESC). European Heart Journal. 2016;**37**:267-315

[51] Windecker S, Kolh P, Alfonso F, et al. 2014 ESC/EACTS Guidelines on myocardial revascularization: The Task Force on Myocardial Revascularization of the European Society of Cardiology (ESC) and the European Association for Cardio-Thoracic Surgery (EACTS) Developed with the special contribution of the European Association of Percutaneous Cardiovascular Interventions (EAPCI). European Heart Journal. 2014 Oct 1;**35**(37):2541-2619

[52] den Uil CA, Akin S, Jewbali LS et al. Short-term mechanical circulatory support as a bridge to durable left ventricular assist device implantation in refractory cardiogenic shock: A systematic review and meta-analysis. European Journal of Cardio-Thoracic Surgery. 2017;**52**:14-25

[53] Tramm R, Ilic D, Davies AR, Pellegrino VA, Romero L, Hodgson C. Extracorporeal membrane oxygenation for critically ill adults. Cochrane Database of Systematic Reviews. 2015 Jan 22;**1**:CD010381

[54] Ouweneel DM, Schotborgh JV, Limpens J, et al. Extracorporeal life support during cardiac arrest and cardiogenic shock: A systematic review and meta-analysis. Intensive Care Medicine. 2016;**42**(12):1922-1934. DOI: 10.1007/s00134-016-4536-8

[55] Yancy CW, Jessup M, Bozkurt B, et al. 2013 ACCF/AHA guideline for the management of heart failure: A report of the American College of Cardiology Foundation/American Heart Association task force on practice guidelines. Journal of the American College of Cardiology. 2013;**62**(16):e147-e239. DOI: 10.1016/j.jacc.2013.05.019

[56] Ariyaratnam P, McLean LA, Cale AR, et al. Extra-corporeal membrane oxygenation for the post-cardiotomy patient. Heart Failure Reviews. 2014;**19**(6):717-725. DOI: 10.1007/s10741-014-9428-9

[57] Karagiannidis C, Brodie D, Strassmann S, et al. Extracorporeal membrane oxygenation: Evolving epidemiology and mortality. Intensive Care Medicine. 2016;**42**:889-896

[58] Ramanathan K, Cosmi J, Harkness SM, French JK, Farkouh ME, Sleeper LA, Dzavik V, Hochman JS. Reversal of systemic hypoperfusion following intra aortic balloon pumping is associated with improved 30-day survival independent of early revascularization in cardiogenic shock complicating an acute myocardial infarction. Circulation. 2003;**108**(suppl I):I-672

[59] Chen EW, Canto JG, Parsons LS, Peterson ED, Littrell KA, Every NR, Gibson CM, Hochman JS, Ohman EM, Cheeks M, Barron HV. Relation between hospital intra-aortic balloon counterpulsation volume and mortality in acute myocardial infarction complicated by cardiogenic shock. Circulation. 2003;**108**:951-957

[60] Sjauw KD, Engström AE, Vis MM, et al. A systematic review and metaanalysis of intra-aortic balloon pump therapy in ST-elevation myocardial infarction: Should we change the guidelines. European Heart Journal. 2009;**30**:459-468

[61] Prondzinsky R, Lemm H, Swyter M, et al. Intra-aortic balloon counterpulsation in patients with acute myocardial infarction complicated by cardiogenic shock: The prospective, randomized IABP SHOCK trial. Critical Care Medicine. 2010;**38**:152-160

[62] Burkhoff D, Cohen H, Brunckhorst C, O'Neill WW. TandemHeart Investigators Group. A randomized multicenter clinical study to evaluate the safetyand efficacy of the TandemHeart percutaneous ventricular assistdevice versus conventional therapy with intraaortic balloon pumping for treatment of cardiogenic shock. American Heart Journal . 2006 Sep;**152**(3):469. e1-8

[63] Thiele H, Sick P, Boudriot E, et al. Randomized comparison of intra-aortic balloon support with a percutaneous left ventricular assist device in patients with revascularized acute myocardial infarction complicated by cardiogenic shock. European Heart Journal. 2005;**26**:1276-1283

[64] Seyfarth M, Sibbing D, Bauer I, et al. A randomized clinical trial to evaluate the safety and efficacy of a percutaneous left ventricular assist device versus intra-aortic balloon pumping for treatment of cardiogenic shock caused by myocardial infarction. Journal of the American College of Cardiology. 2008;**52**:1584-1588

[65] Ouweneel DM, Eriksen E, Sjauw KD, et al. Percutaneous mechanical circulatory support versus intra-aortic balloon pump in cardiogenic shock after acute myocardial infarction. Journal of the American College of Cardiology. 2017;**69**:278-287

[66] Meuwese CL, Ramjankhan FZ, Braithwaite SA, de Jonge N, de Jong M, Buijsrogge MP, Janssen JGD, Klöpping C, Kirkels JH, Donker DW. Extracorporeal life support in cardiogenic shock: Indications and management in current practice. Netherlands Heart Journal. 2018;**26**(2):58-66. DOI: 10.1007/s12471-018-1073-9

[67] Hoefer D, Ruttmann E, Poelzl G, Kilo J, Hoermann C, Margreiter R, Laufer G, Antretter H. Outcome evaluation of the bridge-to-bridge concept in patients with cardiogenic shock. The Annals of Thoracic Surgery. 2006;**82**:28-33

[68] Leshnower BG, Gleason TG, O'Hara ML, Pochettino A, Woo YJ, Morris RJ, Gardner TJ, Acker MA. Safety and efficacy of left ventricular assist device support in postmyocardial infarction cardiogenic shock. The Annals of Thoracic Surgery. 2006;**81**:1365-1370

[69] Dang NC, Topkara VK, Leacche M, John R, Byrne JG, Naka Y. Left ventricular assist device implantation after acute anterior wall myocardial infarction and cardiogenic shock: A two-center study. The Journal of Thoracic and Cardiovascular Surgery. 2005;**130**:693-698

[70] Beurtheret S, Mordant P, Paoletti X, et al. Emergency circulatory support in refractory cardiogenic shock patients in remote institutions: A pilot study (the cardiac-RESCUE program). European Heart Journal. 2013;**34**:112-120

[71] Sheu JJ, Tsai TH, Lee FY, et al. Early extracorporeal membrane oxygenator-assisted primary percutaneous coronary intervention improved 30-day clinical outcomes in patients with ST-segment elevation myocardial infarction complicated with profound cardiogenic shock. Critical Care Medicine. 2010;**38**:1810-1817

[72] Cheng R, Hachamovitch R, Kittleson M, et al. Complications of extracorporeal membrane oxygenation for treatment of cardiogenic shock and cardiac arrest: A meta-analysis of 1,866 adult patients. The Annals of Thoracic Surgery. 2014;**97**:610-616

[73] Aissaoui N, Caudron J, Leprince P, et al. Right-left ventricular interdependence: A promising predictor of successful extracorporeal membrane oxygenation (ECMO) weaning after assistance for refractory cardiogenic shock. Intensive Care Medicine. 2017;**43**(4):592

[74] Aso S, Matsui H, Fushimi K, et al. The effect of Intraaortic balloon pumping under venoarterial extracorporeal membrane oxygenation on mortality of cardiogenic patients: An analysis using a Nationwide inpatient database. Critical Care Medicine. 2016;**44**:1974-1979

[75] Nuding S, Werda K. IABP plus ECMO—Is one and one more than two? Journal of Thoracic Disease. 2017 Apr;**9**(4):961-964 DOI: 10.21037/jtd.2017.03.73

[76] Camboni D, Philipp A, Rottenkolber V, et al. Long-term survival and quality of life after extracorporeal life support: A 10-year report. European Journal of Cardio-Thoracic Surgery. 2017;**52**:241-247

[77] Hochman JS, Sleeper LA, Webb JG, et al. Early revascularization in acute myocardial infarction complicated by cardiogenic shock. SHOCK Investigators. Should we emergently Revascularize occluded coronaries for cardiogenic shock. The New England Journal of Medicine. 1999;**341**:625-634

[78] Hochman JS, Sleeper LA, White HD, et al. One-year survival following early revascularization for cardiogenic shock. Journal of the American Medical Association. 2001;**285**(2):190

[79] Hochman JS, Sleeper LA, Webb JG, et al. Early revascularization and long-term survival in cardiogenic shock complicating acute myocardial infarction. Journal of the American Medical Association. 2006;**295**:2511-2515

[80] Zeymer U. Inhospital mortality in patients with infarct-related cardiogenic shock undergoing coronary angiography treated with and without acute revascularization therapy. German Society of Cardiolology. European Heart Journal. 2017 August 1;**38**(1):ehx502. P2724. https://doi.org/10.1093/eurheartj/ehx502.P2724

[81] Chiu FC, Chang SN, Lin JW, et al. Coronary artery bypass graft surgery provides better survival in patients with acute coronary syndrome or STsegment elevation myocardial infarction experiencing cardiogenic shock after percutaneous coronary intervention: A propensity score analysis. The Journal of Thoracic and Cardiovascular Surgery. 2009;**138**:1326-1330

[82] Rastan AJ, Eckenstein JI, Hentschel B, et al. Emergency coronary artery bypass graft surgery for acute coronary syndrome: Beating heart versus conventional cardioplegic cardiac arrest strategies. Circulation. 2006;**114**:I477-I485

[83] Post F, Gori T, Giannitsis E, et al. Criteria of the German Society of Cardiology for the establishment of chest pain units: Update 2014. Clinical Research in Cardiology. European Heart Journal. 2015 Jun 1;**36**(21):1282-1283

[84] Keeley EC, Boura JA, Grines CL. Primary angioplasty versus intravenous thrombolytic therapy for acute myocardial infarction: A quantitative review of 23 randomised trials. Lancet. 2003;**361**:13-20

[85] Zeymer U, Werdan K, Schuler G, et al. Editor's choice-impact of immediate multivessel percutaneous coronary intervention versus culprit lesion intervention on 1-year outcome in patients with acute myocardial infarction complicated by cardiogenic shock: Results of the randomised IABP-SHOCK II trial. European Heart Journal. Acute Cardiovascular Care. 2017;**6**:601-609

[86] Jaguszewski M, Ghadri JR, Seifert B, et al. Drug-eluting stents vs. bare metal stents in patients with cardiogenic shock: A comparison by propensity score analysis. Journal of Cardiovascular Medicine (Hagerstown, Md.). 2015;**16**:220-229

[87] Ledwoch J, Fuernau G, Desch S, et al. Drug-eluting stents versus baremetal stents in acute myocardial infarction with cardiogenic shock. Heart. 2017;**103**:1177-1184

Long-Term Outcome of High-Risk Percutaneous Coronary Interventions with Extracorporeal Membrane Oxygenation Support for Patients Without Cardiogenic Shock

Vladimir I. Ganyukov, Roman S. Tarasov,
Ivan E. Vereshchagin and Dmitry L. Shukevich

Additional information is available at the end of the chapter

http://dx.doi.org/10.5772/intechopen.75881

Abstract

Percutaneous coronary intervention (PCI) has evolved into the high-risk category in the past 2 decades. Endovascular patients are on average sicker than in the past due to increased age, complex anatomy, reduced global left ventricular systolic function and a greater frequency of surgical refusal. Extracorporeal membrane oxygenation (ECMO) can be taken into account for the management of extremely high-risk PCI without any hemodynamic instability. The rationale for the use of ECMO includes a lower risk of hemodynamic collapse which leads to low perfusion episodes minimization. In the evidence based on ECMO-assisted high-risk PCI, there are no randomized clinical trials but only observational studies and case reports. In this paper, we describe one-year long-term results of ECMO support for PCI in patients without hemodynamic disturbances.

Keywords: elective high-risk PCI, ECMO, stable angina, acute coronary syndrome

1. Introduction

At present, a clear-cut definition of what is a high-risk percutaneous coronary intervention (PCI) is not completely determined. In general, high-risk PCI is an intervention which is likely to cause adverse events that will worsen ischemia and reduced cardiac output culminating into cardiogenic shock. According to the clinical expert consensus statement [1], variables that contribute to an increased risk of PCI can be classified into three groups: (1) lesion specific (Jeopardy Score ≥ 8 [2], calcification, bifurcation, tortuosity, occlusion), (2) clinical presentation specific (cardiogenic shock, acute coronary syndrome (ACS)), and (3) patient specific (age, a history of diabetes mellitus and/or prior myocardial infarction, chronic kidney disease, ejection fraction <35% on the echocardiography assessment). A different combination of these variables can provoke cardiogenic shock in high-risk PCI, whereas the most unfavorable option is a combination of severe left ventricular dysfunction (ejection fraction of the left ventricle (EF) <35% or recent decompensated heart failure) and a technically complicated PCI (left main, last remaining conduit, severe multivessel disease) [1].

In observational studies, extracorporeal membrane oxygenation (ECMO) has an encouraging result for PCI in patients with hemodynamic disturbances [3–6]. A meta-analysis or randomized clinical trials data are not available for ECMO. That is why current European guidelines can only be based on the expert consensus [7–9]: "Short-term mechanical support may be considered in patients with refractory shock" (Class of recommendations IIb, level of evidence C.)" There is no evidence of the ECMO benefits for PCI in patients with stable angina and non–ST-segment elevation acute coronary syndrome (NSTE-ACS) based on long-term results data. We are dealing only with single studies presenting hospital outcomes in small series of patients and case reports [10–13]. Today, only selected NSTE-ACS patients with cardiogenic shock are considered for left ventricular assist devices [7]. Approaches implying the use of circulatory support devices for patients without hemodynamic disturbances who require high-risk PCI are not discussed in the guidelines.

Nowadays, an evolution of PCI to the high-risk category could be observed. Endovascular patients are, on average, sicker than in the past due to increased age, complex anatomy, severity and extent of coronary artery disease, low left ventricular ejection fraction, co-morbidities (renal failure, cerebrovascular disease, peripheral artery disease, diabetes mellitus and chronic obstructive pulmonary disease) and a personal choice of PCI to improve their symptoms [1, 14, 15]. Cardiac surgeons are the biggest providers of patients with high-risk PCI. Because of an elevated surgical risk (high STS score or EuroScore II) as well as elevated ischemic and bleeding risks (in NSTE-ACS patients after P2Y12 inhibitors loading), surgeons could refuse coronary artery bypass graft (CABG) interventions [16–19]. Thus, high-risk PCI is an appropriate revascularization strategy for patients who are not suitable for surgery or have refused CABG.

A patient with co-morbidities and severe stable coronary artery disease (CAD) or NSTE-ACS can have a significantly weakened cardiovascular reserve and be more receptive to low myocardial perfusion stunning. At the same time, an aggressive endovascular approach with technically complex high-risk PCI can be complicated by coronary dissection with vessel closure or no reflow or can require longer and balloon inflations with higher pressure. As a result, a sequence of adverse events can occur, leading to reduced ejection fraction and increased hypoperfusion, resulting in the progression of myocardial ischemia and the development of cardiogenic shock and/or multiple organ failures. The rationale for the use of ECMO includes a decreased risk of hemodynamic collapse which leads to fewer low perfusion episodes. Additionally, a lower risk of hypotensive events could provide an interventional cardiologist with more time to achieve optimal results and complete revascularization. The problem is that it is very difficult to take into account all the unfavorable factors, to correctly assess the complexity of a particular clinical case and to determine the indications for mechanical circulatory support. Having two seemingly comparable patients, we can perform a high-risk PCI procedure without adverse outcomes in one case, and with severe hemodynamic disorders in the other. To resolve the issue we need to conduct a randomized study in the ECMO support PCI versus PCI only but, at the moment, it is not possible due to ethical problems issues and a small number of observations.

Currently, a large number of percutaneous mechanical circulatory support devices is available and has entered clinical practice. These include TandemHeart, intra-aortic balloon pump (IABP), ECMO, Impella [1, 14, 15].

ECMO uses a centrifugal pump for artificial circulation of blood. For the purposes of PCI, veno-arterial ECMO cannulation approach is selected. There are very little data on the use of ECMO in the elective pre-procedural setting: data are limited to reports [12, 13] which demonstrated a single-center experience of high-risk PCI with ECMO support as an adjunct modality. The conclusion of these reports was that elective pre-PCI ECMO is a viable therapeutic alternative capable of ensuring good immediate and mid-term outcomes in high-risk CABG patients.

The reason for choosing ECMO support versus other devices for elective high-risk PCI in patients without cardiogenic shock is given in our earlier publications [20].

Thus, taking into account a high incidence of chronic CAD and ACS [21] as well as an evolution of PCI to the high-risk category there is a strong medical and social need to treat these patients safely. A number of high-risk PCI patients are considered to be at extremely high risk of PCI complications during these complex procedures. Nowadays, the development of cardiac support devices such as ECMO has allowed to introduce a safer approach for the extremely high-risk patient subset. The extracorporeal membrane oxygenation has some advantages over the other types of mechanical circulatory support devices. There is limited evidence data on the safety and efficacy of ECMO-assisted high-risk PCI in patients with stable CAD and NSTE-ACS. The next parts of this chapter are devoted to analyzing immediate and long-term outcomes of ECMO support for high-risk PCI without cardiogenic shock as an adjunct modality in the elective pre-procedural setting.

2. Immediate and long-term outcomes of ECMO support for complex high-risk PCI in stable angina patients: A single-center experience

Elective high-risk PCI with ECMO support in **stable angina** patients with the multivessel disease will be presented in this section. These data are based on the in-hospital and 12-month outcomes of a single-center retrospective observational study in the small series of 16 patients. The purpose of the study was to evaluate the incidence of MACCE (a composite of all-cause death, myocardial infarction (MI), stroke and target vessel revascularization) at 30 days and 12 months. Additionally, bleeding and complete revascularization rates were evaluated. Complete revascularization was defined as the PCI procedure, as a result of which the residual SYNTAX score was ≤2. For the classification of bleeding, the definition of Bleeding Academic Research Consortium (BARC) was used [22]. Hemorrhagic complications of type 3 and higher were taken into account.

High-risk PCI was defined as having two of the three parameters [20]: (1) ejection fraction <35%; (2) Jeopardy Score ≥ 8 [2]; (3) intervention for bifurcation and/or left main and/or chronic total occlusion. An indication for high-risk PCI with ECMO support was based on the heart team decision for those patients, who were not suitable for some types of revascularization (CABG or PCI) and who had two of the three parameters of high-risk PCI.

We started ECMO prior to PCI and used the "RotaFlow System" (by MAQUET). The ECMO cannula was inserted using a surgical technique (9 (56.2%)) and endovascular approach (ProStar XL, 7 (45.8%)). The mean ECMO time was 2.4–3.2 L/min/m^2 (70–100% from the estimated).

The medications during PCI included unfractionated heparin and acetylsalicylic acid. All of the patients received the loading dose of clopidogrel before PCI. Aspirin was prescribed before revascularization (75 mg once daily) for all the study patients and it was continued indefinitely. Unfractionated heparin was used (IV bolus of 100 IU per kilogram of body weight followed by an adjustment according to the target activated clotting time of 250–300 seconds). Antiplatelet regimen routinely included clopidogrel (a loading dose of 300 mg at the time of PCI unless used in advance; then 75 mg daily, the recommended duration of treatment was 12 months).

Baseline clinical and angiographic characteristics of the study patients are shown in **Table 1**. Of note, the mean age was 62.8 ± 6.5 years, and the majority of patients were males (81.2%). Diabetes mellitus was present in 18.7, 75% had a history of myocardial infarction, peripheral artery disease was observed in 50% of patients. Left ventricular ejection fraction (LVEF) was poor: 37.9 ± 17.5%. Our patients had stenotic lesions of two or more significant epicardial arteries and/or large branches (≥2.5 mm) ≥70% and/or stenosis of LMCA ≥50%. The target vessel for PCI was determined taking into account the data on the viability of the myocardium on cardiac magnetic resonance imaging. Fifteen (93.7%) patients had 3 or more affected vessels, significant LMCA stenosis was diagnosed in 7 (43.7%) patients and mean SYNTAX score was 31.4 ± 9.8. In general, stable CAD patients (n = 16) were characterized by a high incidence of a prior MI, very low ejection fraction and severe multivessel disease involving LMCA.

We successfully performed all PCI + ECMO interventions. Procedural characteristics and in-hospital outcomes of the study patients are shown in **Table 2**. The mean bypass/PCI duration was 115.6 ± 43.7/98.6 ± 31.1 minutes. All of the patients were weaned from the system immediately after PCI directly in the cath-lab. Only six (37.5%) patients had a complete revascularization while the mean number/length of implanted stents was 3.6 ± 1.2 and 75.8 ± 23.4 mm, respectively. Only second-generation drug-eluting stents (DES) were implanted. There was one stroke case (6.2%) 5 days after PCI + ECMO which led to the death

Variables	Stable CAD patients PCI+ ECMO (n = 16)
Mean age	62.8 ± 6.5 (51–75)
Male	13 (81.2%)
Mean left ventricular ejection fraction	37.9 ± 17.5
Left ventricular ejection fraction <35	11 (68.7%)
EuroScore II	3.2 ± 2.4
CCS II	6 (37.5%)
CCS III-IV	10 (62.5%)
Chronic kidney disease	4 (25%)
COPD	2 (12.5%)
Diabetes mellitus	3 (18.7%)
Prior myocardial infarction	12 (75%)
Arterial hypertension	134 (89.3%)
Peripheral artery disease	8 (50%)
Prior stroke	1 (6.2%)
SYNTAX Score	31.4 ± 9.8
Jeopardy score [2]	11.3 ± 0.9
Affected vessels: 1, 2	1 (6.2%)
Affected vessels: ≥3	15 (93.7%)
LMCA stenosis ≥50%	7 (43.7%)

BARC: Bleeding Academic Research Consortium, COPD: chronic obstructive pulmonary disease, CCS: Canadian Cardiovascular Society grading of angina pectoris.

Table 1. Baseline characteristics of the study population.

of the patient with carotid artery disease. A BARC bleeding of type 3 or more was observed in 6 (37.5%) patients. The mean hospital stay was 12.6 ± 4.8 days. A significant decrease in hemoglobin levels required blood transfusion in six cases. The blood use averaged 4.2 units of red blood cells.

Long-term outcomes of the study are presented in **Table 2**. About 25% mortality rate was observed at 12 months. The combined endpoint (all-cause death, myocardial infarction (MI), stroke and target vessel revascularization) was observed in 4 (25%) patients. Three (18.7%) deaths occurred in the post-hospitalization period as a result of acute myocardial infarction. Two were due to acute stent thrombosis and one as a consequence of stent restenosis. Myocardial infarctions in the long-term follow-up period (3 (18.7%)) were predominantly new cases after the hospital discharge and led to TVR in two patients. There were no additional stroke cases in the follow-up period.

Variables	Stable CAD patients PCI+ ECMO (n = 16)
In-hospital outcomes	
MACCE	1 (6.2%)
• Death	1 (6.2%)
• Stroke	1 (6.2%)
• MI	0
• TVR	0
Mean bypass duration (min)	115.6 ± 43.7
Mean total time of PCI (min)	98.6 ± 31.1
Mean № of stents	3.6 ± 1.2
Mean diameter of stents	3.25 ± 0.5
Mean length of stents (mm)	75.8 ± 23.4
Bleeding (BARC≥3)	6 (37.5%)
Complete revascularization	6 (37.5%)
Residual SYNTAX score	8.5 ± 10.8
Hospital stay (days)	12.6 ± 4.8
12-month outcomes	
MACCE	4 (25%)
• Death	4 (25%)
• Stroke	1 (6.2%)
• MI	3 (18.7%)
• TVR	2 (12.5%)

BARC: Bleeding Academic Research Consortium, MI: myocardial infarction, TVR: target vessel revascularization.

Table 2. Procedural characteristics and study end points.

This study had patients at high risk of adverse events for any type of revascularization (CABG and PCI). This is the largest series of consecutive high CABG risk chronic CAD patients who underwent ECMO in the elective pre-procedural manner. The main hypothesis of the study was that PCI + ECMO may be a feasible strategy of revascularization for **stable angina** patients at a high risk for CABG or PCI only.

All the patients had severe multivessel disease involving LMCA, poor left ventricular fraction as a result of a prior MI and underwent challenging PCI with ECMO support as an adjunct modality in the elective pre-procedural setting, which allowed to complete a successful revascularization without hemodynamic disturbances and to wean from ECMO immediately after PCI. The hospital results looked satisfactory. There were no serious cardiac adverse outcomes. Hemorrhagic complications were not fatal, although it is necessary to note a high incidence of bleeding and blood transfusions. At the 12-month follow-up, the results became less encouraging. A high number of myocardial infarctions in combination with an in-hospital stroke led to an increased number of cumulative adverse outcomes of 25%. The attention should be drawn to the unsatisfactory effect of implantation of second-generation DES (myocardial infarction and death from myocardial infarction in 18.7% of patients). Nevertheless, our data do not go beyond the results presented in the literature. The long-term all-cause mortality in ischemic cardiomyopathy patients with reduced ejection fraction increased up to 58.9 and 66.1% in the CABG and guideline-directed medical therapy groups, respectively [23, 24]. The main limitation of our analysis is a small number of patients. Therefore, in order to answer the question on the role of ECMO for high-risk PCI in chronic CAD patients, larger trials are required.

In conclusion, our study was designed to report the unique single-center experience in using ECMO to manage high-risk **stable angina** patients in the catheterization laboratory. In-hospital results suggest that PCI with ECMO can be successfully performed and may be a feasible strategy of revascularization in a high-risk cohort of chronic CAD patients with adverse outcomes after any type of revascularization (CABG and PCI). Bleeding control is a critical aspect of care during the PCI + ECMO procedure. The long-term results of PCI with the support of artificial circulation require additional evaluation in larger or/and randomized studies. Particular attention should be paid to factors that increase the risk of stent thrombosis (the number of stents, the quality of stents, the procedure for stent implantation, antiplatelet therapy).

3. PCI + ECMO vs. CABG for NSTE-ACS patients with multivessel disease

We followed NSTE-ACS multivessel coronary artery disease (MVCAD) patients consecutively admitted to our hospital from 2012 to 2015 and undergone revascularization with high-risk PCI + ECMO support or CABG. The study included 53 patients (PCI + ECMO, n = 23, and CABG, n = 30). It was a single-center registry, which compared 12-month outcomes. Inclusion criteria were significant multivessel coronary disease and/or stenosis of the left main coronary artery (LMCA) ≥50%. The PCI + ECMO group of NSTE-ACS patients had an intermediate risk of adverse cardiovascular outcomes (mean GRACE score 117.3 ± 19.4, mean EuroScore II 4.3 ± 3.9%), and a high SYNTAX Score: 33.3 ± 8.3. Significant LMCA stenosis was diagnosed in 60.7% of patients. Every third patient had diabetes mellitus, a prior myocardial infarction was observed in 56.4% cases, peripheral artery disease was diagnosed in 60.7% of patients of the study population. High-risk PCI was defined as having two of the three parameters: (1) left ventricular ejection fraction less than 35%; (2) a large amount of myocardium at risk (Jeopardy Score 8 and more [2]) and (3) complex PCI. An indication for high-risk PCI with ECMO support was based on the heart team decision for those patients, who were not suitable for some types of revascularization (CABG or PCI) and who had two of the three parameters of high-risk PCI.

The CABG group patients also had a moderate risk of adverse cardiovascular outcomes (mean GRACE score 97.5 ± 15.0, mean EuroScore II 2.7 ± 2.1%), and an intermediate-high SYNTAX Score: 29.7 ± 8.3. Significant LMCA stenosis was diagnosed in 36.6% of patients. Diabetes mellitus was present in 16.6% of patients, 60% of patients had a prior myocardial infarction and in every third patient of the study population, peripheral artery disease was diagnosed. Thus, there were no statistically significant differences between the groups in terms of the baseline clinical characteristics, but the PCI + ECMO group had a potentially slightly poorer prognosis compared with the CABG group (**Table 3**).

In order to perform PCI + ECMO, we used 21–23 Fr venous cannula for the right common femoral vein with a surgical technique. For the iliac artery—17-18 Fr arterial cannula was used. The mean ECMO flow was about 2.5 L/min/m2 with a duration of 95.4 ± 25.2 min. During PCI all patients received unfractionated heparin, and acetylsalicylic acid before PCI. About 42%of patients received the loading dose of clopidogrel before PCI. After the surgical cannulation wound closure, the remaining patients received the loading dose of clopidogrel. We connected ECMO ("RotaFlow System" developed by the MAQUET Getinge Groupe, Hirrlingen, Germany) before the start of PCI.

The patients in both groups were waiting for revascularization for about 2 weeks. About 89.9% of the CABG patients had complete revascularization. There were significantly fewer patients having had complete revascularization in the PCI + ECMO group: 30.3% (p = 0.0001).

Variables	PCI + ECMO (n = 23)	CABG (n = 30)	P
Mean age	67.5 ± 8.5 (48–82)	64.4 ± 7 (45–75)	0.125
Male	15 (65.2%)	19 (63.3%)	0.9
Mean left ventricular ejection fraction	47.5 ± 12.8%	54.4 ± 10.0%	0.069
Left ventricular ejection fraction ≤40%	9 (39%)	1 (3.3%)	0.001
Mean GRACE SCORE	117.3 ± 19.4	97.5 ± 15.0	0.205
LMCA stenosis ≥50%	14 (60.7%)	11 (36.6%)	0.08
Diabetes mellitus	8 (34.7%)	5 (16.6%)	0.13
Prior myocardial infarction	13 (56.4%)	18 (60%)	0.8
Arterial hypertension	22 (95.4%)	27 (89.9%)	0.5
Peripheral artery disease	14 (60.7%)	11 (33.3%)	0.049
Prior stroke	2 (8.6%)	2 (6.6%)	0.8
EuroScore II	4.3 ± 3.9%	2.7 ± 2.1	0.01
SYNTAX Score	33.3 ± 8.3	29.7 ± 8.3	0.062
Jeopardy score	10.6 ± 1.8	10.6 ± 1.7	0.876

Table 3. Baseline characteristics of the study groups.

Implanted stents mean length and diameter were 54.6 ± 25.3 mm and 3.28 ± 0.4 mm, respectively. During the PCI procedure, 2.8 ± 1.1 DES were implanted. The average number of grafts in the CABG group was 2.8 ± 0.6.

The study endpoints included death, myocardial infarction, stroke, repeated unplanned revascularization and the combined endpoint of death, myocardial infarction, stroke, and revascularization.

It is important to note, that the in-hospital mortality in the PCI + ECMO group was 4.3% and the combined endpoint of adverse events (MACE) (death, MI, stroke, repeated revascularization) was 8.7%. We observed a high rate of significant hemorrhagic complications (BARC 3) caused by the use of the ECMO cannula: up to 47.8%. Despite this, after 12 months of follow-up, mortality and MACE increased only to 8.7 and 17.4%, respectively. Repeated revascularization was required only in 1 (4.3%) case. These results make it clear that the revascularization approach is justified when PCI is performed on severe stenotic lesions in the large proximal parts of the coronary arteries that supply significant areas of the viable myocardium.

The in-hospital results in the CABG group were characterized by a high mortality level (9.99%). MACE in the hospital period reached 13.3%. Significant hemorrhagic complications (BARC 3–4) occurred in 26.6% of cases, which was the expected outcome in the group of open surgical treatment. Mortality and MACE in the CABG group increased to 13.3 and 23.3%, respectively, after 12 months of follow-up. The analysis of the results shows a high proportion of in-hospital and long-term adverse events, which is caused by a high risk of the open surgery in NSTE-ACS MVCAD patients with a high SYNTAX score. These results should not be considered as unfavorable because according to the data of our Registry [25], the prognosis in this group of patients was extremely poor in the absence of revascularization (mortality rate reached 28%).

The comparison of the PCI + ECMO and CABG results of in NSTE-ACS MVCAD patients showed no significant differences in the study endpoints at 12-month follow-up (**Table 4**) despite a potentially poorer prognosis in the PCI + ECMO group compare to the CABG group based on baseline clinical characteristics.

Thus, PCI + ECMO may be an alternative to the CABG revascularization strategy for NSTE-ACS MVCAD patients with a high surgical risk. Although CABG remains the conventional

Variables	PCI + ECMO (n = 23)	CABG (n = 30)	P
Death	2 (8.7%)	4 (13.3%)	0.27
Myocardial infarction	2 (8.7%)	2 (6.6%)	0.77
Stroke	1 (4.3%)	0	0.26
Revascularization (unplanned)	1 (4.3%)	2 (6.6%)	0.7
MACE (death, MI, stroke, repeated revascularization)	4 (17.4)	7 (23.3%)	0.6

Table 4. Twelve-month outcomes of various treatment strategies.

method of revascularization for patients with complex coronary disease including multivessel and LMCA disease, PCI + ECMO is a technique that improves the access to revascularization for high-risk patients who are often refused a CABG surgery.

In our study, we included patients with a high risk of adverse outcomes for any type of revascularization (CABG and PCI). We assume that PCI + ECMO is a possible strategy of revascularization for high-risk NSTE-ACS patients. These patients usually have diffuse coronary artery disease involving LMCA. PCI with ECMO support makes it possible to perform a successful revascularization with no hemodynamic instability.

The present study had several limitations. First of all, it was not randomized. A very critical clinical and angiographic status of the PCI patient group gave us the opportunity to test ECMO as a method of PCI support in a high-risk cohort of NSTE-ACS patients. It is necessary to conduct randomized trials to answer the question on the role of ECMO support for high-risk PCI in NSTE-ACS patients.

4. Conclusions

Currently, the guidelines approve the use of ECMO support in cardiogenic shock or cardiac arrest patients. There are limited data on the use of ECMO support for PCI in stable angina and NSTE-ACS patients without hemodynamic disturbances. However, the use of ECMO for PCI support has a theoretical and practical rationale and showed encouraging results in our single-center observation. Our single-center experience demonstrated that PCI supported by ECMO may be an alternative for high-risk revascularization (CABG and PCI) for both stable angina and NSTE-ACS patients. The extremely poor prognosis in high-risk patients treated with a pharmacological approach who are often refused a CABG surgery or standard PCI makes PCI + ECMO method very promising as it improves the access to revascularization.

Our experience in this study allowed us to come to the following conclusions. A detailed assessment of the viable myocardium in a group of patients with stable coronary artery disease can improve the 12-month results as a more accurate selection of patients for PCI + ECMO support will be done. A particular attention should be paid to factors that increase the probability of stent thrombosis. The role of this revascularization method for NSTE-ACS patients is more obvious. PCI + ECMO is a life-saving technique that significantly improves hospital and 12-month survival of patients who were refused a CABG surgery or standard PCI. Unfortunately, we do not know the exact indications for ECMO in the elective pre-procedural setting, therefore, we need to develop a methodology (calculator) to immediately assess the need for mechanical circulatory support devices during high-risk PCI. In the end, selection of mechanical circulatory support devices is a matter of a personalized approach and should be based on the results of upcoming large randomized comparative studies.

Author details

Vladimir I. Ganyukov[1]*, Roman S. Tarasov[2], Ivan E. Vereshchagin[1] and Dmitry L. Shukevich[3]

*Address all correspondence to: ganyukov@mail.ru

1 Interventional Cardiology Laboratory, State Research Institute for Complex Issues of Cardiovascular Diseases, Kemerovo, Russia

2 Reconstructive Surgery Laboratory, Cardiac Surgery Department, State Research Institute for Complex Issues of Cardiovascular Diseases, Kemerovo, Russia

3 Critical Conditions Laboratory, State Research Institute for Complex Issues of Cardiovascular Diseases, Kemerovo, Russia

References

[1] Rihal CS, Naidu SS, Givertz MM, et al. SCAI/ACC/HFSA/STS clinical expert consensus statement on the use of percutaneous mechanical circulatory support devices in cardiovascular care (endorsed by the American Heart Association, the Cardiological Society of India, and Sociedad Latino Americana de Cardiología Intervencionista; affirmation of value by the Canadian Association of Interventional Cardiology—Association Canadienne de Cardiologie d'intervention). Journal of the American College of Cardiology. 2015;**65**(19):2140-2141

[2] Califf RM, Phillips HR, Hindman MC, et al. Prognostic value of a coronary artery jeopardy score. Journal of the American College of Cardiology. 1985;**5**:1055-1063

[3] Ghodsizad A, Singbartl K, Loebe M, et al. Extracorporeal membrane oxygenation (ECMO): An option for cardiac Reccovery from advanced cardiogenic shock. The Heart Surgery Forum. 2017;**20**(6):E274-E277. DOI: 10.1532/hsf.1635

[4] van den Brink FS, Magan AD, Noordzij PG, et al. Veno-arterial extracorporeal membrane oxygenation in addition to primary PCI in patients presenting with ST-elevation myocardial infarction. Netherlands Heart Journal. 2017. DOI: 10.1007/s12471-017-1068-y [Epub ahead of print]

[5] Basir MB, Schreiber T, Dixon S, et al. Feasibility of early mechanical circulatory support in acute myocardial infarction complicated by cardiogenic shock: The Detroit cardiogenic shock initiative. Catheterization and Cardiovascular Interventions. 2017. DOI: 10.1002/ccd.27427 [Epub ahead of print]

[6] Tsao NW, Shih CM, Yeh JS, et al. Extracorporeal membrane oxygenation-assisted primary percutaneous coronary intervention may improve survival of patients with acute myocardial infarction complicated by profound cardiogenic shock. Journal of Critical Care. 2012;**27**(5):530.e1-530.11

[7] Roffi M, Patrono C, Collet JP, et al. 2015 ESC Guidelines for the management of acute coronary syndromes in patients presenting without persistent ST-segment elevation. Task Force for the Management of Acute Coronary Syndromes in Patients Presenting without Persistent ST-Segment Elevation of the European Society of Cardiology (ESC). European Heart Journal. 2016;**37**(3):267-315. DOI: 10.1093/eurheartj/ehv320

[8] Windecker S, Kolh P, Alfonso F, et al. Task force members, 2014 ESC/EACTS guidelines on myocardial revascularization: The task force on myocardial revascularization of the European Society of Cardiology (ESC) and the European Association for Cardio-Thoracic Surgery (EACTS) developed with the special contribution of the European Association of Percutaneous Cardiovascular Interventions (EAPCI). European Heart Journal. 2014;**35**(37):2541-2619

[9] Ibanez B, James S, Agewall S, et al. 2017 ESC guidelines for themanagement of acutemyocardial infarction in patients presenting with ST-segment elevation. European Heart Journal. 2017;**00**:1-66. DOI: 10.1093/eurheartj/ehx393

[10] Arlt M, Philipp A, Voelkel S, et al. Early experiences with miniaturized extracorporeal life support in the catheterization laboratory. European Journal of Cardio-Thoracic Surgery. 2012;**42**:858-863

[11] Liu S, Ravandi A, Kass M, et al. A case of awake percutaneous extracorporeal membrane oxygenation for high-risk percutaneous coronary intervention. Cureus. 2017;**9**(4):e1191. DOI: 10.7759/cureus.1191

[12] Galassi AG, Ganyukov V, Tomasello SD, et al. Successful antegrade revascularization by the innovation of composite core dual coil in a three-vessel total occlusive disease for cardiac arrest patient using extracorporeal membrane oxygenation. European Heart Journal. 2014;**35**(30):2009

[13] Tomasello SD, Boukhris M, Ganyukov V, et al. Outcome of extracorporeal membrane oxygenation support for complex high-risk elective percutaneous coronary interventions: A single-center experience. Heart & Lung. 2015;**44**(4):309-313

[14] Vetrovec GW. Hemodynamic support devices for shock and high-risk PCI: When and which one. Current Cardiology Reports. 2017;**19**:100. DOI: 10.1007/s11886-017-0905-3

[15] Myat A, Patel N, Tehrani S, et al. Percutaneous circulatory assist devices for high-risk coronary intervention. JACC. 2015;**8**:229-244

[16] Chalmers J, Pullan M, Fabri B, et al. Validation of EuroSCORE II in a modern cohort of patients undergoing cardiac surgery. European Journal of Cardio-Thoracic Surgery. 2013;**43**(4):688-694

[17] Shahian DM, O'Brien SM, Filardo G, et al. Society of Thoracic Surgeons quality measurement task F. The Society of Thoracic Surgeons 2008 cardiac surgery risk models: Part 3: Valve plus coronary artery bypass grafting surgery. The Annals of Thoracic Surgery. 2009;**88**(1 Suppl):S43-S62

[18] Held C, Asenblad N, Bassand JP, et al. Ticagrelor versus clopidogrel in patients with acute coronary syndromes undergoing coronary artery bypass surgery: Results from the PLATO (platelet inhibition and patient outcomes) trial. Journal of the American College of Cardiology. 2011;**57**:672-684

[19] Smith PK, Goodnough LT, Levy JH, et al. Mortality benefit with prasugrel in the TRITON-TIMI 38 coronary artery bypass grafting cohort: Risk-adjusted retrospective data analysis. Journal of the American College of Cardiology. 2012;**60**:388-396

[20] Ganyukov VI, Tarasov RS, Shukevich DL. Extracorporeal membrane oxygenation support for complex PCI in patients without cardiogenic shock. In: Fistenberg MS, editor. Book: Extracorporeal Membrane Oxygenation Advances in Therapy. Croatia: InTech; 2016. p. 127

[21] Benjamin EJ, Blaha MJ, Chiuve SE, et al. Heart disease and stroke statistics—2017 update: A report from the American Heart Association. Circulation. 2017;**135**:e146-e603

[22] Mehran R, Rao SV, Bhatt DL, et al. Standardized bleeding definitions for cardiovascular clinical trials: A consensus report from the bleeding academic research consortium. Circulation. 2011;**123**:2736-2747

[23] Carson P, Wertheimer J, Miller A, et al. The STICH trial (surgical treatment for ischemic heart failure): Mode-of-death results. JACC: Heart Failure. 2013;**1**(5):400-408

[24] Petrie MC, Jhund PS, She L, et al. Ten-year outcomes after coronary artery bypass grafting according to age in patients with heart failure and left ventricular systolic dysfunction: An analysis of the extended follow-up of the STICH trial (surgical treatment for ischemicheart failure). Circulation. 2016;**134**(18):1314-1324

[25] Barbarash LS, Ganyukov VI, Popov VA, et al. Hospital results of treatment of acute coronary syndrome without ST-segment elevation in multivessel coronary artery disease. Depending on the Kardiologicheskij Vestnik. 2013;**8**(2):17-23

Chapter 4

Severe Acute Respiratory Distress Syndrome

Carmen Silvia Valente Barbas,
Roberta Fittipaldi Palazo and
Gustavo Faissol Janot de Matos

Additional information is available at the end of the chapter

http://dx.doi.org/10.5772/intechopen.77071

Abstract

Acute respiratory distress syndrome is characterized by an increase of the permeability of the lungs' alveolar-capillary membranes, leading to the extravasation of liquid rich in proteins inside the alveolar spaces that turns air-filled lungs into heavy high-osmotic pressure liquid-filled lungs. The consequence is the collapse of the lowermost lung regions, shunt, refractory hypoxemia, decrease in lungs' compliance and increase in dead spaces that are more pronounced with the severity of the permeability changes of the pulmonary alveoli-capillary membrane. According to the recent Berlin definition, severe acute respiratory distress syndrome is defined by bilateral pulmonary infiltrates of recent onset (less than 1 week) in a patient with a risk factor for ARDS that has a PaO_2/FIO_2 equal or less than 100 with a positive end-expiratory pressure equal or more than 5 cm H_2O with no evidence of cardiac failure or hypervolemia. Severe ARDS patients present a higher mortality ratio, a more difficult mechanical ventilatory support (higher airway pressures with low tidal ventilation and higher $PaCO_2$ levels) and benefits for adjunctive ventilatory support therapy. The recommended mechanical ventilatory support in severe ARDS is with low tidal ventilation (less than 6 mL/Kg predicted body weight) with driving inspiratory pressures less than 15 cm H_2O, respiratory rate sufficient to keep adequate minute ventilation and $PaCO_2$ levels. PEEP higher than 15 cm H_2O and prolonged prone position are recommended for more severe patients to improve their survival. Adjunctive recruitment maneuvers can be used to improve oxygenation and allow more homogeneous ventilation and PEEP titration. In refractory hypoxemia and especially in younger patients with prognosis, extra-corporeal veno-venous membrane oxygenation support can be used.

Keywords: ARDS, mechanical ventilation, ECMO, hypoxemia

1. Diagnosing and evaluating the severe acute respiratory distress syndrome

Acute respiratory distress syndrome is characterized by an increase of the permeability of the lungs alveolar-capillary membranes leading to the extravasation of the intravascular plasma of the lungs capillary network surrounding the alveoli to the alveolar spaces that were previously filled by air. This accumulation of liquid rich in proteins inside the alveolar spaces turns an air-filled lungs into a heavy high-osmotic pressure liquid-filled lungs and the consequent collapse of the lowermost lung regions, shunt, refractory hypoxemia, decrease in lungs compliance and increase in dead space that are more pronounced the more severe the permeability changes of the pulmonary alveoli-capillary membrane. Regarding the physiopathology of ARDS, the hallmark mechanism of injury is inflammation leading to increased endothelial and epithelial permeability and liberation of receptors for angiopoietin-2 and advanced glycation end products (RAGE) [1–4].

2. Severe ARDS according to Berlin definition

According to the recent Berlin definition, severe acute respiratory distress syndrome is defined by bilateral pulmonary infiltrates of recent onset (less than 1 week) in a patient that have a PaO_2/FIO_2 equal or less than 100 with a positive end-expiratory pressure equal or more 5 cm H_2O with no evidence of cardiac failure or hypervolemia. The patient also needs to present a risk factor for ARDS development as respiratory infection, gastric content aspiration, lungs contusion, blood products transfusion, sepsis, high-risk trauma, high-risk surgery, shock, and pancreatitis [1–4].

3. The hole of extravascular lung water and pulmonary vascular index in the evaluation of severe ARDS

The extravascular lung water index (EVLWi) is calculated as the intra-thoracic total volume minus the intra-thoracic blood volume indexed by predicted body weight measured using a transpulmonary thermodilution method. The pulmonary vascular permeability index (PVPI) was calculated as extravascular lung water divided by the pulmonary blood volume [5]. Theoretically, the greater the EVLWi and PVPi, the greater the severity of ARDS. Recently, Kushimoto and colleagues [5] evaluated the relationship among the severity categories of ARDS as defined by the Berlin definition, EVLWi and PVPi to confirm their predictive validity for severity of ARDS. They measured EVLWi and PVPi in 195 patients with an EVLWi of ≥10 mL/kg, which fulfilled the Berlin definition of ARDS in 23 intensive care units for three consecutive days. Patients with moderate and severe ARDS had higher acute physiology and chronic health evaluation II (APACHE II) and sequential organ failure assessment scores (SOFA) on the day of enrollment compared to patients with mild ARDS. Patients with severe

ARDS had higher EVLWi (severe, 19.1; moderate, 17.2; mild, 16.1; $P < 0.05$) and PVPI (3.2; 3.0; 2.7; $P < 0.05$). When the authors evaluated 495 independent measurements over three consecutive days, they observed a moderative and negative correlation between PaO_2/FIO_2 ratio and EVLWi (r = −0.355, $P < 0.001$) and PaO_2/FIO_2 and PVPi (r = −0.345, $P < 0.001$ The authors observed an association between ARDS severity according to Berlin definition and 28-day mortality rate: severe, the odds ratio 4.167 relative to mild.

4. The hole of pulmonary arterial hypertension and right ventricular dysfunction in ARDS severity stratification

Hemodynamic data from the ARDSnet Fluids and Catheter Therapy Trial (FACCT) [6] that analyzed 475 patients randomized to receive a pulmonary artery catheter for ARDS management, none of the baseline measures of cardiopulmonary dysfunction distinguished survivors from nonsurvivors. When the authors measured the transpulmonary gradient (TGP), they observed that 73% of the ARDS patients monitored with the Swan-Ganz had an elevated TGP (>12 mm Hg). Patients with a TPG > 12 mm Hg had a significantly greater mortality rate than patients with a TPG < 12 mm Hg (30 vs. 19%; $P = 0.02$). In multivariate analysis, an elevated TPG and a high PVRi remained an independent predictor of an adverse outcome in this ARDS population. In a recent, prospective and observational study in an academic medical intensive care unit in France [7], 226 consecutive patients with moderate to severe ARDS ventilated who received a protective ventilation (plateau pressure less than 30 cm H_2O and mean PEEP of 8.8 ± 3.6 cm H_2O, underwent transesophageal echocardiography (TEE) within the first 3 days after the diagnosis of ARDS. Cor pulmonale (dilated right ventricle associated with septal dyskinesia), was detected in 49 patients (prevalence of 22%; 95% confidence interval, 16–27%). Patients who had cor pulmonale presented a significantly higher 28-day mortality rate (60 vs. 36%, $P < 0.01$) compared with the ARDS patients without cor pulmonale. Sepsis and higher values of driving pressure were associated with the presence of cor pulmonale that was an independent risk factor for 28-day mortality in their population. Taking these results into consideration, a subgroup of ARDS severity stratification: ARDS with right ventricular dysfunction should be proposed especially because different ventilatory strategies (prone position, low driving pressures, titrated PEEP levels), distinct pharmacologic therapy (pulmonary artery vasodilators) should be tested in order to improve prognosis of this subgroup of ARDS patients [4].

5. The hole of low respiratory system compliance in ARDS severity stratification

Other factors that are associated with severe ARDS are respiratory system compliance of less than 20 mL/cm H_2O, pulmonary dead space fraction greater than 0.60, as well as high APACHE II and SAPS II score as well as multiple organ failures (the higher the organ failures, the higher the patient mortality) [1–4].

Ichikado [8] showed that fibroproliferation signs in high-resolution CT evaluation of early ARDS patients were correlated with higher mortality and ventilator dependency. The lung SAFE study [3], an international, multicenter, prospective cohort study of patients undergoing invasive or noninvasive ventilation, conducted in 459 ICUs from 50 countries across five continents showed that 2.377 out of 29.144 patients developed ARDS in the first 48 h and whose respiratory failure was managed with invasive mechanical ventilation. The period prevalence of mild ARDS was 30.0% (95% CI, 28.2–31.9%); of moderate ARDS, 46.6% (95% CI, 44.5–48.6%); and of severe ARDS, 23.4% (95% CI, 21.7–25.2%). The cumulative frequency distribution of tidal volume was similar in patients in each severity category, with 65% of patients with acute respiratory distress syndrome (ARDS) receiving a tidal volume of 8 mL/kg of predicted body weight or less. In contrast, a right shift of the cumulative frequency distribution curves of plateau pressures was seen for increasing ARDS severity category, with plateau pressure of more than 30 cm H_2O in 8.5% of patients for which these data were available. There was a lower likelihood of survival to day 28 with increasing severity of acute respiratory distress syndrome (ARDS) at day 1. Patients with a driving pressure of greater than 14 cm H_2O on day 1 of ARDS criteria had a higher mortality. Taking into consideration, these data that tidal volume ventilation was similar across the ARDS severity but inspiratory driving pressure less than 14 cm H_2O was associated with decreased mortality of those patients one could argue that in the future tidal volume should be titrated according to the derived driving inspiratory pressure.

Amato and colleagues [9] analyzed individual data from 3562 patients with ARDS enrolled in nine previously published randomized clinical trials of mechanical ventilation using a multilevel mediation analysis. They observed a strong association between driving pressure and ARDS survival even though all the ventilator settings that were used were lung protective (RR of death: 1.36, 95% CI 1.17–1.58, $P < 0.001$). These observations suggest that tidal volume might be adjusted to the resultant airway driving pressure in addition to the adjustment to the predicted body weight. They also observed that airway driving pressures higher than 15 cm H_2O were associated with increasing rates of mortality in ARDS patients. Recently, Villar and colleagues [10] analyzed the data from two observational studies enclosing 778 patients with moderate and severe ARDS. They assessed the risk of hospital death based on quantiles of tidal volume, positive end-expiratory pressure, plateau inspiratory pressure and airway driving pressure evaluated 24 h after ARDS diagnosis while the patients were ventilated with lung protective ventilation. The authors verified that positive end expiratory pressure and tidal volume that were set according to a protective lung ventilation strategy had no impact on mortality while a plateau pressure higher than 29 cm H_2O and a driving pressure higher than 19 cm H_2O were associated with a higher hospital mortality.

As respiratory system driving pressure does not account for variable chest wall compliance or different degrees of intra-abdominal pressures or even more to the presence of inspiratory efforts or asynchrony, esophageal manometry can be used to measure transpulmonary pressure that represents the lungs parenchyma stress during tidal volume ventilation. Recently, Baedorf and colleagues examined the relationships between respiratory system and transpulmonary driving pressure measured at baseline, 5 min and 24 h after PEEP titration and

28-day mortality in 56 ARDS patients. They observed that PEEP titration to target positive end-expiratory transpulmonary pressures resulted in both improved elastance and driving pressures and was associated with improved 28-day mortality.

However, future studies regarding the evaluation of respiratory system and transpulmonary driving pressure in ARDS patients with normal and increased abdominal pressure and various degrees of respiratory system compliance is still needed in order to establish the value of both as a bedside ventilator target as well as a prognosticator of evolution and mortality of those patients.

6. The hole of increased dead space, high $PaCO_2$ and multiple organ failure in severe ARDS

Increased dead space in the first day of mechanical ventilation, increased $PaCO_2$ levels with protective ventilation and multiple organ failure are all associated with higher mortality in severe ARDS. However, specific therapeutic aiming to decrease dead space fraction, decrease $PaCO_2$ levels or even multimodal therapeutic approach to treat multiple organ failure still need to be defined and tested [4].

7. Does the risk factor for ARDS influence the patient mortality rate?

Recently, Villar and colleagues [11] showed in a cohort of 778 patients that severe ARDS occurred in about 37.5% at ARDS diagnosis and after 24 h of ARDS onset 20.8% and moderate to severe ARDS had an overall mortality of 38.8%. They also showed that the underlying cause of ARDS influence in the mortality ratio (the mortality ratio was higher in pancreatitis and progressively lower in sepsis, pneumonia and trauma).

8. Treating the severe ARDS patient

Low-tidal ventilation (≤6 mL/kg of predicted body weight) must be initiated as soon as the ARDS patient is intubated and mechanically ventilated. The predicted body weight (PBW) can be calculated as follows: for women, PBW = 45.5 + 0.91 (height in centimeters—152.4) and for men, PBW = 50.0 + 0.91 (height in centimeters—152.4). It is well documented that lower tidal volumes (6 mL/kg of predicted body weight) compared to higher tidal volumes (12 mL/kg of predicted body weight) associated with PEEP levels titrated by a PEEP/FIO_2 table reduced mortality in a randomized, clinical trial that analyzed 861 ARDS patients (ARMA trial) [12].

It is crucial to adjust tidal volume to lung size that depends of the height and sex, but more importantly is to adjust the tidal volume to functional lung size that depends on the ARDS severity (lung compliance), sex, height, and chest wall compliance. The patient with severe

ARDS and a low compliance will be ventilated with high airway pressures if ventilated with 6 mL/predicted body weight. Amato and colleagues [9], in 2015, reported that driving pressure (ΔP), that can be also be represented by tidal volume (VT)/respiratory system compliance (CRS), in which VT is intrinsically normalized to functional lung size, was a ventilatory variable more strongly associated with survival than VT or PEEP in patients who are not actively breathing. Using a statistical tool known as multilevel mediation analysis to study individual data from 3562 patients with ARDS enrolled in nine previously reported randomized trials, they examined ΔP as an independent variable associated with survival. In the mediation analysis, they estimated the isolated effects of changes in ΔP resulting from randomized ventilator settings while minimizing confounding due to the baseline severity of lung disease. The authors observed that among ventilation variables, ΔP was most strongly associated with survival. A 1-SD increment in ΔP (approximately 7 cm of water) was associated with increased mortality (relative risk, 1.41; 95% confidence interval [CI], 1.31–1.51; $P < 0.001$), even in patients receiving "protective" plateau pressures and VT (relative risk, 1.36; 95% CI, 1.17–1.58; $P < 0.001$). Individual changes in VT or PEEP after randomization were not independently associated with survival; they were associated only if they were among the changes that led to reductions in ΔP (mediation effects of ΔP, $P = 0.004$ and $P = 0.001$, respectively). They concluded that ΔP was the ventilation variable that best stratified risk. Decreases in ΔP owing to changes in ventilator settings were strongly associated with increased survival.

Moreover, recent evidences [13] showed that in severe ARDS patients, inspiratory efforts during assisted ventilation could worsen ventilator lung injury induced by the mechanical ventilation during the ventilatory support of the ARDS patients. This associated and added injury could explain the results of a phase IV randomized controlled trial in moderate-severe ARDS patients ($PaO_2/FIO_2 < 150$), comparing cisatracurium to placebo for 48 h showed an improved adjusted 90-day survival rate and increased ventilator-free in the cisatracurium group without a significant increase in muscle weakness. Short-term paralysis may facilitate patient-ventilator synchrony in the setting of lung protective ventilation. Short-term paralysis would eliminate patient triggering and expiratory muscle activity. In combination, these effects may serve to limit regional overdistention and cyclic alveolar collapse. Paralysis may also act to lower metabolism and overall ventilatory demand [14]. Recently, Sottile and colleagues [15] showed that the use of neuromuscular blockade in ARDS patients receiving low tidal volume ventilation and a PaO_2/FIO_2 ratio less than 120 were associated with decreased biomarkers of epithelial (serum surfactant protein-D) and endothelial (serum Von Willebrand factor) lung injury and systemic inflammation (serum interleukin 8).

At the same time, that an adequate sedation, an adequate short-term paralysis and low tidal volume were set in severe ARDS patients [16], an adequate respiratory rate must be concurrently set in order to keep a minute ventilation around 7–8 L/min and a $PaCO_2$ around 40–60 mm Hg and a pH above 7.2. In the more severe ARDS patients, sometimes after the adjustment of a minute ventilation around 7–8 L/min with tidal volumes lesser than 6 mL/kg of predicted body weight, the $PaCO_2$ levels stay above 80 mm Hg and pH less than 7.2 (specially patients with septic shock and metabolic acidosis). In these cases, the VCO_2 must be assessed and be kept as least as possible (fever control, low carbohydrate intake) and hemodialysis can be initiate (especially in ARDS patients with concomitant acute renal failure) in order to help control the metabolic acidosis. Efforts must be taken to decrease the pulmonary dead space by means of recruitment maneuvers and PEEP titration, tidal volume and respiratory rate adjustments or even the initiation of prone ventilation. In the most difficult cases, tracheal gas insufflation or extracorporeal CO_2 removal or extracorporeal oxygenation should be started in order to keep the protective low tidal volume ventilation [17].

Permissive hypercapnia can carry potential harmful consequences including pulmonary vasoconstriction and pulmonary hypertension, proarrhythmic effects of increased discharge of catecholamines and cerebral vasodilation yielding increased intracranial pressure. When applying protective ventilation in patients with severe ARDS, special attention should be given to patients with pulmonary hypertension and right ventricular dysfunction that could not tolerate high $PaCO_2$ and low pH levels. Nonetheless, permissive hypercapnia should probably be used with caution in patients with heart disease and is relatively contraindicated in those with elevated intracranial pressure. In ARDS cases with pulmonary hypertension and right ventricular dysfunction, prone position ventilation should be preferred [17].

Recently, three large clinical trials [18–20], including acute lung injury/ARDS patients ventilated with low tidal-volume, have compared different PEEP strategies (high vs. low), but none of them could show a significant difference in mortality. Moreover, a recent meta-analysis [21] has pooled those trials, revealing some combined benefits of the high PEEP strategy; still, the survival benefit was modest and limited to the subgroup of ARDS patients with $PaO_2/FIO_2 < 200$ (moderate and severe ARDS according to Berlin definition). Conceptually, one could argue that none of the "high-PEEP" strategies was designed to test the "open-lung hypothesis" postulated by Lachmann, that is, the hypothesis that most of the collapsed lung tissue observed in early ARDS can be reversed at an acceptable clinical cost, potentially resulting in better lung protection [22–24]. According to a recent study by Borges and colleagues [25], a straight test of the "open-lung hypothesis" would certainly require more aggressive recruiting maneuvers in association with individualized, decremental PEEP titration. Recently, de Matos and colleagues [26] reported the experience with maximal recruitment strategy (MRS) in 51 patients with ARDS. MRS consisted of 2-min steps of pressure-controlled ventilation, fixed driving pressure of 15 cm H_2O, respiratory rate of 10 breaths/min, inspiratory/expiratory ratio of 1:1, and stepwise increments in PEEP levels from 10 to 45 cm H_2O (recruitment phase). After that, PEEP was decreased to 25 cm H_2O and, then, from 25 to 10 cm H_2O (PEEP titration phase) in steps of 5 cm H_2O, each one lasting 4 min monitored by thoracic tomography images. At each of the steps, computer tomography image sequences from the carina to the diaphragm were acquired during an expiratory pause of 6–10 s. Visual inspection of the images was performed during the tomographic examination in order to assess the lung collapse in the lungs bases for immediate clinical decision, and after an offline quantitative analysis was realized. Nonaerated parenchyma decreased significantly from 53.6% (interquartile range (IQR): 42.5–62.4) to 12.7% (IQR: 4.9–24.2) ($P < 0.0001$) after MRS. The opening plateau pressure observed during the recruitment protocol was 59.6 (±5.9 cm H_2O), and the mean PEEP titrated after MRS was 24.6 (±2.9 cm H_2O). The mean PaO_2/FiO_2 ratio increased from 125 (±43) to 300 (±103; $P < 0.0001$) after MRS and was sustained above 300 throughout 7 days. MRS showed a statistically significant decrease in nonaerated areas of the ARDS lungs that was accompanied by a significant increment in oxygenation. The potentially recruitable lung was estimated at 45% (IQR: 25–53). ICU mortality was 28% and hospital mortality was 32%. The independent risk factors associated with mortality were older age and higher driving pressures. There were no significant clinical complications with MRS or barotrauma. A better evolution of these ARDS patients with less necessity of oxygen supplementation in the recovery phase of the disease and a better quality of life were observed in these patients [26].

A recent systematic review and meta-analysis [27] that analyzed the effects of recruitment maneuvers for adult patients with acute respiratory distress syndrome showed an overall pool effect of a significant decrease on mortality in these patients and no associated increase in barotrauma. However, soon after, a large prospective, multicenter and controlled trial (ART trial) [28] that compared recruitment maneuver and best-compliance PEEP titration in 501 ARDS patients with 509 ARDS patients ventilated with low PEEP showed an increased 6-month mortality in both groups, but higher in the recruitment and PEEP titration group (65.3 vs. 59.9%, respectively, $P = 0.04$). However, in our opinion, the recruitment maneuver tested in ART trial was abrupt and short (started at 25 cm H_2O PEEP, duration of 1 s and not imaging monitored) what could have contributed to the higher levels of observed barotrauma and mortality [29]. When we combined the results of the systematic review and meta-analysis with the ART results, we observed a total of 1144 patients undergoing recruitment maneuvers and PEEP titration and 1179 controls with standard ventilation with a final result of no significant differences in mortality relatite risk of 0.91 [95% CI, 0.74–1.13]. The most effective recruitment maneuver and PEEP titration in ARDS remain to be determined [29].

Our group is used to apply maximal recruitment strategy maneuvers in our severe ARDS patients with PEEP titration with thoracic tomography with good results. Here, we present a case of a 47-year-old man, previously asymptomatic, that started with cough, dyspnea, and an acute hypoxemic respiratory failure. The chest-X-ray showed a bilateral pulmonary infiltrate that predominates in the lower lungs fields (**Figure 1**). SpO_2 in ambient air was 77% and after oxygen mask of 100% SpO_2 was 88% and he needed intubation and mechanical ventilation. Arterial pressure is of 11 × 7 cm Hg and HR of 110 rpm. Hemocultures and tracheal secretion were collected as well as a nasopharyngeal swab for respiratory viruses. Oseltamivir, clarithromycin and ceftriaxone were initiated. A transthoracic echocardiogram showed normal right and left ventricular function and a normal arterial pulmonary pressure. A protective mechanical ventilation was initiated with tidal volume of 6 mL/kg/predicted body weight (420 mL), RR of 20 rpm, PEEP of 15 cm H_2O, FIO_2 of 100%, SpO_2 de 90% and an arterial blood gas analysis showed a pH of 7,35, $PaCO_2$ of 50 mm Hg, PaO_2 of 60 mm Hg, sodium bicarbonate of 23 and base excess of −1, lactate of 10 mg/dL, SvO_2 of 70 mm Hg, Hb of 13 g/dL, 12,000 leucocytes, platelets of 250,000, reactive C-protein of 120 mg/L, BNP of 40 pg/mL. He was submitted to maximal recruitment strategy maneuvers and PEEP titration of 25 cm H_2O in the tomography room (**Figure 2**). The PaO_2/FIO_2 ratio increased from 60 to 200, and after 3 days, he was with PEEP of 15 cm H_2O and a PaO_2/FIO_2 of 300. After 10 days, he was extubated and presented in ambient air a SpO_2 of 95% and an expressive improvement in chest X-ray (**Figure 3**). All the collect cultures and the nasopharyngeal swab for respiratory viruses were negative. The thoracic tomography performed 3 days after extubation showed an important improvement of the lungs infiltrates (**Figure 4**).

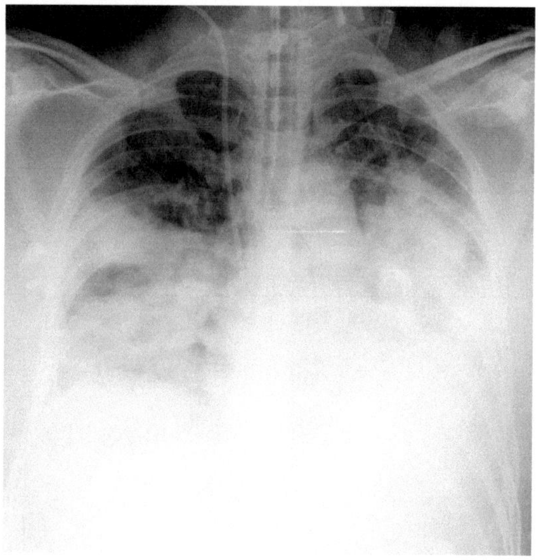

Figure 1. Chest X-ray showing bilateral pulmonary infiltrates that predominate in lower lungs fields.

Recent evidence showed that prolonged prone position ventilation (16 h) must be used in early ARDS with PaO_2/FIO_2 < than 150 with PEEP levels of or more than 5 cm H_2O in order to significantly improved 90-day mortality compared to supine ventilation (PROSEVA trial) [30].

Recent meta-analysis also showed that in the era of low tidal ventilation, the prone position use improved mortality of moderate/severe ARDS patients that needed invasive mechanical ventilatory support [31]. If PEEP titration during prone position, ventilation should improve survival of ARDS patients, which is still a matter of debate.

For patients in whom gas exchange is refractory to conventional ventilation and other advanced therapies, extracorporeal membrane oxygenation (ECMO) may be appropriate as salvage therapy. Venovenous ECMO may be able to support refractory hypoxemia in the setting of severe ARDS. It may also be used for carbon dioxide removal when respiratory system compliance is severely compromised and efforts to maintain plateau airway pressures within acceptable parameters lead to unsustainable levels of hypercapnia and respiratory acidosis.

Prospective randomized controlled trial of ECMO in severe ARDS, reported in 2009, was the Conventional Ventilation or ECMO for Severe Adult Respiratory Failure (CESAR) trial [32], in which 180 subjects with severe ARDS were randomized to conventional mechanical ventilation or referral to a specialized center for consideration of ECMO. The United Kingdom randomized and prospective clinical trial (CESAR) revealed a survival advantage in the ECMO group; the ECMO group had a 63% survival after 6 months, while the control group had a 47% survival rate. The study was criticized because there was no standardized protocol management for the control group and some patients in the ECMO group did not receive the proposed treatment. The authors demonstrated that this strategy is also likely to be cost-effective in settings with similar services to those in the United Kingdom. Patients should be considered for weaning

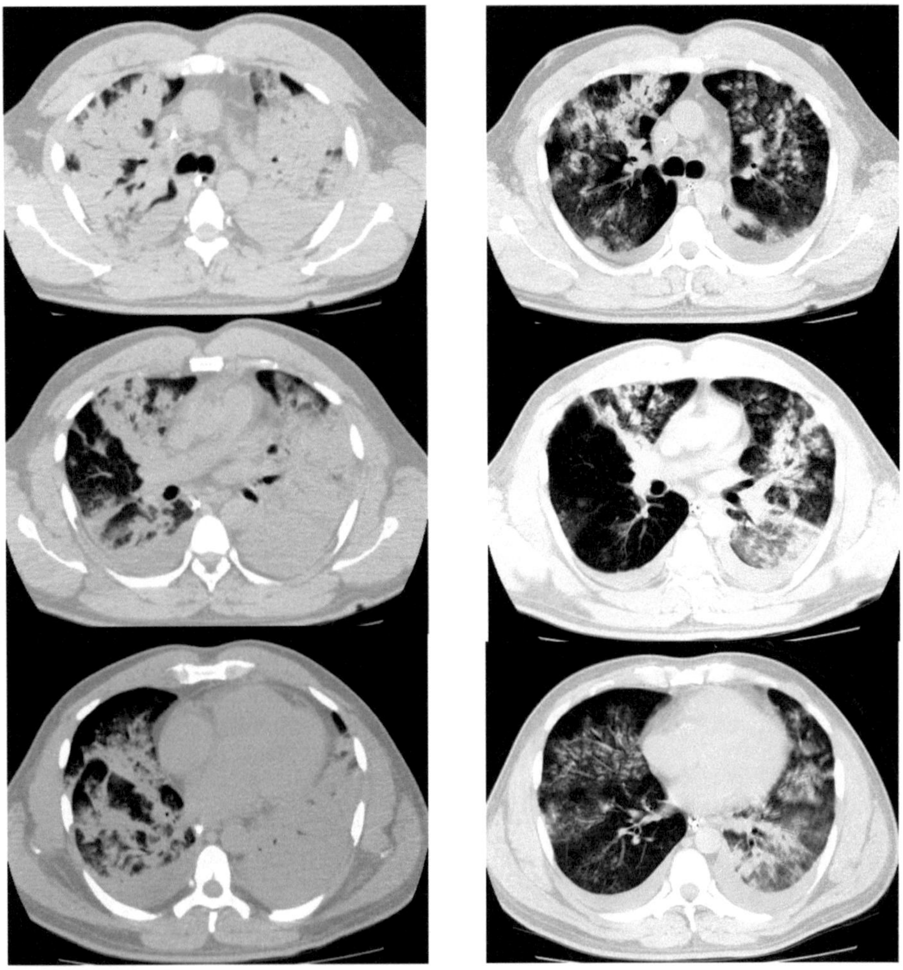

Figure 2. Thoracic tomography before and after maximal recruitment maneuvers and PEEP titration. Pre-recruitment PEEP of 10 cm H_2O. Pos-recruitment PEEP of 25 cm H_2O.

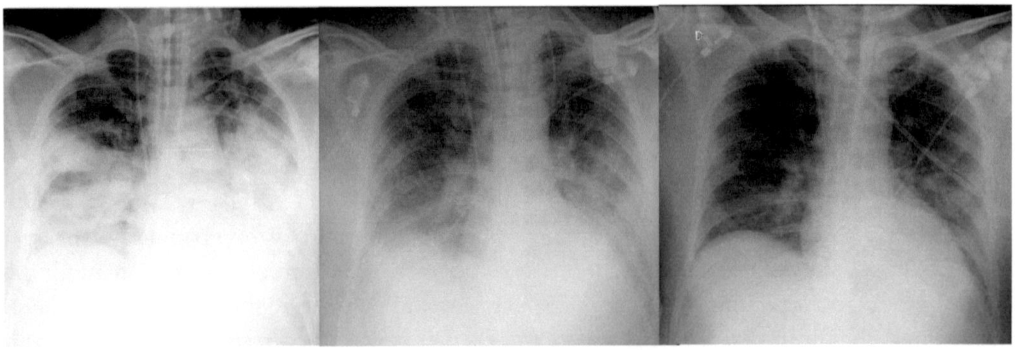

Figure 3. Chest-X-ray day 1, day 3, and day 10 after admission (day of extubation).

http://dx.doi.org/10.5772/intechopen.77071

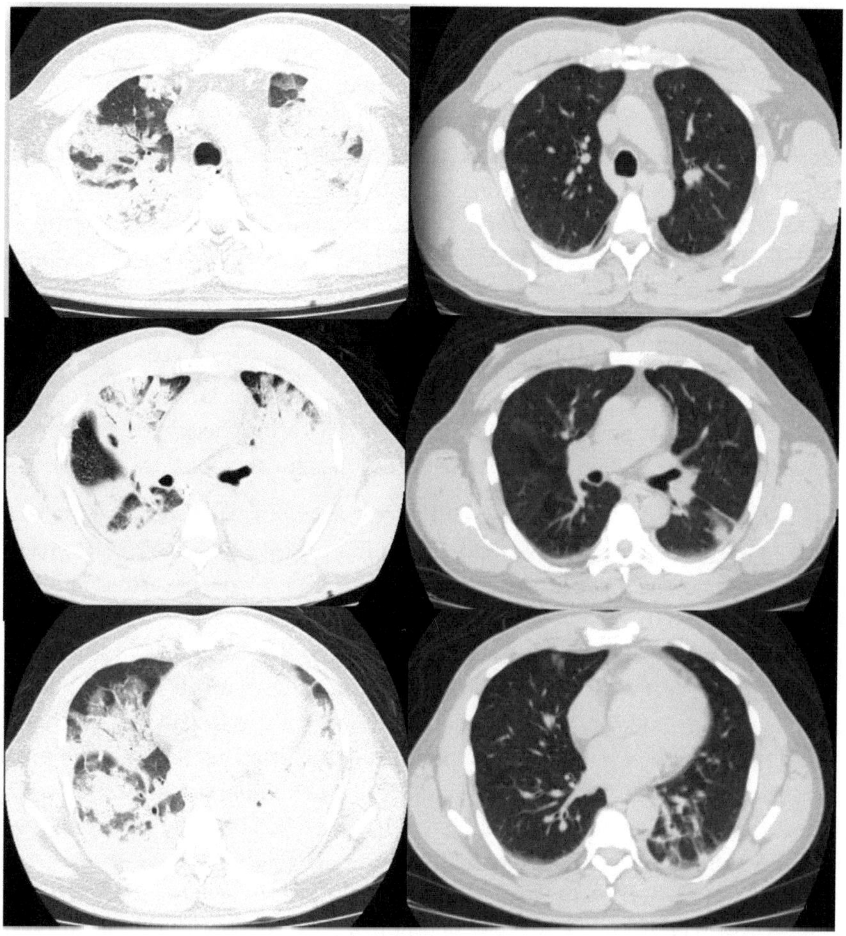

Figure 4. Thoracic tomography at first day after admission and thoracic tomography 3 days after extubation.

from venovenous ECMO once the underlying disease process for which ECMO was initiated has sufficiently resolved so that they can be safely and adequately supported by protective ventilatory strategy and oxygenation support without evidence of excessive respiratory work of breathing. Markers of sufficient native lung function recovery include adequate gas exchange reserve, acceptable respiratory system compliance, and improvement in chest images [32].

Another recent approach for application of extracorporeal carbon dioxide removal new devices (ECMO-R) in ARDS patients is the observation in thoracic tomography of ARDS patients that in severe ARDS, even the low tidal volume ventilation with 6 mL/kg of predicted body weight can cause tidal hyperdistension in the nondependent regions of the lungs accompanied by plateau airway pressures greater than 28 cm H_2O and elevated plasma markers of inflammation. Application of ECMO-R in these severe ARDS patients could allow the authors to decrease the tidal volume to less than 6 mL/kg with a consequent plateau pressure less than 25 cm H_2O that was associated with lower levels of lung-derived inflammatory cytokines and a lower radiographic index of lung injury [33], but prognostic implications of ECMO-R devices application in clinical practice are still under investigation [34]. Pumpless interventional lung assist (iLA) is also used in patients with ARDS and is aimed at improving extracorporeal gas exchange with a membrane integrated in a passive arteriovenous shunt. iLA can be used in severe ARDS patients as an extracorporeal device to remove CO_2 enabling low tidal volume and a reduced inspiratory plateau pressure in the mechanical ventilator in extremely severe ARDS patients. iLA device was used in 51 severe ARDS patients by Zimmermann and colleagues with a decrease in $PaCO_2$ allowing the ultraprotective ventilation (lower tidal volume and plateau inspiratory pressures) with a hospital mortality of 49% [35]. More recently, the use of an ultraprotective strategy using 4 mL/kg of predicted body weight associated with low flow extracorporeal carbon removal in 15 moderate ARDS patients was described by Faneli and coworkers [36]. Additional data to the use of ECMO in ARDS patients will be added with the publication of EOLIA trial (ClinicalTrials.gov Identifier: NCT01470703), a prospective and randomized trial that evaluated the role of ECMO in severe ARDS that has finished but not published yet.

In conclusion, the severe ARDS is defined as an acute bilateral pulmonary infiltrate onset, in a patient with a PaO_2/FIO_2 equal or less than 100 with a positive end expiratory pressure equal or more than 5 cm H_2O that have an ARDS risk factor with no signs of cardiac failure or hypervolemia. Thus, when an intensivist evaluates an ARDS patient severity, he/her has to take into consideration the patient's age, cause of ARDS, the PaO_2/FIO_2 ratio, response to PEEP, prone position, $PaCO_2$ with protective ventilation (6 mL/predicted body weight), right ventricular function and level of pulmonary artery pressure, presence of shock (and necessity of vasoactive drugs), APACHE II score, number of organ failures (specially renal failure). The severe ARDS patients present a higher mortality ratio and required an extremely careful and specialized treatment. The cause of ARDS initiation should be addressed and promptly treated. These patients present a more difficult mechanical ventilatory support (higher airway pressures with low tidal ventilation and higher $PaCO_2$ levels). They should be adequately monitored (airway and esophageal pressure measurements, bedside echocardiography and lung ultrasound, if possible). Protective ventilatory strategy must be offered and monitored (low tidal volume (less than 6 mL/kg of predicted body weight) and low distending inspiratory driving pressures (less than 15 cm H_2O) with adequate PEEP levels, and early prone position applied for more than 16 h. The possible benefits for adjunctive ventilatory support therapy (higher PEEP, recruitment maneuvers, inhalatory nitric oxide, ECMO and continuous hemodialysis) in the refractory cases should be offered, observing and monitoring the cross-talking among the multiple organ dysfunctions and guiding and changing the treatment according to the patients' responses. The more difficult cases must be treated in specialized centers with expertise supervision [4, 17, 26, 37, 38].

Author details

Carmen Silvia Valente Barbas[1,2]*, Roberta Fittipaldi Palazo[2] and Gustavo Faissol Janot de Matos[2]

*Address all correspondence to: carmen.barbas@gmail.com

1 University of São Paulo, Brazil

2 Adult ICU, Hospital Israelita Albert Einstein, São Paulo, SP, Brazil

References

[1] Ranieri VM, Rubenfeld GD, Thompson BT, Ferguson ND, Caldwell E, Fan E, Camporota L, Slutsky AS. Acute respiratory distress syndrome: The Berlin definition. ARDS definition task force. JAMA. 2012;**307**(23):2526-2533

[2] Caser EB, Zandonade E, Pereira E, Gama AM, Barbas CS. Impact of distinct definitions of acute lung injury on its incidence and outcomes in Brazilian ICUs: prospective evaluation of 7,133 patients. Critical Care Medicine. 2014;**42**(3):574-582

[3] Bellani G, Laffey JG, Pham T, Fan E, Brochard L, Esteban A, Gattinoni L, van Haren F, Larsson A, McAuley DF, Ranieri M, Rubenfeld G, Thompson BT, Wrigge H, Slutsky AS, Pesenti A, LUNG SAFE investigators; ESICM trials group. Epidemiology, patterns of care, and mortality for patients with acute respiratory distress syndrome in intensive care units in 50 countries. JAMA. 2016;**315**(8):788-800

[4] Barbas CS, Isola AM, Caser EB. What is the future of acute respiratory distress syndrome after the Berlin definition? Current Opinion in Critical Care. 2014;**20**(1):10-16

[5] Kushimoto S, Endo T, Yamanouchi S, Sakamoto T, Ishikura H, Kitazawa Y, Taira Y, Okuchi K, Tagami T, Watanabe A, Yamaguchi J, Yoshikawa K, Sugita M, Kase Y, Kanemura T, Takahashi H, Kuroki Y, Izumino H, Rinka H, Seo R, Takatori M, Kaneko T, Nakamura T, Irahara T, Saito N. The Picco Pulmonary Edema Study Group. Relationship between extravascular lung water and severity categories of acute respiratory distress syndrome by the Berlin definition. Critical Care. 2013;**17**(4):R132

[6] Wiedemann HP, Wheeler AP, Bernard GR, Thompson BT, Hayden D, deBoisblanc B, Connors AF Jr, Hite RD, Harabin AL. Comparison of two fluid-management strategies in acute lung injury. New England Journal of Medicine. 2006;**354**(24):2564-2575

[7] Boissier F, Katsahian S, Razazi K, Thille AW, Roche-Campo F, Leon R, Vivier E, Brochard L, Vieillard-Baron A, Brun-Buisson C, Mekontso Dessap A. Prevalence and prognosis of cor pulmonale during protective ventilation for acute respiratory distress syndrome. Intensive Care Medicine. 2013;**39**(10):1725-1733

[8] Ichikado K. The Berlin definition and clinical significance of high resolution CT (HRCT) imaging in acute respiratory distress syndrome. Masui. 2013;**62**(5):522-531

[9] Amato MB, Meade MO, Slutsky AS, Brochard L, Costa EL, Schoenfeld DA, Stewart TE, Briel M, Talmor D, Mercat A, Richard JC, Carvalho CR, Brower RG. Driving pressure and survival in the acute respiratory distress syndrome. The New England Journal of Medicine. 2015;**372**(8):747-755

[10] Villar J, Martín-Rodríguez C, Domínguez-Berrot AM, Fernández L, Ferrando C, Soler JA, Díaz-Lamas AM, González-Higueras E, Nogales L, Ambrós A, Carriedo D, Hernández M, Martínez D, Blanco J, Belda J, Parrilla D, Suárez-Sipmann F, Tarancón C, Mora-Ordoñez JM, Blanch L, Pérez-Méndez L, Fernández RL, Kacmarek RM. Spanish initiative for epidemiology, stratification and therapies for ARDS (SIESTA) investigators network. A quantile analysis of plateau and driving pressures: Effects on mortality in patients with acute respiratory distress syndrome receiving lung-protective ventilation. Critical Care Medicine. 2017;**45**(5):843-850

[11] Villar J, Martínez D, Mosteiro F, Ambrós A, Añón JM, Ferrando C, Soler JA, Montiel R, Vidal A, Conesa-Cayuela LA, Blanco J, Arrojo R, Solano R, Capilla L, Del Campo R, Civantos B, Fernández MM, Aldecoa C, Parra L, Gutiérrez A, Martínez-Jiménez C, González-Martín JM, Fernández RL, Kacmarek RM. Stratification and outcome of acute respiratory distress syndrome (STANDARDS) network. Is overall mortality the right composite endpoint in clinical trials of acute respiratory distress syndrome? Critical Care Medicine. Feb 7, 2018. DOI: 10.1097/CCM.0000000000003022. [Epub ahead of print]

[12] The Acute Respiratory Distress Syndrome Network. Ventilation with lower tidal volumes as compared with traditional tidal volumes for acute lung injury and the acute respiratory distress syndrome. The New England Journal of Medicine. 2000;**342**:1301-1308

[13] Yoshida T, Torsani V, Gomes S, De Santis RR, Beraldo MA, Costa EL, Tucci MR, Zin WA, Kavanagh BP, Amato MB. Spontaneous effort causes occult pendelluft during mechanical ventilation. American Journal of Respiratory and Critical Care Medicine. 2013;**188** (12):1420-1427

[14] Papazian L, Forel JM, Gacouin A, et al. Neuromuscular blockers in early acute respiratory distress syndrome. The New England Journal of Medicine. 2010;**363**(12):1107-1116

[15] Sottile PD, Albers D, Moss MM. Neuromuscular blockade is associated with the attenuation of biomarkers of epithelial and endothelial injury in patients with moderate-to-severe acute respiratory distress syndrome. Critical Care. 2018;**22**:63

[16] Barbas CSV. In: Chiumello D, editor. Acute Respiratory Distress Syndrome (ARDS). Switzerland: Springer International Publishing; 2017. pp. 29-39

[17] Barbas CS, Matos GF, Amato MB, Carvalho CR. Goal-oriented respiratory management for critically ill patients with acute respiratory distress syndrome. Critical Care Research and Practice. 2012;**2012**:952168

[18] Brower RG, Lanken PN, MacIntyre N, Matthay MA, Morris A, Ancukiewicz M, Schoenfeld D, Thompson BT. Higher versus lower positive end-expiratory pressures in patients with the acute respiratory distress syndrome. The New England Journal of Medicine. 2004;**351**:327-336

[19] Mercat A, Richard JC, Vielle B, Jaber S, Osman D, Diehl JL, Lefrant JY, Prat G, Richecoeur J, Nieszkowska A, Gervais C, Baudot J, Bouadma L, Brochard L. Expiratory pressure (express) study group. Positive end-expiratory pressure setting in adults with acute lung injury and acute respiratory distress syndrome: A randomized controlled trial. JAMA. 2008;**299**:646-655

[20] Meade MO, Cook DJ, Guyatt GH, Slutsky AS, Arabi YM, Cooper DJ, Davies AR, Hand LE, Zhou Q, Thabane L, Austin P, Lapinsky S, Baxter A, Russell J, Skrobik Y, Ronco JJ, Stewart TE. Lung open ventilation study investigators. Ventilation strategy using low tidal volumes, recruitment maneuvers, and high positive end-expiratory pressure for acute lung injury and acute respiratory distress syndrome: A randomized controlled trial. JAMA. 2008;**299**:637-645

[21] Briel M, Meade M, Mercat A, Brower RG, Talmor D, Walter SD, Slutsky AS, Pullenayegum E, Zhou Q, Cook D, Brochard L, Richard JC, Lamontagne F, Bhatnagar N, Stewart TE, Guyatt G. Higher vs. lower positive end-expiratory pressure in patients with acute lung injury and acute respiratory distress syndrome: Systematic review and meta-analysis. JAMA. 2010;**303**:865-873

[22] Lachmann B. Open up the lung and keep the lung open. Intensive Care Medicine. 1992;**18**:319-321

[23] Barbas CS, de Matos GF, Pincelli MP, da Rosa Borges E, Antunes T, de Barros JM, Okamoto V, Borges JB, Amato MB, de Carvalho CR. Mechanical ventilation in acute respiratory failure: Recruitment and high positive end-expiratory pressure are necessary. Current Opinion in Critical Care. 2005;**11**:18-28

[24] Papadakos PJ, Lachmann B. The open lung concept of mechanical ventilation: The role of recruitment and stabilization. Critical Care Clinics. 2007;**23**:241-250

[25] Borges JB, Okamoto VN, Matos GF, Caramez MP, Arantes PR, Barros F, Souza CE, Victorino JA, Kacmarek RM, Barbas CS, Carvalho CR, Amato MB. Reversibility of lung collapse and hypoxemia in early acute respiratory distress syndrome. American Journal of Respiratory and Critical Care Medicine. 2006;**174**:268-278

[26] de Matos GF, Stanzani F, Passos RH, Fontana MF, Albaladejo R, Caserta RE, Santos DC, Borges JB, Amato MB, Barbas CS. How large is the lung recruitability in early acute respiratory distress syndrome: A prospective case series of patients monitored by computed tomography. Critical Care. 2012;**16**(1):R4

[27] Goligher EC, Hodgson CL, Adhikari NKJ, Meade MO, Wunsch H, Uleryk E, Gajic O, Amato MPB, Ferguson ND, Rubenfeld GD, Fan E. Lung recruitment maneuvers for adult patients with acute respiratory distress syndrome. A systematic review and meta-analysis. Annals of the American Thoracic Society. 2017;**14**(4):S304-S311

[28] Writing Group for the Alveolar Recruitment for Acute Respiratory Distress Syndrome Trial (ART) Investigators, Cavalcanti AB, Suzumura ÉA, Laranjeira LN, Paisani DM, Damiani LP, Guimarães HP, Romano ER, Regenga MM, Taniguchi LNT, Teixeira C, Pinheiro de Oliveira R, Machado FR, Diaz-Quijano FA, Filho MSA, Maia IS, Caser EB, Filho WO, Borges MC, Martins PA, Matsui M, Ospina-Tascón GA, Giancursi TS, Giraldo-Ramirez ND, Vieira SRR, Assef MDGPL, Hasan MS, Szczeklik W, Rios F, Amato MBP, Berwanger O, Ribeiro de Carvalho CR. Effect of lung recruitment and titrated positive end-expiratory pressure (PEEP) vs. low PEEP on mortality in patients with acute respiratory distress syndrome: A randomized clinical trial. Journal of the American Medical Association. 2017;**318**(14):1335-1345

[29] Barbas CSV, Nemer SN. Lung recruitment and positive end-expiratory pressure titration in patients with acute respiratory distress syndrome. Journal of the American Medical Association. 2018;**319**(9):933

[30] Guérin C, Reignier J, Richard JC, Beuret P, Gacouin A, Boulain T, Mercier E, Badet M, Mercat A, Baudin O, Clavel M, Chatellier D, Jaber S, Rosselli S, Mancebo J, Sirodot M,

Hilbert G, Bengler C, Richecoeur J, Gainnier M, Bayle F, Bourdin G, Leray V, Girard R, Baboi L, Ayzac L. PROSEVA study group. Prone positioning in severe acute respiratory distress syndrome. The New England Journal of Medicine. 2013;**368**(23):2159-2168

[31] Beitler JR, Shaefi S, Montesi SB, Devlin A, Loring SH, Talmor D, Malhotra A. Prone positioning reduces mortality from acute respiratory distress syndrome in the low tidal volume era: A meta-analysis. Intensive Care Medicine. 2014;**40**(3):332-341

[32] Peek GJ, Mugford M, Tiruvoipati R, et al. Efficacy and economic assessment of conventional ventilatory support versus extracorporeal membrane oxygenation for severe adult respiratory failure (CESAR): A multicentre randomised controlled trial. The Lancet. 2009;**374**(9698):1351-1363

[33] Ranieri VM, Terragni PP, Del Sorbo L, et al. Tidal volume lower than 6 ml/kg enhances lung protection: Role of extracorporeal carbon dioxide removal. Anesthesiology. 2009;**111**(4):826-835

[34] Costa EL, Amato MB. Ultra-protective tidal volume: How low should we go? Critical Care. 2013;**17**(2):127

[35] Zimmermann M, Bein T, Arlt M, et al. Pumpless extracorporeal interventional lung assist in patients with acute respiratory distress syndrome: A prospective pilot study. Critical Care. 2009;**13**(1):2009, R10

[36] Fanelli V, Ranieri MV, Mancebo J, Moerer O, Quintel M, Morley S, Moran I, Parrilla F, Costamagna A, Gaudiosi M, Combes A. Feasibility and safety of low-flow extracorporeal carbon dioxide removal to facilitate ultra-protective ventilation in patients with moderate acute respiratory distress sindrome. Critical Care. 2016;**20**(1):36

[37] Fan E, Brodie D, Slutsky AS. Acute respiratory distress syndrome: Advances in diagnosis and treatment. JAMA. 2018;**319**(7):698-710

[38] Gattinoni L, Marini JJ, Quintel M. Time to rethink the approach to treating acute respiratory distress syndrome. Journal of the American Medical Association. 2018;**319**(7):664-666

Chapter 5

Extracorporeal Membrane Oxygenation Use in Asphyxiated Newborns Treated with Hypothermia: Review of the Current Evidence

Asim Al Balushi, Samara Zavalkoff and
Pia Wintermark

Additional information is available at the end of the chapter

http://dx.doi.org/10.5772/intechopen.78761

Abstract

Asphyxiated newborns may be hemodynamically unstable during their first days of life. They often present with severe persistent pulmonary hypertension and/or cardiac dysfunction, which may require aggressive supportive management to maintain homeostasis and prevent further brain injury. In the most severe cases, extracorporeal membrane oxygenation (ECMO) may be required to ensure adequate oxygenation, ventilation and cardiac output. However, due to the risk of irreversible brain injury, clinicians often are concerned about offering ECMO to these newborns. Therapeutic hypothermia during the first days of life has become the standard of care for these newborns to improve their prognosis; however, this treatment in itself has been associated with increased hemodynamic instability and coagulopathy. An additional concern with using ECMO in these newborns is the potential increased bleeding risk when continuing the hypothermia treatment during the ECMO course. This chapter reviews the reported feasibility of performing hypothermia during ECMO. We also review the reported outcomes of asphyxiated newborns treated with hypothermia and ECMO and highlight their potential survival without neurodevelopmental impairments. Thus, ECMO should be considered as a therapeutic option for asphyxiated newborns treated with hypothermia.

Keywords: birth asphyxia, brain, extracorporeal membrane oxygenation, hemodynamics, neonatal encephalopathy, therapeutic hypothermia

1. Introduction

Neonatal encephalopathy secondary to perinatal asphyxia is a common condition, with a global incidence varying between 1.3 and 6.6‰ depending on birth location [1]. It is associated with significant mortality (i.e., 23% of all neonatal deaths worldwide) and long-term morbidity, including cerebral palsy and global developmental delay [2–4]. In developed countries, therapeutic hypothermia has become the standard treatment for newborns born at 36 or more weeks of gestational age who have suffered from birth asphyxia and who present with moderate to severe encephalopathy in the first hours of life [5]. Hypothermia treatment has been shown to reduce the risk of death and long-term disability in these newborns [6, 7].

Hemodynamic instability can develop after birth asphyxia and during hypothermia [8], and may be so severe that some of these asphyxiated newborns treated with hypothermia require support with extracorporeal membrane oxygenation (ECMO) [9–11]. First, transient myocardial ischemia and papillary muscle dysfunction due to subendocardial ischemia occur in one-third of asphyxiated newborns [12, 13]. Second, pulmonary vascular resistances in these newborns are high due to hypoxia-induced pulmonary vasoconstriction, and thus pulmonary hypertension frequently co-exists along with the cardiac dysfunction. Acute pulmonary hypertension may lead to a reduction in the right ventricular function, which, if left untreated, subsequently can impair the left ventricular filling, and hence explain a lower cardiac output [14]. In addition, therapeutic hypothermia results in a lower heart rate in these newborns and a reduction of cardiac output, which reflect the adaptation to the decreased tissue demand during hypothermia treatment [15]. Evidence is accumulating that this hemodynamic instability (including hypotension and persistent pulmonary hypertension) and associated metabolic acidosis and hypoxemia have the potential to worsen brain injury in these newborns [16–18], and thus deserve early and optimal management. Therefore, optimizing the hemodynamic profile of these newborns as early as possible is of the utmost importance for decreasing their risk of further brain injury, even if this requires initiation of ECMO.

2. General aspects of neonatal ECMO

The first reported successful use of neonatal ECMO was in 1975 with a newborn who had meconium aspiration syndrome [19]. Since then, the neonatal ECMO field has evolved rapidly along with the indications and contraindications for this therapy. Broadly, ECMO usually is indicated in newborns for disease processes—believed to be reversible—associated with high mortality.

One of the largest randomized clinical trials of ECMO with newborns was undertaken by the United Kingdom collaborative ECMO trial group [20]. This study enrolled a total of 185 newborns with gestational age ≥35 weeks and birth weight ≥2 kg. The main indication for ECMO in this study was severe respiratory failure with an oxygenation index ≥40. The primary diagnosis was persistent pulmonary hypertension, meconium aspiration, congenital diaphragmatic hernia, sepsis, and idiopathic respiratory distress. The results suggested significant survival benefits for the newborns, who received ECMO, with a relative risk reduction of 0.55 (95% CI 0.39–0.77) ($p = 0.0005$). These results translate into four newborns, who needed to be treated with ECMO for one newborn to benefit from a reduction in mortality.

As of mid-2017, the international extracorporeal life support organization (ELSO) registry reported a total of 35,598 neonatal runs of ECMO worldwide in active centers [21]. The majority of these neonatal ECMO runs were for pulmonary indications (75%) and a smaller proportion for cardiac indications (20%); extracorporeal cardiopulmonary resuscitation (ECPR) constituted only 5% of the total neonatal ECMO runs [21].

Several studies have reported on the short- and long-term outcomes of newborns treated with ECMO (22, 23). Some of these studies have found that newborns treated with ECMO are at an increased risk of death and neurodevelopmental impairments [22, 23]. However, a population-based study, which reported the outcomes of 224 newborns treated with ECMO for various indications between 1993 and 2000, showed that 86% of these newborns survived, and 49% had a normal development in the motor, cognitive, and behavioral domains at 5 years of age. The survival and long-term outcomes of newborns, who received ECMO, have been shown to depend significantly on the underlying disease and the indication for ECMO [24, 25]. For example, newborns with congenital diaphragmatic hernia had lower survival rates and a higher incidence of long-term neurodevelopmental impairments, compared to newborns treated with ECMO for other indications, such as meconium aspiration syndrome [25].

ECMO-related brain injury is a multifactorial process in which factors related to the pre-ECMO illness and events during the ECMO course (including cannulation) play a role [26–30]. During cannulation, a period occurs of decreased blood flow and potential hypoxia when the neck vessels need to be ligated. In veno arterial (VA) ECMO, the lack of pulsatile blood flow may lead to endothelial dysfunction, which could contribute to the lack of brain autoregulation [29, 30]. In veno-venous (VV) ECMO, even if the carotid artery is spared, a concern exists about venous congestion due to the obstructive nature of the cannula, which can lead to systemic venous congestion and a higher incidence of posterior fossa hemorrhage, compared to patients who are treated with VA ECMO [27, 28]. Thus, although neonatal ECMO has significantly improved the prognosis of some critically ill newborns, it still is associated with a non-negligible risk for brain injury in the treated newborns.

3. ECMO and therapeutic hypothermia

Clinicians raise concern about increased bleeding risk when providing therapeutic hypothermia during ECMO support. However, several studies have reported the short- and long-term outcomes of newborns treated with ECMO and hypothermia without bleeding complications. Hichiba et al. [31] found that newborns with a body weight between 2 and 5 kg, who were treated with ECMO for severe respiratory failure, could receive hypothermia treatment down to 34°C for 12 h while on ECMO without worsening their survival rate, hemodynamic instability, bleeding risk, and thromboembolic complications. Horan et al. [32] found that newborns who were more than 33 weeks of gestation and who were treated with ECMO for severe respiratory failure could receive hypothermia treatment down to 34°C for 48 h during ECMO without worsening their cardiovascular status, nor having major bleeding. Of note, newborns with severe encephalopathy were excluded from both studies. The safety of maintaining hypothermia down to 34°C during ECMO also was observed in 37 newborns after cardiac surgery by Lou et al. [33]; none of the newborns treated with ECMO and hypothermia developed intracranial hemorrhage or a worsening of hemodynamic instability. In addition, Field et al. [22, 34] found that mild hypothermia down to 34°C could be safely maintained during ECMO for 72 h with newborns with meconium aspiration, persistent pulmonary hypertension, or severe cardiorespiratory failure. When they compared the outcomes at 2 years of age of their 45 newborns treated with mild hypothermia to 34°C for 48–72 h during ECMO to the outcomes of their 48 newborns treated only with ECMO, the mild hypothermia treatment did not improve the outcomes of these 45 newborns [22]. However, given the heterogeneity of the initial diagnoses in this studied population of newborns, these results cannot be extrapolated directly to asphyxiated newborns, in whom hypothermia, not in the context of ECMO, has been shown to be of benefit [6, 7]. Therefore, as of now, no evidence exists that the incidence of significant bleeding and the need for inotropes were worsened when hypothermia was provided to newborns during the ECMO course.

4. Feasibility of ECMO with asphyxiated newborns treated with hypothermia

The major complications during an ECMO course are hemorrhagic and/or thromboembolic, with an increased risk of intracranial hemorrhage. Asphyxiated newborns treated with hypothermia are already at an increased risk of hemodynamic instability, thrombocytopenia, and coagulopathy, which are risk factors for intracranial bleeding [35, 36] and further brain injury [10, 17] (**Figure 1**). These complications may be due to the primary asphyxial event or the consequence of the therapeutic hypothermia [8]. Thus, questions have been raised about whether providing ECMO treatment for these asphyxiated newborns may worsen their outcome and increase their risk of intracranial bleeding.

To date, only a limited number of studies reported on the use of ECMO with asphyxiated newborns treated with hypothermia [9–11]. The Cuevas Guaman et al. [10] study is the largest of these studies, which included 187 asphyxiated newborns treated with ECMO. They did not find any difference in the incidence of bleeding or mortality in the 78 asphyxiated newborns treated with hypothermia during the ECMO course, compared to the 109 not-cooled asphyxiated newborns treated only with ECMO. These two groups also did not differ in their incidence of cardiopulmonary, renal, neurological, and metabolic complications. Therefore, according to the currently limited available evidence, it appears that ECMO therapy may be run safely with asphyxiated newborns treated with hypothermia.

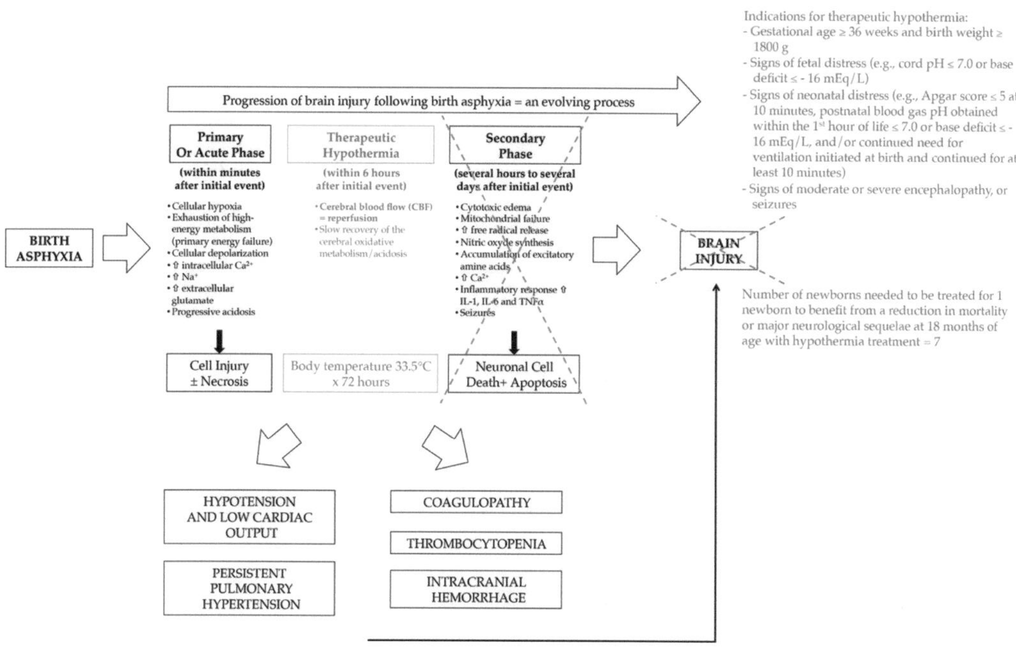

Figure 1. Schematic explaining indications of hypothermia treatment, and potential complications of birth asphyxia and hypothermia.

5. Short- and long-term outcomes in asphyxiated newborns treated with hypothermia and ECMO

Hypothermia treatment has improved the prognosis of asphyxiated newborns, making neonatal encephalopathy a "reversible" condition in one of seven treated newborns [37, 38]. However, due to their risk of irreversible brain injury, clinicians often are concerned about offering ECMO to these newborns [39]. Data on the outcome of asphyxiated newborns who received ECMO during the first 72 h of life are scarce [9–11] (**Table 1**). Shah et al. [11] reported on two asphyxiated newborns treated with hypothermia and ECMO who survived, but they did not mention their outcome. Massaro et al. [9] reported on five asphyxiated newborns treated with hypothermia and ECMO: they all survived and three of them were developmentally age appropriate at follow-up at 6–21 months; one had increased tone at 3 months but then was lost to follow up; and one had significant motor and cognitive delay. Cuevas Guaman et al. [10] studied 78 asphyxiated newborns treated with hypothermia and ECMO and reported a 15% mortality, 22% neurological complications (e.g., brain hemorrhage or infarction), and 12% seizure rate; however, they did not report on the long-term outcomes of these newborns. Thus, current evidence suggests that the outcome of asphyxiated newborns treated with hypothermia and ECMO is not always poor.

In addition, to achieve optimal results, early rather than later consideration of ECMO during the course of therapeutic hypothermia is probably important for these critically ill newborns,

Reference	Number of newborns	Survival rate	Outcomes
Shah et al. [11]	Two asphyxiated newborns treated with hypothermia and ECMO	2/2 (100%) survived	Long-term neurodevelopmental outcome not known
Massaro et al. [9]	Five asphyxiated newborns treated with hypothermia and ECMO	5/5 (100%) survived	• 3/5 (60%) developmentally age appropriate at follow-up at 6–21 months; • 1/5 (20%) increased tone at 3 months but then was lost to follow up; • 1/5 (20%) significant motor and cognitive delay
Cuevas Guaman et al. [10]	Seventy-eight asphyxiated newborns treated with hypothermia and ECMO	66/78 (85%) survived	Long-term neurodevelopmental outcome not known Short-term outcome included: • 17/78 (22%) neurological complications (e.g., brain hemorrhage or infarction) • 9/78 (12%) seizure rate

Table 1. Outcomes in asphyxiated newborns treated with hypothermia and extracorporeal membrane oxygenation (ECMO).

since a prolonged duration of metabolic acidosis, inotropic support, and a need for inhaled nitric oxide prior to ECMO initiation have been associated with a higher rate of bleeding complications [40, 41], and since hemodynamic instability has been associated with worsened brain injury in those newborns [16]. In addition, it may be safer to start ECMO, if required, before the rewarming phase following the 72-h hypothermia treatment, so to allow hemodynamic support during this time-period when pulmonary hypertension crises are more likely to occur [11].

6. Considerations for using ECMO in asphyxiated newborns treated with hypothermia

ECMO is an expensive and labor-intensive, life-sustaining modality. The ideal candidate for ECMO is a patient with a reversible disease condition for whom standard treatments have failed to reverse the disease process and for whom mortality risk is high. The most common contraindications for neonatal ECMO currently include a gestational age less than 34 weeks, weight of less than 2 kg, significant coagulopathy, significant intraventricular hemorrhage, and an underlying genetic condition with a poor prognosis [42]. Severe metabolic acidosis prior to ECMO also is considered a relative contraindication for ECMO, since this has been associated previously with higher mortality and brain injury [43]. However, the successful use of ECMO has been reported for a newborn with persistent pulmonary hypertension, presumed sepsis, and a pre-ECMO pH of less than 6.6 [44]. Thus, asphyxiated newborns treated with hypothermia—if they do not present with intraventricular hemorrhage or proven severe and irreversible brain injury at the time of cannulation—should be eligible for ECMO.

http://dx.doi.org/10.5772/intechopen.78761

If started in an optimal timeframe, ECMO associated with hypothermia treatment may ensure adequate oxygenation, treat catecholamines-resistant hypotension, and minimize further brain injury in these newborns, without causing intracerebral hemorrhage if coagulopathy can be kept under control.

7. Conclusions

In conclusion, ECMO might thus be considered as a therapeutic option for asphyxiated newborns treated with hypothermia, if they need it respiratory or hemodynamic support, if they have no proven irreversible brain injury visible at the time of starting ECMO.

Acknowledgements

We thank Mr. Wayne Ross Egers for his professional English correction of the manuscript.

Conflict of interest

The authors declare no competing financial interests. No honorarium, grant, or other form of payment was received for the preparation of this manuscript.

Funding

Pia Wintermark receives research grant funding from the FRSQ Clinical Research Scholar Career Award Junior 2 and a CIHR Operating Grant.

Author details

Asim Al Balushi[1], Samara Zavalkoff[2] and Pia Wintermark[3]*

*Address all correspondence to: pia.wintermark@bluemail.ch

1 Division of Pediatric Cardiology, Stollery Children's Hospital, Edmonton, Canada

2 Division of Pediatric Intensive Care Unit, Department of Pediatrics, Montreal Children's Hospital, Montreal, Canada

3 Division of Newborn Medicine, Department of Pediatrics, Montreal Children's Hospital, Montreal, Canada

References

[1] Maulik PK, Darmstadt GL. Childhood disability in low- and middle-income countries: Overview of screening, prevention, services, legislation, and epidemiology. Pediatrics. 2007;**120**(Suppl 1):S1-S55

[2] Lawn J, Shibuya K, Stein C. No cry at birth: Global estimates of intrapartum stillbirths and intrapartum-related neonatal deaths. Bulletin of the World Health Organization. 2005;**83**:409-417

[3] Bryce J, Boschi-Pinto C, Shibuya K, Black RE, Group WHOCHER. WHO estimates of the causes of death in children. Lancet. 2005;**365**:1147-1152

[4] American Academy of Pediatrics, Committee on Fetus and Newborn and ACOG Committee on Obstetric Practice. Guidelines for Perinatal Care. 8th ed. Itasca: American Academy of Pediatrics and American College of Obstetrics and Gynecology; 2017. 691p. ISBN-13: 978-1-61002-088-6

[5] Jacobs SE, Berg M, Hunt R, Tarnow-Mordi WO, Inder TE, Davis PG. Cooling for newborns with hypoxic ischaemic encephalopathy. The Cochrane Database of Systematic Reviews. 2013;**1**:CD003311. DOI: 10.1002/14651858.CD003311.pub3

[6] Gluckman PD, Wyatt JS, Azzopardi D, Ballard R, Edwards AD, Ferriero DM, Polin RA, Robertson CM, Thoresen M, Whitelaw A, Gunn AJ. Selective head cooling with mild systemic hypothermia after neonatal encephalopathy: Multicentre randomised trial. Lancet. 2005;**365**:663-670

[7] Shankaran S, Laptook AR, Ehrenkranz RA, Tyson JE, McDonald SA, Donovan EF, Fanaroff AA, Poole WK, Wright LL, Higgins RD, Finer NN, Carlo WA, Duara S, Oh W, Cotten CM, Stevenson DK, Stoll BJ, Lemons JA, Guillet R, Jobe AH, National Institute of Child Health and Human Development Neonatal Research Network. Whole-body hypothermia for neonates with hypoxic-ischemic encephalopathy. The New England Journal of Medicine. 2005;**353**:1574-1584

[8] Giesinger RE, Bailey LJ, Deshpande P, McNamara PJ. Hypoxic-ischemic encephalopathy and therapeutic hypothermia: The hemodynamic perspective. The Journal of Pediatrics. 2017;**180**:22 e2-30 e2. DOI: 10.1016/j.jpeds.2016.09.009

[9] Massaro A, Rais-Bahrami K, Chang T, Glass P, Short BL, Baumgart S. Therapeutic hypothermia for neonatal encephalopathy and extracorporeal membrane oxygenation. The Journal of Pediatrics. 2010;**157**:499.e1-501.e1. DOI: 10.1016/j.jpeds.2010.04.011

[10] Cuevas Guaman M, Lucke AM, Hagan JL, Kaiser JR. Bleeding complications and mortality in neonates receiving therapeutic hypothermia and extracorporeal membrane oxygenation. American Journal of Perinatology. 2018;**35**:271-276. DOI: 10.1055/s-0037-1607197

[11] Shah SK, Khan AM, Cox CS Jr. Pulmonary hypertensive crisis requiring ECMO associated with re-warming from whole body hypothermia for hypoxic ischemic encephalopathy: Clinical observations from a case series. European Journal of Pediatric Surgery. 2010;**20**:205-206. DOI: 10.1055/s-0029-1241872

[12] Dattilo G, Tulino V, Tulino D, Lamari A, Falanga G, Marte F, Patanè S. Perinatal asphyxia and cardiac abnormalities. International Journal of Cardiology. 2011;**147**:e39-e40. DOI: 10.1016/j.ijcard.2009.01.032

[13] Kanik E, Ozer EA, Bakiler AR, Aydinlioglu H, Dorak C, Dogrusoz B, et al. Assessment of myocardial dysfunction in neonates with hypoxic-ischemic encephalopathy: Is it a significant predictor of mortality? The Journal of Maternal-Fetal & Neonatal Medicine. 2009;**22**:239-242. DOI: 10.1080/14767050802430834

[14] Lapointe A, Barrington KJ. Pulmonary hypertension and the asphyxiated newborn. The Journal of Pediatrics. 2011;**158**:e19-e24. DOI: 10.1016/j.jpeds.2010.11.008

[15] Gebauer CM, Knuepfer M, Robel-Tillig E, Pulzer F, Vogtmann C. Hemodynamics among neonates with hypoxic-ischemic encephalopathy during whole-body hypothermia and passive rewarming. Pediatrics. 2006;**117**:843-850

[16] More KS, Sakhuja P, Giesinger RE, Ting JY, Keyzers M, Sheth JN, Lapointe A, Jain A, Moore AM, Miller SP, PJ MN. Cardiovascular associations with abnormal brain magnetic resonance imaging in neonates with hypoxic-ischemic encephalopathy undergoing therapeutic hypothermia and rewarming. American Journal of Perinatology. 2018. DOI: 10.1055/s-0038-1629900. [Epub ahead of print]

[17] Al Balushi A, Barbosa Vargas S, Maluorni J, Sanon PN, Rampakakis E, Saint-Martin C, Wintermark O. Hypotension and brain injury in asphyxiated newborns treated with hypothermia. American Journal of Perinatology. 2018;**35**:31-38. DOI: 10.1055/s-0037-1604392

[18] Al Balushi A, Guilbault MP, Wintermark P. Secondary increase of lactate levels in asphyxiated newborns during hypothermia treatment: Reflect of suboptimal hemodynamics (a case series and review of the literature). AJP Reports. 2016;**6**:e48-e58. DOI: 10.1055/s-0035-1565921

[19] Bartlett RH, Gazzaniga AB, Jefferies MR, Huxtable RF, Haiduc NJ, Fong SW. Extracorporeal membrane oxygenation (ECMO) cardiopulmonary support in infancy. Transactions - American Society for Artificial Internal Organs. 1976;**22**:80-93

[20] UK collaborative randomised trial of neonatal extracorporeal membrane oxygenation. UK Collaborative ECMO Trail Group. Lancet. 1996;**348**:75-82

[21] The Extracorporeal Life Support Organization. 2018. Available from: www.elso.org [Accessed: March 28, 2018]

[22] Field D, Juszczak E, Linsell L, Azzopardi D, Cowan F, Marlow N, Edwards D, NEST Study Collaborative Group. Neonatal ECMO study of temperature (NEST): A randomized controlled trial. Pediatrics. 2013;**132**:e1247-e1256. DOI: 10.1542/peds.2013-1754

[23] Raets MM, Dudink J, Ijsselstijn H, van Heijst AF, Lequin MH, Houmes RJ, Wildschut ED, Reiss IK, Govaert P, Tibboel D. Brain injury associated with neonatal extracorporeal membrane oxygenation in the Netherlands: A nationwide evaluation spanning two decades. Pediatric Critical Care Medicine. 2013;**14**:884-892. DOI: 10.1097/PCC.0b013e3182a555ac

[24] Bernbaum J, Schwartz IP, Gerdes M, D'Agostino JA, Coburn CE, Polin RA. Survivors of extracorporeal membrane oxygenation at 1 year of age: The relationship of primary diagnosis with health and neurodevelopmental sequelae. Pediatrics. 1995;**96**:907-913

[25] Nijhuis-van der Sanden MW, van, der Cammen-van Zijp MH, Janssen AJ, Reuser JJ, Mazer P, van Heijst AF, Gischler SJ, Tibboel D, Kollée LA. Motor performance in five-year-old extracorporeal membrane oxygenation survivors: A population-based study. Critical Care. 2009;**13**:R47. DOI: 10.1186/cc7770

[26] Klein MD, Lessin MS, Whittlesey GC, Chang CH, Becker CJ, Meyer SL, Smith AM. Carotid artery and jugular vein ligation with and without hypoxia in the rat. Journal of Pediatric Surgery. 1997;**32**:565-570

[27] Bulas DI, Taylor GA, Fitz CR, Revenis ME, Glass P, Ingram JD. Posterior fossa intracranial hemorrhage in infants treated with extracorporeal membrane oxygenation: Sonographic findings. AJR. American Journal of Roentgenology. 1991;**156**:571-575

[28] Brunberg JA, Kewitz G, Schumacher RE. Venovenous extracorporeal membrane oxygenation: Early CT alterations following use in management of severe respiratory failure in neonates. AJNR. American Journal of Neuroradiology. 1993;**14**:595-603

[29] Ingyinn M, Rais-Bahrami K, Evangelista R, Hogan I, Rivera O, Mikesell GT, Short BL. Comparison of the effect of venovenous versus venoarterial extracorporeal membrane oxygenation on renal blood flow in newborn lambs. Perfusion. 2004;**19**:163-170

[30] Ingyinn M, Lee J, Short BL, Viswanathan M. Venoarterial extracorporeal membrane oxygenation impairs basal nitric oxide production in cerebral arteries of newborn lambs. Pediatric Critical Care Medicine. 2000;**1**:161-165

[31] Ichiba S, Killer HM, Firmin RK, Kotecha S, Edwards AD, Field D. Pilot investigation of hypothermia in neonates receiving extracorporeal membrane oxygenation. Archives of Disease in Childhood. Fetal and Neonatal Edition. 2003;**88**:F128-F133

[32] Horan M, Ichiba S, Firmin RK, Killer HM, Edwards D, Azzopardi D, Hodge R, Kotecha S, Field D. A pilot investigation of mild hypothermia in neonates receiving extracorporeal membrane oxygenation (ECMO). The Journal of Pediatrics. 2004;**144**:301-308

[33] Lou S, MacLaren G, Paul E, Best D, Delzoppo C, d'Udekem Y, Butt W. Safety of therapeutic hypothermia in children on veno-arterial extracorporeal membrane oxygenation after cardiac surgery - CORRIGENDUM. Cardiology in the Young. 2015;**25**:1374. DOI: 10.1017/S1047951115001316

[34] Field DJ, Firmin R, Azzopardi DV, Cowan F, Juszczak E, Brocklehurst P, NEST Study Group. Neonatal ECMO study of temperature (NEST)—A randomised controlled trial. BMC Pediatrics. 2010;**10**(24). DOI: 10.1186/1471-2431-10-24

[35] Al Yazidi G, Srour M, Wintermark P. Risk factors for intraventricular hemorrhage in term asphyxiated newborns treated with hypothermia. Pediatric Neurology. 2014;**50**:630-635. DOI: 10.1016/j.pediatrneurol.2014.01.054

[36] Al Yazidi G, Boudes E, Tan X, Saint-Martin C, Shevell M, Wintermark P. Intraventricular hemorrhage in asphyxiated newborns treated with hypothermia: A look into incidence, timing and risk factors. BMC Pediatrics. 2015;**15**:106. DOI: 10.1186/s12887-015-0415-7

[37] Edwards AD, Brocklehurst P, Gunn AJ, Halliday H, Juszczak E, Levene M, Strohm B, Thoresen M, Whitelaw A, Azzopardi D. Neurological outcomes at 18 months of age after moderate hypothermia for perinatal hypoxic ischaemic encephalopathy: Synthesis and meta-analysis of trial data. BMJ. 2010;**340**:c363. DOI: 10.1136/bmj.c363

[38] Jacobs SE, Tarnow-Mordi WO. Therapeutic hypothermia for newborn infants with hypoxic-ischaemic encephalopathy. Journal of Paediatrics and Child Health. 2010;**46**: 568-576. DOI: 10.1111/j.1440-1754.2010. 01880

[39] Cashen K, Reeder RW, Shanti C, Dalton HJ, Dean JM, Meert KL, Eunice Kennedy Shriver National Institute of Child Health and Human Development Collaborative Pediatric Critical Care Research Network (CPCCRN). Is therapeutic hypothermia during neonatal extracorporeal membrane oxygenation associated with intracranial hemorrhage? Perfusion. 2017;**33**:354-362. DOI: 10.1177/0267659117747693

[40] Hardart GE, Fackler JC. Predictors of intracranial hemorrhage during neonatal extracorporeal membrane oxygenation. The Journal of Pediatrics. 1999;**134**:156-159

[41] de Mol AC, van Heijst AF, de Haan TF, van, der Staak FH, Liem KD. The effect of inhaled nitric oxide on the course of extracorporeal membrane oxygenation and the occurrence of hemorrhagic complications. ASAIO Journal. 2009;**55**:213-216. DOI: 10.1097/MAT.0b013e31819901a5

[42] Frenckner B, Radell P. Respiratory failure and extracorporeal membrane oxygenation. Seminars in Pediatric Surgery. 2008;**17**:34-41

[43] Thiagarajan RR, Laussen PC, Rycus PT, Bartlett RH, Bratton SL. Extracorporeal membrane oxygenation to aid cardiopulmonary resuscitation in infants and children. Circulation. 2007;**116**:1693-1700

[44] Boon Lim JK, Lee JH, Mok YH, Chan YH. Successful use of extracorporeal membrane oxygenation in a neonate with arterial pH less than 6.6. World Journal for Pediatric and Congenital Heart Surgery. 2015;**6**:466-469. DOI: 10.1177/2150135114558849

Chapter 6

Percutaneous Mechanical Circulatory Support Devices: Systems and Clinical Options

Antonio Loforte, Giuditta Coppola, Carlo Mariani,
Gregorio Gliozzi, Francesco Grigioni and
Giuseppe Marinelli

Additional information is available at the end of the chapter

http://dx.doi.org/10.5772/intechopen.76925

Abstract

Cardiogenic shock (CS) still remains a leading cause of hospital death. The adoption of percutaneous ventricular assist devices (pVADs) as treatment of CS is an option which continues to rise. Several types of pVADs have been developed by time to provide full cardiac support with few related complications and easy implantation settings. pVADs are used to support the failing heart as a bridge to recovery, decision, durable device or heart transplantation. None of these devices adopted in the clinical practice is ideal for all patients. Disadvantages may be related to the risk of limb/arm ischaemia or cerebral stroke or haemolysis. The most important choice is to identify the best device for each patient depending on haemodynamics, clinical scenario and patient anatomical/pathological issues. This chapter discusses the current pVAD options to treat CS patients.

Keywords: pVADs, IABP, ECMO, cardiogenic shock, refractory end-stage heart failure, bridge-to-bridge therapy

1. Introduction

Cardiogenic shock (CS) still remains a leading cause of hospital death [1–5]. So far the most common cause of CS is myocardial infarction. However, acute regurgitant valve failure, myocarditis, post-cardiotomy shock and acute on chronic heart failure also may present with end-organ dysfunction from hypoperfusion due to cardiac pump failure, the hallmark of this syndrome. The adoption of percutaneous ventricular assist devices (pVADs) as treatment of CS is an option which continues to rise [1–5]. Several types of pVADs have been developed by time to provide full cardiac support with few related complications and easy implantation settings. There are only few randomized trials on pVADs, and the current use of them depends on single centre experience [1–5]. pVADs are used to support the failing heart as a bridge to recovery, decision, durable device or heart transplantation (Htx). Improvement in haemodynamic parameters by pVADs has clearly been demonstrated though without mortality benefit in the limited studies to date [1–5]. Early versus late implementation of support may prevent or ameliorate systemic inflammation and end-organ dysfunction in CS syndrome [1–5].

None of these devices used in the clinical practice is ideal for all patients. Disadvantages may be related to the risk of limb/arm ischaemia or cerebral stroke or haemolysis [1–5]. The most important choice is to identify the best device for each patient depending on haemodynamics, clinical scenario and patient anatomical/pathological issues.

This chapter discusses the current pVAD options to treat CS patients.

2. Intra-aortic balloon pump

The intra-aortic balloon pump (IABP) device has been available since 1968 [1–5], and it remains the most used pVAD in clinical practice. It consists of a cylindrical polyethylene balloon that is inserted through the femoral artery and placed into proximal descending aorta distal to the

Device	IABP	TandemHeart	Impella 2.5	Impella CP	Impella 5.0	Peripheral ECMO
Cannula size	7.9 Fr	21 Fr inflow; 15–17 Fr outflow	13 Fr	14 Fr	22 Fr	Centrifugal
Pump mechanism	Pneumatic	Centrifugal	Axial flow	Axial flow	Axial flow	Centrifugal
Insertion technique	Descending aorta via the femoral artery	21 Fr inflow cannula into the left atrium via the left femoral vein and transseptal puncture and 15–17 Fr outflow cannula into the femoral artery	12 Fr catheter placed retrograde across the aortic valve via the femoral artery	14 Fr catheter placed retrograde across the aortic valve via the femoral artery	22 Fr catheter placed retrograde across the aortic valve via a surgical cutdown of the femoral, axillary or subclavian artery	Inflow cannula into the right atrium via the femoral vein, outflow cannula into the femoral artery or axillary artery
Maximum haemodynamic support	0.5–1.0 L/min	4 L/min	2.5 L/min	3.7 L/min	5.0 L/min	>4.5 L/min
Implantation time	+	+++	++	++	++++	++
Risk of leg (or arm) ischaemia	+	+++	++	++	++	+++
Anticoagulation	+	+++	+	+	+	+++

Table 1. Comparison of percutaneous support devices [1–5].

subclavian artery. The balloon inflates during diastole and increases the perfusion of coronary arteries via retrograde flow. The antegrade displacement of the blood caused by the inflation of the balloon increases the mean arterial pressure (MAP) and the flow to the body. The onset of ventricular systole leads to a rapid deflation of the balloon with the drop of the pressure in the aorta and consequently the forward flow with a reduction in afterload, left ventricular end-diastolic pressure (LVEDP) and rise in stroke volume and cardiac output. The decrease of left ventricular wall tension, coronary microvascular resistance and LVEDP along with the rise of diastolic pressure reduces the oxygen consumption and therefore myocardial ischaemia [1–5]. It usually provides a marginal increase in cardiac output of up to 0.5 l/min (**Table 1**). The placement of the device is quite easy to perform. A radiopaque tip is inserted through the arterial access and placed under fluoroscopy, confirmed by the use of the X-ray. To be effective, it requires some level of left ventricular function of the patient and stable electrical rhythm. It should not be used in patients with more than mild aortic insufficiency because of the eventual increase of the diastolic retrograde flow. There are several potential complications due to the IABP placement like balloon rupture, leak or entrapment, infection, limb ischaemia and cerebral stroke. Rarely, it may be the cause of aortic dissection or rupture. The use of the IABP has been tested in several studies [6–9]. The SHOCK trial demonstrated a decrease of hospital mortality in patients with myocardial infarction associated with the thrombolytic therapy or early interventional/surgical revascularization [6, 7]. Nevertheless, there is an increased risk of complications like stroke and bleeding and no improvement in mortality in several meta-analyses when IABP is used for CS due to myocardial infarction [6, 7]. In spite of this, IABP use is widely common and has Class II indications in the current guidelines [8].

3. TandemHeart

The TandemHeart (CardiacAssist, Inc., Pittsburgh, PA) is a continuous-flow centrifugal assist device that was first studied by Thiele et al. [1–5, 9, 10] who randomized 41 patients with CS after acute myocardial infarction (AMI) to IABP or TandemHeart and showed an improvement in cardiac output, power index, pulmonary capillary wedge pressure and mean pulmonary arterial pressure in the second group. On the other side, there was an increased risk of limb ischaemia and coagulopathy [9, 10]. TandemHeart transfers oxygenated blood from the left atrium to the iliac arteries and perfuses the aorta retrogradely [1–5, 9–12]. It provides up to 5 L of haemodynamic support (**Table 1**). One cannula is introduced through the femoral vein up to the right atrium and by means of a transseptal puncture to the left atrium (**Figure 1**). Hence, the oxygenated blood from the left atrium is directed to the pump, and by means of a second cannula into the femoral artery, it can be delivered to the body. It requires very good expertise in transseptal puncture. Contraindications are aortic insufficiency, peripheral vascular diseases, the presence of thrombus in the right and left atrium and coagulopathy. The possible dangerous complications due to the placement of the device are cardiac perforation and tamponade, infection and embolic events including limb ischaemia and cerebral stroke. The TandemHeart device is approved for up to 6 hours of extracorporeal support for cardiopulmonary bypass [1–4, 9–12]. The placement of the device requires between 30 and 45 minutes with

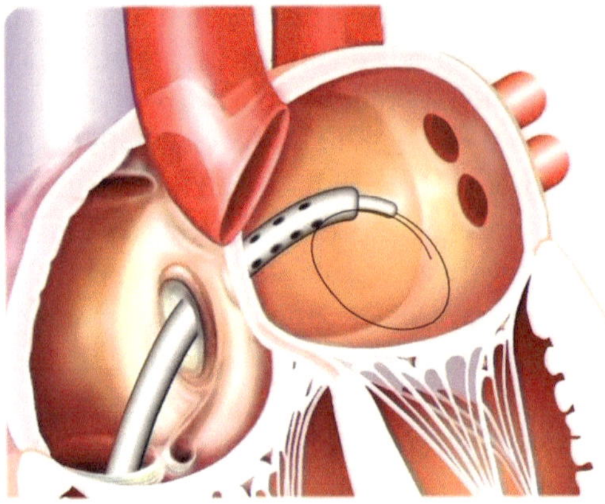

Figure 1. TandemHeart inflow cannula across the atrial septum.

full systemic heparinization [1–4, 9–12]. The left ventricle preload, the filling pressures and the wall stress are reduced, and the peripheral tissue perfusion is increased. Several studies demonstrate a better support and improved haemodynamics than the IABP, but the mortality benefit is the same [9–12]. The Texas Heart Institute experience analyzed 117 patients with severe CS refractory to pharmacological therapy and/or IABP and found a significant improvement in cardiac index and systolic blood pressure [11, 12]. In the 2015 Guidelines for Heart failure, the TandemHeart may be considered in severe left ventricle dysfunction or recent decompensated heart failure with associated technically challenging or prolonged percutaneous intervention (PCI) and continued deterioration of CS patient despite IABP and/or Impella [8].

4. Impella

The Impella Recover LP (Abiomed Inc., Danvers, MA) is a microaxial pump that moves the blood continuously from the LV to the ascending aorta [1–5] (**Figure 2**). There are three classes (**Table 1**) currently available—the Impella 2.5, Impella CP and Impella 5.0—depending on the level of LV support (2.5, 3.5 and 5 L/min, respectively). The Impella 2.5 and CP are the most commonly used [1–5]. The system is composed of three major components: catheter, purge system and automated controller. An impeller and the adjacent motor are positioned near the outlet area in the ascending aorta. Thanks to the rotation, the negative pressure draws the ventricular blood into the inlet area and through the cannula. The Impella 2.5 is used for up to 6 hours for high-risk PCI to prevent haemodynamic instability, while the CP model is indicated for up to 6 hours for partial circulatory support when the cardiopulmonary bypass is not required. Like the TandemHeart, the Impella devices have superior haemodynamics if compared to the IABP in patients with ischaemic cardiogenic shock [1–5]. The Impella 5.0 was developed initially for femoral artery, but nowadays it is positioned through the axillary or subclavian artery. There are two clinical effects provided by this device: the unloading of the cardiac ventricle and the increase in forward flow. The left ventricle wall tension and the

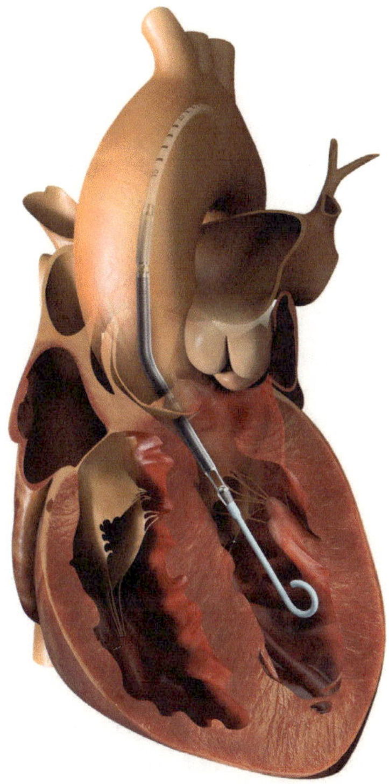

Figure 2. Impella recover left ventricular support.

myocardial oxygen demand are decreased. There is also evidence of improved coronary perfusion pressure and decrease of microvascular resistances [1–5]. The most important limitation of Impella adoption is the size of peripheral vessels to accommodate the large bore catheters. Anticoagulation is required, so the presence of coagulopathy or recent hemorrhage may prohibit the use of this device. Other contraindications to the use of Impella are the presence of a mechanical aortic valve prosthesis or a left ventricle (LV) mural thrombus. The improper positioning or inadequate LV volume may cause suction. Hence, the correct Impella position has to be confirmed with imaging. Case studies [1–5, 13–15] demonstrated successful use of the Impella 5.0 as bridge from ECMO to durable device, during acute rejection in Htx, LV support in RV failure as bridge to durable left ventricular assist device (LVAD), bridge to recovery in patients with myocarditis and bridge to heart transplantation. There are several potential complications due to the use of this device. They include bleeding, infection, vascular injury, stroke, haemolysis, cardiac tamponade and damage to the aortic valve. The PROTECT II trial randomized 452 symptomatic patients with complex multivessel disease or unprotected left main disease and severely depressed LV function, thus showing the superiority of IMPELLA compared with the IABP support [13–15]. Additionally, the catheter-based ventricular assist device (cVAD) registry, which is an observational, multicentre, retrospective registry of patients supported with Impella, reflects the device real-world use and suggests greater survival with pre-PCI Impella insertion than pre-PCI IABP and/or pharmacotherapy alone [13–15].

5. Extracorporeal membrane oxygenation

Extracorporeal membrane oxygenation (ECMO), as being a heparin-coated closed circuit, is a model of mechanical pulmonary or cardiopulmonary support that can be used for a prolonged period [1–5, 16–20]. There are two types of ECMO support: venovenous (VV) and venoarterial (VA). The first one provides only respiratory support since the blood is taken from the right atrium and then oxygenated and CO_2 removed prior to being returned to the right atrium. Both the inflow and the outflow cannulae are positioned through a venous access. It works only for gas exchange in a respiratory failure clinical scenario. The exception is when the outflow cannula is placed in the pulmonary artery to unload and support the right ventricle (RV). In contrast, the VA ECMO provides both haemodynamic/cardiac and respiratory supports. It is used during left ventricular or biventricular failure. The inflow cannula is placed into the right atrium or inferior vena cava, and the blood after gas exchange is delivered back into the arterial vascular system at either peripheral or central cannulation sites. It can provide flows up to 6 L/min without any intrinsic activity of the heart (**Table 1**). The components of ECMO system are drainage and perfusion cannulae, centrifugal or roller pump, membrane oxygenator and heart exchanger. ECMO is important in the case of the need of haemodynamic support for patients with CS or requiring a salvage treatment while on cardiac arrest. It decreases the preload of both right and left ventricles, increases the mean arterial pressure (MAP) and improves end-organ perfusion. Since it increases the LV afterload, the myocardial oxygen consumption is not reduced. The amount of flow depends on the size of the cannulae and the speed of the pump. Even ECMO requires full systemic heparinization [1–5, 16–19]. Contraindications are the presence of an irreversible clinical process, severe multiple organ failure, aortic dissection, peripheral arterial disease and aortic regurgitation. Potential complications are bleeding, injury of vascular vessels, limb or arm ischaemia and thromboembolic events. There are no large randomized trials on the use of ECMO. The Extracorporeal Life Support Organization (ELSO) registry demonstrated a 27% survival to hospital discharge [16, 20]. Recently, a 49% survival was reached with the use of other types of mechanical support systems plus ECMO in a bridge-to-bridge setting as treatment of CS [1–5, 16–20]. Current guidelines recommend the use of ECMO when concomitant hypoxaemia and RV failure are present [1–5, 8, 16–20].

6. Right ventricular assist devices

For several decades the volume administration to maintain RV preload, the vasodilators to decrease RV afterload and the inotropes to ameliorate RV contractility have been used in clinical practice [1–5, 21–27]. The in-hospital mortality is high in patients with RV failure that is refractory to maximal medical treatment [1–5, 21–27]. With the TandemHeart, the percutaneous right ventricular assist device (RVAD) support has become a reality [21]. The TandemHeart is used to provide RV support in such conditions as RV infarction and severe pulmonary hypertension and temporary RV support after placement of a long-term LVAD. In this version the TandemHeart cannulae are positioned into the right atrium and the pulmonary

http://dx.doi.org/10.5772/intechopen.76925

artery [21]. One model of Impella device, the RP, is approved by the Food and Drug Administration (FDA) for humanitarian device exemption for patients who develop acute right heart failure or decompensation after LVAD implantation, AMI and Htx [22]. The device is implanted into the femoral vein for inflow through the inferior vena cava to reach the outlet area in the pulmonary artery (**Figure 3**). The RECOVER RIGHT trial was a prospective multicentre study that was conducted in 2014 to evaluate the safety and efficacy of the Impella RP [22]. There was successful implantation in 90% of patients who suffered from RV failure with an increase of cardiac index and 73% successful survival to either 30 days or to hospital discharge [22]. Contraindications to the use of this device include severe regurgitation, stenosis or replacement of the tricuspid or pulmonic valves, the presence of filter in the inferior vena cava or the presence of thrombus in the right atrium or in the inferior vena cava. Possible complications are tamponade, vascular injury, liver failure, injury to the tricuspid and pulmonic valves. The other extracorporeal devices used in the clinical practice are the Levitronix CentriMag (Abbott), currently, while the Rotaflow (Maquet) and the Abiomed AB 5000 (Abiomed), historically [23–27]. It is important to choose the adequate sizing for inflow and

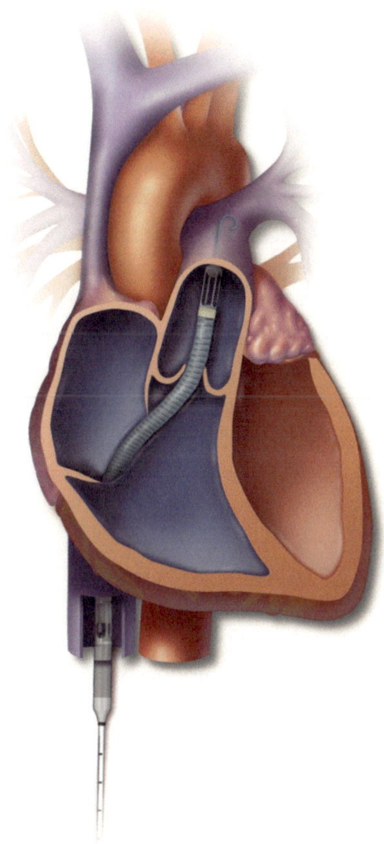

Figure 3. Impella RP setting.

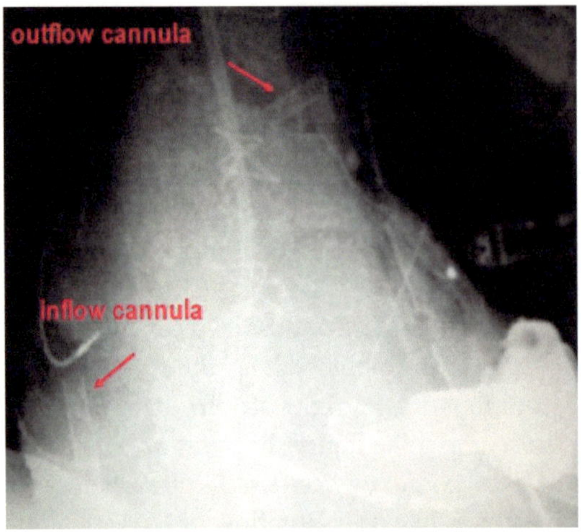

Figure 4. Percutaneous temporary right ventricular assist device placement post-long-term left ventricular assist device insertion.

outflow cannulae to achieve the proper venous drainage and maintain a flow up to 7–8 L/min. Several approaches for RVAD circuit setting arrangement exist nowadays [23–27]. The standard approach requires a full median sternotomy. The inflow cannula is positioned in the right atrium and the outflow in the main pulmonary artery, both secured by double purse-string sutures. The explantation of the device, at the time of RV recovery, requires a re-sternotomy approach. Additionally, alternative effective minimally invasive approaches for RVAD placement exist [23–27]. The one reported by Cohn et al. [25] needs vessel grafts with bedside removal because the cannulas are inserted from outside the chest of the patient and reach the right atrium and the pulmonary artery through the attached grafts. The grafts are firmly secured around their cannulas with heavy sutures. When RV support is no more necessary, the pump lines are clamped, the redundant portions from inside are exposed, the tapes are cut and the cannulas removed, without reopening the chest [25]. A modified transcutaneous technique has been described by Strauch et al. [26]. A minithoracotomy approach may be used in the case of post-LVAD RV failure [23, 24] (**Figure 4**). According to this Berlin technique, the main pulmonary artery cannula is located through a transthoracic needle under transesophageal echo (TEE) guidance. The venous cannula of RVAD is advanced through the inferior vena cava into the right atrium by Seldinger approach. This technique is difficult in the case of severe adhesions related to previous cardiothoracic surgery [23, 24].

Disclosures

No funding sources and relevant disclosures to declare.

http://dx.doi.org/10.5772/intechopen.76925

Author details

Antonio Loforte*, Giuditta Coppola, Carlo Mariani, Gregorio Gliozzi, Francesco Grigioni and Giuseppe Marinelli

*Address all correspondence to: antonioloforte@yahoo.it

Department of Cardiothoracic, Transplantation and Vascular Surgery, S. Orsola Hospital, Bologna University, Bologna, Italy

References

[1] Basra SS, Loyalka P, Kar B. Current status of percutaneous ventricular assist devices for cardiogenic shock. Current Opinion in Cardiology. 2011;**26**(6):548-554

[2] Naidu SS. Novel percutaneous cardiac assist devices. Circulation. 2011;**123**:533-543

[3] Ergle K, Parto P, Krim SR. Percutaneous ventricular assist devices: A novel approach in the management of patients with acute cardiogenic shock. The Ochsner Journal. 2016; **16**(3):243-249

[4] Werdan K, Gielen S, Ebelt H, Hochman JS. Mechanical circulatory support in cardiogenic shock. European Heart Journal. 2014;**35**(3):156-167

[5] Touchan J, Guglin M. Temporary mechanical circulatory support for cardiogenic shock. Current Treatment Options in Cardiovascular Medicine. 2017;**19**(10):77

[6] Sanborn TA, Sleeper LA, Bates ER, et al. Impact of thrombolysis, intra-aortic balloon pump counterpulsation, and their combination in cardiogenic shock complicating acute myocardial infarction: A report from the SHOCK Trial Registry. Should we emergently revascularize occluded coronaries for cardiogenic shock? Journal of the American College of Cardiology. 2000;**36**:1123-1129

[7] Thiele H, Schueler G, Neumann FJ, et al. Intraaortic balloon counterpulsation in acute myocardial infarction complicated by cardiogenic shock: Design and rationale of the Intraaortic balloon pump in cardiogenic shock II (IABP-SHOCK II) trial. American Heart Journal. 2012;**163**(6):938-945

[8] Rihal CS, Naidu SS, Givertz MM, et al. SCAI/ACC/HFSA/STS clinical expert consensus statement on the use of percutaneous mechanical circulatory support devices in cardiovascular care: Endorsed by the American Heart Association, the Cardiological Society of India, and Sociedad Latino Americana de Cardiologia Intervencion; affirmation of value by the Canadian Association of Interventional Cardiology-Association Canadienne de Cardiologie d'intervention. Journal of the American College of Cardiology. 2015, 2015;**65**(19):e7-e26

[9] Thiele H, Sick P, Boudriot E, et al. Randomized comparison of intra-aortic balloon support with a percutaneous left ventricular assist device in patients with revascularized acute myocardial infarction complicated by cardiogenic shock. European Heart Journal. 2005; **26**(13):1276-1283

[10] Burkhoff D, Cohen H, Brunckhorst C, O'Neill WW, the TandemHeart Investigators. A randomized multicenter clinical study to evaluate the safety and efficacy of the TandemHeart percutaneous ventricular assist device versus conventional therapy with intraaortic balloon pumping for treatment of cardiogenic shock. American Heart Journal. 2006;**152**(3):469 e1-8

[11] Gregoric ID, Basra SS, et al. The percutaneous ventricular assist device in severe refractory cardiogenic shock. Kar B, Journal of the American College of Cardiology. 2011;**57**:688-696

[12] Bruckner BA, Jacob LP, Gregoric ID, et al. Clinical experience with the TandemHeart percutaneous ventricular assist device as a bridge to cardiac transplantation. Texas Heart Institute Journal. 2008;**35**(4):447-450

[13] O'Neill WW, Kleiman NS, Moses J, et al. A prospective, randomized clinical trial of hemodynamic support with Impella 2.5 versus intraaortic balloon pump in patients undergoing high-risk percutaneous coronary intervention: The PROTECT II study. Circulation. 2012;**126**:1717-1727

[14] Dangas GD, Kini AS, Sharma SK, et al. Impact of hemodynamic support with Impella 2.5 versus intraaortic balloon pump on prognostically important clinical outcomes in patients undergoing high-risk percutaneous coronary intervention (from the PROTECT II randomized trial). The American Journal of Cardiology. 2014;**113**:222-228

[15] Cohen MG, Ghatak A, Kleiman NS, et al. Optimizing rotational atherectomy in high-risk percutaneous coronary interventions: Insights from the PROTECT IotaIota study. Catheterization and Cardiovascular Interventions. 2014;**83**:1057-1064

[16] Rousse N, Juthier F, Pincon C, et al. ECMO as a bridge to decision: Recovery, VAD, or heart transplantation? International Journal of Cardiology. 2015;**187**:620-627

[17] Abrams D. Extracorporeal membrane oxygenation in cardiopulmonary disease in adults. Journal of the American College of Cardiology. 2014;**63**(25):2769-2778

[18] Thiagarajan RR, Brogan TV, Scheurer MA, et al. Extracorporeal membrane oxygenation to support cardiopulmonary resuscitation in adults. The Annals of Thoracic Surgery. 2009; **87**:778-785

[19] Takayama H, Truby L, Koekort M, et al. Clinical outcome of mechanical circulatory support for refractory cardiogenic shock in the current era. The Journal of Heart and Lung Transplantation. 2013;**32**(1):106

[20] Abrams D, Garan AR, Abdelbary A, et al. International ECMO Network (ECMONet) and The Extracorporeal Life Support Organization (ELSO). Position paper for the organization

of ECMO programs for cardiac failure in adults. Intensive Care Medicine; 2018 Feb 15. DOI: 10.1007/s00134-018-5064-5. [Epub ahead of print]

[21] Kapur NK, Paruchuri V, Korabathina R, et al. Effects of a percutaneous mechanical circulatory support device for medically refractory right ventricular failure. The Journal of Heart and Lung Transplantation. 2011;**30**(12):1360-1367

[22] Anderson MB, Goldstein J, Milano C, et al. Benefits of a novel percutaneous ventricular assist device for right heart failure: The prospective RECOVER RIGHT study of the Impella RP device. The Journal of Heart and Lung Transplantation. 2015;**34**(12):1549-1560

[23] Stepanenko A, Kukucka M, Vierecke J, et al. Right ventricular recovery induced by temporary right ventricular assist device support. Thoracic and Cardiovascular Surgeon. 2015;**63**(Suppl 1):88

[24] Loforte A, Stepanenko A, Potapov EV, et al. Temporary right ventricular mechanical support in high-risk left ventricular assist device recipients versus permanent biventricular or total artificial heart support. Artificial Organs. 2013;**37**(6):523-530

[25] Cohn WE, Gregoric ID, La Francesca S, Frazier OH. Bedside right ventricular assist device removal in the conscious patient. The Annals of Thoracic Surgery. 2007;**83**(4):1556-1557

[26] Strauch JT, Franke UF, Madershahian N, Wahlers T. Right ventricular assist device implantation: A new transcutaneous approach. The Thoracic and Cardiovascular Surgeon. 2004;**52**(6):378

[27] Loforte A, Grigioni F, Marinelli G. The risk of right ventricular failure with current continuous-flow left ventricular assist devices. Expert Review of Medical Devices. 2017; **14**(12):969-983

Chapter 7

Mechanical Circulatory Support (MCS) for Primary Graft Dysfunction (PGD)

Luiz Fernando Caneo and Vitor Barzilai

Additional information is available at the end of the chapter

http://dx.doi.org/10.5772/intechopen.76697

Abstract

Primary graft dysfunction is the main cause of early mortality after heart transplantation (HT). Preventive strategies to avoid primary graft dysfunction (PGD) have been focused on better donor choice and maintenance, heart preservation methods in long-distance retrievals with prolonged ischemia time, and better myocardial protection during implantation, among others. Hemodynamic deterioration, caused by cardiogenic shock due to pump failure unresponsive to inotropes, has a catastrophic progression if not corrected in time. Severe PGD without response to inotropes and heart rhythm control in the absence of cardiac tamponade should be treated promptly with mechanical circulatory support. Extracorporeal life support (ECLS) should be installed early, before the occurrence of multiorgan dysfunction or prior to cardiac arrest, as highlighted in the literature. The aim of this chapter is to discuss the use of mechanical circulatory support (MCS) and its impact on the success to survival for patients with PGD.

Keywords: extracorporeal membrane oxygenation, mechanical circulatory support, primary graft dysfunction, orthotopic heart transplantation, heart failure, heart-assist devices

1. Introduction

Heart transplantation (HT) remains the preferred treatment for end-stage heart disease that currently affects 5.1 million people in the United States, with an estimated growth of 25% by 2030 [1]. More than 4000 patients undergo HT annually worldwide for this condition [2, 3], with an improved survival rate in the last two decades. Through the years, the advent of multiple platforms of mechanical circulatory support (MCS) as an arm of transplantation has made it possible to rescue patients that were too sick to be treated without the help of devices.

Despite surgical advances and improved long-term survival, heart transplant patients are still at significant risk to develop early graft dysfunction (EGD), leading to significant perioperative morbidity and mortality [2, 4, 5]. Notwithstanding the better results of HT, mortality from EGD varies among centers and over the years. In addition, the different set of criteria jeopardize comparison for incidence and mortality.

There are two basic entities that compose of EGD: primary graft dysfunction (PGD) and secondary graft dysfunction (SGD). The latter is based on pathology-proven rejection, clear surgical complications, or hemodynamic parameters. A postoperative transpulmonary gradient greater than 15 mmHg, associated with low cardiac output, was considered as graft dysfunction secondary to pulmonary hypertension classified as SGD. The aim of this chapter is to discuss exclusively cardiogenic shock due to PGD and its management. Secondary graft dysfunction is not the scopes of this chapter.

2. Primary graft dysfunction

2.1. Definitions and classification

Primary graft dysfunction is reported as dysfunction affecting the right ventricle (RV), left ventricle (LV), or both, according to echocardiographic findings. Primary graft dysfunction (PGD) is common and ranges from 2.3 to 28.2% depending on the definition [6–10].

The diagnosis of PDG should be considered if any dysfunction is observed at the end of cardiopulmonary bypass, restricted to the first 24 h after surgery and based on echocardiographic and/or hemodynamic criteria, as summarized in **Table 1**.

Severe PGD is defined as the need for MCS—other than an intra-aortic balloon pump—to maintain an adequate organ perfusion following HT and is the leading cause of early mortality after transplantation [5]. Hemodynamic deterioration caused by cardiogenic shock due to pump failure unresponsive to inotropes has a catastrophic progression if not addressed in time. For this reason, heart transplant patients should be routinely monitored by a pulmonary artery catheter. It provides continuous information about cardiac output and other real-time hemodynamics parameters required for therapeutic decision-making, in combination with other clinical variables, such as tissue perfusion. In a PGD after HT, the amount of inotropes and vasopressors—vasotropic score—the patient is on and micro- and macro-hemodynamics help to decide whether to rely on medical management or choose MCS.

Intraoperative transesophageal echocardiography (TEE) is recommended routinely upon the discontinuation of cardiopulmonary bypass. It provides useful information about ventricular dimensions and function, blood volume, residual surgical defects, and helps to de-air cavities. If the diagnosis of postoperative shock is challenging, both operating room (OR) and bedside echocardiography are informative and should be performed whenever cardiac dysfunction

http://dx.doi.org/10.5772/intechopen.76697

PGD-LV	Mild - meets one of the following criteria:	Echocardiography: LVEF < 40% OR Hemodynamics: CVP > 15 mmHg, PCWP > 20 mmHg, CI < 2 L/min/m2 lasting for 1 hour and requiring low-dose inotropes
	Moderate - meets one criterion from 1 and another criterion from 2:	1. Echocardiography: LVEF < 40% OR Hemodynamics: CVP > 15 mmHg, PCWP > 20 mmHg, CI < 2 L/min/m2, hypotension with MAP < 70 mmHg 2. Inotrope score > 10 or intra-aortic balloon pump
	Severe	Dependence on mechanical circulatory support, excluding intra-aortic balloon pump
PGD-RV	Requires 1 + 2, or 3 alone	1. CVP > 15 mmHg, PCWP < 15 mmHg, CI < 2 L/min/m2 2. TPG < 15 mmHg AND/OR SBP < 50 mmHg 3.Requirement of right circulatory assistance

PGD-LV: left ventricular primary graft dysfunction; LVEF: left ventricular ejection fraction; CVP: central venous pressure; PCWP: pulmonary capillary wedge pressure; CI: cardiac index; MAP: mean arterial pressure; PGD-RV: right ventricular primary graft dysfunction; TPG: transpulmonary pressure gradient; SBP: systolic blood pressure.

Table 1. Classification of primary graft dysfunction after heart transplantation.

and hemodynamic parameters indicate cardiogenic shock. **Figure 1** shows a suggested algorithm to rule out PGD post-heart transplantation.

In a recent consensus on April 23, 2013, during the annual meeting of the International Society of Heart and Lung Transplantation (ISHLT) [5], PGD was defined as any graft dysfunction that occurs up to 24 h after transplantation. This agreement formulates guidelines to better define the diagnosis and management of patients with primary graft dysfunction (PGD) in heart transplantation. Before the conference, an online survey was used to obtain contemporary thoughts on diagnosis and management of PGD patients from transplant centers. A total of 47 transplant centers responded and the results are summarized in **Table 1**. Epidemiology factors were set as the baseline. Parameters such as the requirement of inotropic support, left ventricular ejection fraction (LVEF), and requirement of cardiac mechanical support were put as possible criteria for PGD. The purpose of this consensus was to initiate a standardization of the study of PGD and serve as a guide for the heart transplant community regarding diagnosis, management, and risk stratification of post-transplanted PGD, thus permitting uniform comparisons among centers and studies.

During implant		
	Optimize protection during bypass:	
		Maximize myocardial protection during bypass according to the type of Cardioplegia
		LV Venting to avoid rapidly rewarming
After implant		
	Optimise inotropes before weaning	
	Rule out air in coronary arteries	
	Rule out Kinking of pulmonary arteries	
	Start Reperfusion at least 30 min before weaning bypass	
		If difficult to wean bypass, extends reperfusion.
	Exclude RV disfunction after increased PVR	
End of bypass		
	Unable to wean bybass, higher vasoative-inotropic score:	
		Consider PGD
		Consider IABP, prepare for MCS/ECLS.
		Consider a myocardial biopsy sample

Figure 1. Ruling out secondary graft dysfunction in heart transplantation.

The conference had 71 participants— including cardiologists, cardiac surgeons, pathologists, and immunologists—representing 42 heart transplant centers from North America, Australia, Europe, and Asia, that had published on PGD or had vast clinical experience in heart transplantation.

Additionally, the moment to start support is not well stablished. A high inotropic score seems to be related with worst prognosis. Beside high inotropic score, the need of vasotropic agents to sustain hemodynamics plays an important rule in chose for ECLS in PGD. It is important to acknowledge that a vasoactive-inotropic score (**Figure 2**), rather only the inotropic score, may determine better the prognosis and initiation of support. In Cardiogenic shock patients, a high vasoactive-inotropic score during the first 48 hours was related with increased in-hospital mortality [11, 12].

Inotrope Score (IS)

IS = Dopamine dose (mcg/kg/min) + Dobutamine dose + 100 x Epinephrine dose (mcg/kg/min)

Vasoactive-Inotropic Score (VIS)

VIS = IS + 10 x Milrinone dose (mcg/kg/min) + 10,000 x Vosopressein dose (units/kg/min) + 100 x Norepinephrine dose (mcg/kg/min)

Figure 2. Vasoactive-ionotrophic criteria: The need of a vasoactive score higher than 85 seems to determine worst prognosis in cardiogenic shock patients [11].

2.2. Etiology and pathogeneses

The etiology of PGD is likely to be multifactorial. Donor, procedure and recipient causes are involved. Brain death and its sequelae in the donor, hypothermic ischemia during transport, warm ischemia during implant surgery, and reperfusion injury after the release of the aortic cross-clamp in the recipient can negatively affect the donor's heart. In addition, systemic factors in the recipient may create a "hostile" environment that further compromises its function after reperfusion and contributes to the development of PGD.

It is important to say that PDG is a phenomenon not correlated with hyperacute rejection. The results of the International Society of Heart and Lung Transplantation (ISHLT) autopsy survey pre-consensus showed that less than 4% of biopsies had some kind of antibody-mediated rejection and 7% had evidence of cellular rejection [5].

2.2.1. Donor aspects

Donor's brain death is associated with a series of events that result in impaired myocardial contractility and sensitize the heart to ischemia–reperfusion injury [13]. These events include an intense release of endogenous norepinephrine that results in mitochondrial and cytosolic calcium overload that may activate autophagy, apoptosis, or necrosis. Calcium overload of the contractile proteins leads to contracture and is associated with a characteristic histologic appearance known as "contraction band necrosis." Administration of exogenous catecholamines during donor resuscitation may contribute to desensitization of myocardial β-receptor signaling after brain death. Many other donor-related aspects leading to PGD are described, including ischemic preconditioning insults related to older donors [14].

Most donor hearts are transported and stored in a cold preservation solution and that slows but does not effectively arrest cellular metabolism. Consequently, a progressive ischemic injury is an inevitable consequence of prolonged static storage.

Furthermore, the reperfusion of the heart with oxygenated blood leads to further calcium overload and an initial burst of oxygen-derived free radicals that bind to and disrupt the function of multiple cellular enzymes. The combination of Ca^{+} overload and high oxidant stress in an energy-depleted cardiac myocyte activates the formation of the mitochondrial permeability transition pore (MPTP)—a non-specific channel that forms in the mitochondrial membrane allowing pro-apoptotic factors, such as cytochrome C, to be released into the cell cytoplasm [15]. Water that enters by the MPTP causes mitochondrial swelling and may lead to membrane rupture, triggering necrotic cell death. Currently, there is an increasing interest in ex-vivo perfusion of the donor's heart in order to preserve the organ, minimize the above-mentioned negative impact of preimplantation ischemia, and increase availability [16].

2.2.2. *Recipient aspects*

Vasoplegia has a catastrophic result on any heart surgery, particularly in heart transplant, in which it seems to affect the donor's heart impairing its ability to adapt to this hostile environment. Many aspects of the receptor are involved in the genesis of this phenomenon. Risk factors include mechanical circulatory support before transplantation, prolonged cross-clamp time, and significant transfusion requirements. The activation of systemic inflammatory response in the recipient results in a vasodilated systemic circulation that is refractory to conventional vasopressor support that seems to lead to PGD. It probably involves the concerted action of multiple pro-inflammatory cytokines leading to upregulation of inducible nitric oxide synthase or indoleamine dioxygenase, with overproduction of nitric oxide or other endogenous vasodilators.

2.3. Risk factors

Transplanted hearts are at risk of ischemia/reperfusion injury, damage from proinflammatory cytokines, and beats on decreased donor cortisol and thyroid hormone levels [17–21]. Recipient-related factors include age, increased pulmonary vascular resistance (PVR), and recipient inflammatory cytokines, which can worsen vasoplegia, as well as oxidative stress in the transplanted heart [22–30]. In addition, transplant recipient dependence on pre-transplantation inotropic support and mechanical ventilation has been associated with increased incidence of PGD [24, 31–34].

In a single-center study, Segovia et al. [26] developed a predictive model for the development of PGD. The risk factors were included in the model and used to calculate a predictive score are recipient age ≥ 60 years, recipient diabetes mellitus, recipient inotrope dependence, right atrial pressure ≥ 10 mm Hg, donor age ≥ 30 years, and ischemic time ≥ 4 h (RADIAL score) [26]. This model was later validated in a separate cohort of HT performed at programs in Spain between 2006 and 2010 [35]. In the latter study, PGD occurred with an incidence of 22%. Isolated RV dysfunction was present in 45% of patients with PGD, whereas isolated LV PGD occurred in 8% of patients and combined biventricular PGD in 47%. The RADIAL score was higher in patients with PGD and stratified patients into groups with incremental PGD incidence [35].

Nicoara et al. [36] conducted a single-center retrospective cohort study to evaluate the incidence, trends, and independently associated risk factors for PGD after HT. In addition, they explored the performance of the RADIAL score variables in this study population. Of the 317 patients who underwent HT over the study period and met inclusion criteria, 99 (31.23%) developed PGD defined according to the ISHLT consensus statement [5]. Isolated PGD-LV occurred in 60 patients (18.9%), 22 patients (7%) had biventricular PGD and 17 patients (5.3%) had isolated PGD-RV. Risk factors independently associated with the type of PGD included ischemia time, recipient African American race, and recipient pre-transplantation treatment with amiodarone [36].

Several studies previously identified a variety of donor, recipient, and procedural risk factors associated with PGD, with a high variability of results giving different definitions, use of single-center or multi-center databases, and different time periods analyzed [37, 38–41]. Most consistently among these are donor age [22], donor high dose of inotropic support [24], cause of brain death [24], recipient age [24, 36], recipient inotropic support [26], mechanical support [22, 24], ischemia time [24, 36], and donor-recipient weight mismatches [32]. Several studies [36–37, 42] identified ischemia time as an independent risk factor associated with PGD development, with each additional hour of ischemia time almost doubling the risk of PGD.

2.3.1. Amiodarone use

Recipient treatment with amiodarone pre-transplantation has been controversially discussed, with divergent results regarding early graft failure, morbidity, and mortality after heart transplantation [43–46]. Nicoara et al. [36] found that recipient pre-transplantation's use of amiodarone was an independent factor that increases the risk of PGD development, by 67%. The 30-s official adult heart transplantation report from the registry of ISHLT did not find amiodarone independently associated with early graft failure. However, we had a higher incidence of early graft failure and in-hospital graft dysfunction among patients treated with amiodarone, suggesting that it may play a role in early post-transplantation outcomes or may be associated with an unmeasured indicator an ill patient population [3]. A recent retrospective cohort analysis of adult HT recipients from the ISHLT registry found that amiodarone use before HT has increased over time and is associated with increased 1-year mortality [46]. The long half life of amiodarone combined with its pharmacological effects—negative chronotropic and inotropic, calcium channel blockage, and α- and β-receptor blockade—may be responsible for its effects or an unidentified interaction with oxidative stress leading to worsening ischemia–reperfusion injury, but this is speculative [46].

2.3.2. Congenital heart disease

Over the last decade, the advances in the medical and surgical management of patients with congenital heart disease (CHD) have led to an improvement in their life expectancy with 85% of children surviving till adulthood [47]. However, some patients will develop late myocardial dysfunction resulting in heart failure with 10–20% of them requiring heart transplantation [48, 49]. Adults with congenital heart diseases recipients (ACHDR) pose unique challenges due to complex anatomy, multiple prior procedures, preformed human leucocyte antigen (HLA) antibodies, pulmonary hypertension, and malnutrition [50]. Because of these complexities, ACHDR has a higher operative [51, 52] and a 1-year mortality [2, 53].

In ACHDR, graft dysfunction was seen more commonly when compared to non-cardiac recipients (NCR) (9.9% vs. 7.4%, $p < 0.01$).

United Network for Organ Sharing (UNOS) database reports three categories of graft dysfunction: primary non-function, that is, primary graft dysfunction (PGD), acute rejection, and chronic rejection. PGD was significantly higher in ACHDR compared to NCR (4.3% vs. 2.6%, $p < 0.01$); however, there was no difference in acute and chronic rejection rates [49]. PGD continues to be a significant cause of morbidity in the most recent era [54].

Graft and cardiovascular dysfunction in ACHDR were the top two causes of early mortality and most likely related to the presence of elevated PVR, allosensitization, and longer donor organ ischemic times [30, 55–59]. The ACHDR were more likely to have longer-than-4-h ischemic times, peak panel-reactive antibody (PRA) class II >10%, and were found to have a higher rate of graft failure due to primary graft dysfunction. Thompson et al. showed that early graft survival was directly related to the number of HLA-DR (class-II) mismatches [59]. Graft dysfunction and postoperative bleeding are more likely to cause death in ACHDR compared to non-cardiac recipients (NCR) [49, 53, 60]. Because of graft dysfunction and young age, the re-transplant rate is higher among ACHDR compared to NCR [49, 55]. Improvement in the graft dysfunction rate in recent times can be attributed to better medical management of mild PGD with the use of levosimendan, nitric oxide, and phosphodiesterase inhibitors. The short-term survival for ACHDR is poorer as compared to NCR, and primary graft dysfunction remains a significant issue affecting short-term survival in ACHDR. The fact that the ACHDR who survives the first post-transplant year have better long-term survival than NCR indicates that perioperative mortality and morbidity is most likely the Achilles heel for cardiac transplantation in ACHDR [54]. Management of severe PGD with early intervention and short-term mechanical support appears to have improved survival [5].

3. Mechanical circulatory support

MCS may be provided by VA-ECMO or the implantation of a temporary paracorporeal ventricular assistance device (VAD) and the choice depends on the knowledge about devices and shelf-available items. There's no manual or evidence-based decision-making protocol to choose one or another. Nevertheless, ECLS management may determinate success to discharge of patients experiencing PGD.

Advances in durable MCSs (LVADs) made its use reliable in patients with heart failure as a bridge to heart transplant, as well as postoperative support with ECLS in PGD HT to allow organ recovery. Although an LVAD is usually the choice for consistent outcomes in patients supported while waiting for a heart transplant, ECLS may be used in patients in whom LVADs, BiVADs, or TAH (total artificial hearts) are not reliable or available. It includes patients who are likely to receive a heart transplant within a short time period after listing.

ECLS use in heart transplant PGD continues to be the first line of support with some recent evidence of improved outcomes. There is some evidence on the use of short-term VAD but with limited results in a real-world setting [61]. Although further studies are necessary to understand the optimal role of ECLS in heart transplantation the objective of this chapter is to discuss its role in PGD, that accounts for 40–50% early mortality after heart transplantation according to studies using the International Society of Heart and Lung Transplantation (ISHLT) registry [5]. Mechanical circulatory support may be provided by VA-ECMO or implantation of a temporary VAD. In a recent analysis of 54 patients supported on ECMO for PGD in a large French center, 36 patients (67%) were weaned from the assisting device and 27 of the patients supported with ECMO (50%) were discharged from the hospital [62].

http://dx.doi.org/10.5772/intechopen.76697

The overall conditional survival was 73% at 1 year and 66% at 5 years. The authors concluded that ECMO support is a reliable therapeutic option for severe, early graft failure after cardiac transplantation. Furthermore, patients treated with ECMO had the same 1-year conditional survival as patients who did not suffer from PGD. In this study, the authors found no difference in weaning when comparing peripheral ECMO and central ECMO (50%) but a higher rate of vascular complications (18%) in patients supported on peripheral ECMO.

The device of choice and timing of insertion varies among institutions, and the use of mechanical circulatory support tends to be more liberal for early support in high-volume centers with a potentially positive effect on graft recovery [63]. Although ECMO has been traditionally favored due to the ease installation, and the ability to provide oxygenation following a prolonged cardiopulmonary bypass, its use is associated with increased risk of bleeding, insufficient LV unloading, and the chance of intracardiac thrombosis in patients with minimal sistolic function [64, 65].

Takeda and colleagues from Columbia University performed an analysis of patients requiring mechanical support for PGD following heart transplant [66]. Of the 597 patients who received a heart transplant during the study period, severe PGD developed in 44 (7.4%). Within 24 h of transplant, 17 of these patients received support via a continuous-flow external VAD, and 27 received VA-ECMO support. The patients who received a VAD were more likely to have a longer support time, major bleeding requiring chest re-exploration, and renal failure requiring renal replacement therapy after surgery. In-hospital mortality was 41% for VAD patients and 19% for VA-ECMO patients. A total of 10 patients (59%) were weaned from VAD support, and 24 patients (89%) were removed from VA-ECMO support after adequate graft function recovery. The 3-year post-transplant survival was 41% in the VAD group and 66% in the VA-ECMO group, leading to the conclusion that for severe PGD, support with VA-ECMO appears to result in better clinical outcomes than VAD support. ECMO in patients with PGD or allograft failure due to other causes seems to be associated with better outcomes than ECMO support for other reasons. Tran and colleagues [67], from UCLA, demonstrated that patients requiring ECMO for graft failure after heart transplant had lower mortality (51.6%) when compared with patients who needed ECMO for other etiologies (69.1%).

ECLS/ECMO seems to be the best way to support PGD patients in almost all scenarios for many reasons. It can provide safe maximum flow and pulmonary support with different cannulation strategies—percutaneously, hybrid, or by central access. It is rapidly installed, and cost of disposable equipment is relatively inexpensive compared with other devices. In basic settings, veno-arterial (VA) ECMO is considered the main strategy. Central access is preferable due to fast installation, direct evaluation of the heart decompression, and easiest way to install a left-side drainage cannula in the left atrium or left ventricle if it remains distended.

A total of 16% of our PGD patients had a left cannula installed as a venting strategy to guarantee LV resting. Our preference is to use central VA ECMO. Patients may be extubated as any other heart surgery postoperatively after recovering from anesthesia. Cannulas may be positioned inferiorly through the thoracic wall and the chest fully closed to facilitate mobility and ambulation. Extubation may be done even if only the skin is closed—not sutured sternum. In this case, the care team has to ensure a sealed bandage around the cannulas to avoid pneumothorax formation.

Full support is sufficient when hemodynamic variables and microperfusion are normalized—VA ECMO usually provides normal oxymetric parameters if the patient is well supported. MAP goal usually is around 70, CVP < 15, SVO_2 > 60%, serum lactate <2.0 mmol/L, and O_2 saturation > 95%. Since the pulmonary flow is shunted throw the ECLS system, pulmonary artery pressures are expected to be very low, and most of the times cardiac index cannot be measured. Pulsatile waveforms are almost invisible or show a very low pulse pressure gradient (less than 20 mm Hg).

Usually, in the range of 3–7 days, it is possible to see some degree of heart recovery. Pulse pressure may rise above 20 mmHg, CI may be measurable through PAC, pulmonary pressures may rise, and the patient may be hemodynamically stable with a lower flow on ECLS system. At this point, the weaning protocol should require an echocardiographic evaluation to reassess biventricular function. In adults, patients showing aortic time-velocity integral (VTI) ≥10 cm, left ventricular ejection fraction (LVEF) >20–25%, and lateral mitral annulus peak systolic velocity (TDSa) ≥6 cm/s at minimal ECMO flow were all successfully weaned [68].

Although ECMO may provide adequate support, it has limitations such as insufficient LV unloading, limited time of support, and risks of thromboembolic and vascular complications. High pressures in left chambers may not be easily documented, and the patient may run with hemodynamic instability. Non-treatable low flow related to sequestration of stroke volume in the lungs, secondary of left chambers distention, and inability of the heart to decompress from ECMO post-load augmentation may be seen. A documented left-side heart high pressure requires an immediately strategy to unload left chambers and re-establish the desired flow. A drainage cannula in left atrium or ventricle that allows a fast connection on the ECMO circuit permits good drainage and is a feasible choice. It is important to note that, in this case, optimum flow will be achieved after a left-side drainage cannula insertion.

In case of recovery of the left ventricle's ability to unload, the left cannula may be removed before starting the weaning protocol or just reducing the ECMO to allow filing up the ventricle and considering weaning. Intra-aortic balloon pump has been documented, but in a different scenario setting, as a way to reducing systemic vascular resistance, helping to prevent LV distention, during the VA ECMO run [69]. More recently, in the largest US-based retrospective study, the addition of Impella to VA-ECMO for patients with refractory cardiogenic shock was associated with lower all-cause 30-day mortality, lower inotrope use, and comparable safety profiles as compared with VA-ECMO alone. This study reinforces the importance of LV decompression as an important factor to improve outcomes during VA ECMO in severe ventricular dysfunction [70].

If recovery is not noted on PGD, other strategies should be considered and palliative care may be an option. Although we were able to prolong ECMO support in an infant up to 44 days until recovery, a biventricular support including a durable VAD or a total artificial heart may be an option in selected patients. Since there is lack of evidence to support use of those alternatives on PGD, the selection of a device should be made according to the patient's clinical condition and the center's experience.

3.1. Personal experience

Between January 2007 and December 2013, a total of 71 heart transplantations were performed in patients with advanced heart failure and 11 (15.5%) of these patients presented PGD [71].

All patients had advanced heart failure and 2 (18.2%) patients were in a priority state before the transplantation. As for the etiology of the cardiomyopathy, 5 (45.4%) were due to Chagas disease, 3 idiopathic dilated cardiomyopathy, 1 from secondary to valvular cardiomyopathy, 1 had restrictive cardiomyopathy, and 1 was associated with peripartum cardiomyopathy. None of the patients had PRAc—preformed antibodies calculated panel—above 10%.

In our experience, the causes of PGD were not associated with severe rejection, as documented by routine endomyocardial biopsy in the first week, with only one patient presenting cellular rejection greater than 2R. Donors were predominantly male (n = 7; 63.6%) and had an average age of 26.6 ± 12.3 years (ranging from 15 to 48 years). The causes of death among donors included head trauma in 7 cases (63.6%), hemorrhagic stroke in 3 (27.3%), and cerebral tumor in 1. A total of 7 cases (63.6%) received continuous infusion of norepinephrine >0.1 mcg/kg/min at the time of the retrieval. Retrievals took place in the same hospital of the implantation in 6 (54.5%) cases and at a distant center in the 5 remaining cases. The average ischemia time was 151 ± 82 min (ranging from 73 to 270 min), with 82.8 ± 14.2 min in the local retrievals and 233 ± 35.4 min in distant retrievals ($p < 0.0001$). The cold ischemia "limit" of 4 h was exceeded in 2 (18.2%) patients.

In this group of patients, the use of ECMO met the desired goals, promoting cardiac recovery in most cases, with acceptable complication rates, considering the severity of the clinical condition of patients [71]. We were successful in removing the ECMO, with cardiac recovery in 81.8% of the patients after an average of 76 h. The main postoperative problems that we found were acute renal failure, stroke, and requirement for surgical revision of hemostasis. The first is a frequent complication [72] and is secondary to multiple insulting factors—shock, nephrotoxic drugs, and systemic venous congestion—and pre-transplant cardiorenal syndrome. Renal function recovered in all patients after a few sessions of hemodialysis, as described by Listijono et al. [73]. The last two are complications related to the requirement of anticoagulation during ECMO, which is difficult to control. Complicating factors are recent heart surgery, the presence of shock with concomitant hepatic dysfunction, and, eventually, disseminated intravascular coagulation. Excessive use of blood products complicates immunological sensitization, systemic congestion—including liver congestion, which increases bleeding—and pulmonary hypertension. The use of heparin-coated circuits, antifibrinolytics, careful surgical technique, maintenance of hemodynamic stability with systemic venous decompression, and synthetic derivatives of coagulation factors are important to minimize these complications. Although patients who developed stroke showed increased hospital mortality, those who survived had full recovery of motor activity without limitation in their quality of life.

4. Conclusion(s)

The aim of circulatory assistance in PGD is always cardiac recovery. Thus, the characteristics of the ideal device must comply with the following requirements: ability to be quickly installed, allowing the rapid re-establishment of cardiac output in order to maintain adequate tissue perfusion and reverse multiorgan dysfunction, reducing ventricular filling pressures, promoting myocardial protection with increased coronary flow, and having a low complication rate.

Heart decompression is important for a successful recovery since intracavitary hypertension curtails subendocardial coronary perfusion, especially in those patients who had no electrical activity or lacked sufficient contractile activity for adequate LV decompression.

Regardless of showing complete recovery, patients with PGD have a higher mortality when multiple organs were involved. Hence, there is need for strengthened intensive care in this population, systematically focused on the management of organs and systems and on the prevention of sepsis.

The rapid hemodynamic deterioration due to PGD shows that the earlier the implantation (operation room), the best are the outcomes for weaning and survival. Patients in whom ECMO was initiated due to cardiac arrest had a poor outcome, and the appropriate timing was certainly neglected.

Acknowledgements

We are grateful to Rodolfo A. Neirotti, M.D., Ph.D., for his expertise, mentoring, valuable suggestions, and help with the review of this chapter.

Conflict of interest

The authors declare no conflicts of interest with outside companies.

All funding was provided internally.

Author details

Luiz Fernando Caneo[1*] and Vitor Barzilai[2]

*Address all correspondence to: luiz.caneo@incor.usp.br

1 Pediatric Cardiac Surgery – Heart Institute, University of São Paulo Medical School, São Paulo, Brazil

2 Instituto de Cardiologia do Distrito Federal (ICDF), Brasília, DF, Brazil

References

[1] Go AS, Mozaffarian D, Roger VL, et al. Heart disease and stroke statistics–2014 update: A report from the American Heart Association. Circulation. 2014;**129**(3):e28-e292. DOI: 10.1161/01.cir.0000441139.02102.80

[2] Stehlik J, Edwards LB, Kucheryavaya AY, et al. The registry of the International Society for Heart and Lung Transplantation: 29th official adult heart transplant report–2012.

The Journal of Heart and Lung Transplantation. 2012;**31**(10):1052-1064. DOI: 10.1016/j.healun.2012.08.002

[3] Lund LH, Edwards LB, Kucheryavaya AY, et al. The registry of the International Society for Heart and Lung Transplantation: Thirtieth official adult heart transplant report–2013; focus theme: Age. The Journal of Heart and Lung Transplantation. 2013;**32**(10):951-964. DOI: 10.1016/j.healun.2013.08.006

[4] Iyer A, Kumarasinghe G, Hicks M, et al. Primary graft failure after heart transplantation. Journal of Transplantion. 2011;**2011**:175768. DOI: 10.1155/2011/175768

[5] Kobashigawa J, Zuckermann A, Macdonald P, et al. Report from a consensus conference on primary graft dysfunction after cardiac transplantation. The Journal of Heart and Lung Transplantation. 2014;**33**(4):327-340. DOI: 10.1016/j.healun.2014.02.027

[6] Blume ED, Rosenthal DN, Rossano JW, et al. Outcomes of children implanted with ventricular assist devices in the United States: First analysis of the pediatric interagency registry for mechanical circulatory support (PediMACS). The Journal of Heart and Lung Transplantation. 2016;**35**(05):578-584. DOI: 10.1016/j.healun.2016.01.1227

[7] Kirklin JK, Naftel DC, Pagani FD, et al. Seventh INTERMACS annual report: 15,000 patients and counting. The Journal of Heart and Lung Transplantation. 2015;**34**(12):1495-1504. DOI: 10.1016/j.healun.2015.10.003

[8] Cabrera AG, Sundareswaran KS, Samayoa AX, et al. Outcomes of pediatric patients supported by the HeartMate II left ventricular assist device in the United States. The Journal of Heart and Lung Transplantation. 2013;**32**(11):1107-1113. DOI: 10.1016/j.healun.2013.07.012

[9] Burki S, Adachi I. Pediatric ventricular assist devices: Current challenges and future prospects. Vascular Health and Risk Management. 2017;**13**:177 185. DOI: 10.2147/VHRM.S82379

[10] Gregoric ID, Cohn WE, Frazier OH. Diaphragmatic implantation of the HeartWare ventricular assist device. The Journal of Heart and Lung Transplantation. 2011;**30**(04):467-470. DOI: 10.1016/j.healun.2010.11.014. [pub ahead of print]

[11] Na SJ et al. Vasoactive inotropic score as a predictor of mortality in adult patients with cardiogenic shock: Medical therapy versus ECMO. Revista Española de Cardiología. 2018. DOI: 10.1016/j.rec.2018.01.003

[12] Gaies MG, Jeffries HE, Niebler RA, Pasquali SK, Donohue JE, Yu S, et al. Vasoactive-inotropic score is associated with outcome after infant cardiac surgery: An analysis from the pediatric cardiac critical care consortium and virtual PICU system registries. Pediatric Critical Care Medicine. 2014 Jul;**15**(6):529-537. DOI: 10.1097/PCC.0000000000000153

[13] Cooper DK, Novitzky D, Wicomb WN. The pathophysiological effects of brain death on potential donor organs, with particular reference to the heart. Annals of the Royal College of Surgeons of England. 1989;**71**(4):261-266

[14] Ryan JB, Hicks M, Cropper JR, et al. Functional evidence of reversible ischemic injury immediately after the sympathetic storm associated with experimental brain death.

The Journal of Heart and Lung Transplantation. 2003;**22**(8):922-928. DOI: 10.1016/S1053-2498(02)00558-2

[15] Halestrap AP. The mitochondrial permeability transition: Its molecular mechanism and role in reperfusion injury. Biochemical Society Symposium. 1999;**66**:181-203

[16] Messer S, Ardehali A, Tsui S. Normothermic donor heart perfusion: Current clinical experience and the future. Transplant International. 2014 Jul 7;**28**(6):634-642. DOI: 10.1111/tri.12361

[17] Pratschke J, Wilhelm MJ, Kusaka M, Hancock WW, Tilney NL. Activation of proinflammatory genes in somatic organs as a consequence of brain death. Transplantation Proceedings. 1999;**31**(1-2):1003-1005. DOI: 10.1016/S0041-1345(98)02095-8

[18] D'Amico TA, Meyers CH, Koutlas TC, et al. Desensitization of myocardial beta-adrenergic receptors and deterioration of left ventricular function after brain death. The Journal of Thoracic and Cardiovascular Surgery. 1995;**110**(3):746-751. DOI: 10.1016/S0022-5223(95)70107-9

[19] Novitzky D, Cooper DK, Rosendale JD, Kauffman HM. Hormonal therapy of the brain-dead organ donor: Experimental and clinical studies. Transplantation. 2006;**82**(11):1396-1401. DOI: 10.1097/01.tp.0000237195.12342.f1

[20] Yellon DM, Hausenloy DJ. Myocardial reperfusion injury. The New England Journal of Medicine. 2007;**357**(11):1121-1135. DOI: 10.1056/NEJMra071667

[21] Hicks M, Hing A, Gao L, Ryan J, Macdonald PS. Organ preservation. Methods in Molecular Biology. 2006;**333**:331-374. DOI: 10.1385/1-59745-049-9:331

[22] Russo MJ, Iribarne A, Hong KN, et al. Factors associated with primary graft failure after heart transplantation. Transplantation. 2010;**90**(4):444-450. DOI: 10.1097/TP.0b013e3181e6f1eb

[23] Marasco SF, Kras A, Schulberg E, Vale M, Lee GA. Impact of warm ischemia time on survival after heart transplantation. Transplantation Proceedings. 2012;**44**(5):1385-1389. DOI: 10.1016/j.transproceed.2011.12.075

[24] D'Alessandro C, Golmard JL, Barreda E, et al. Predictive risk factors for primary graft failure requiring temporary extra-corporeal membrane oxygenation support after cardiac transplantation in adults. European Journal of Cardio-Thoracic Surgery. 2011;**40**(4):962-969

[25] D'Ancona G, Santise G, Falletta C, et al. Primary graft failure after heart transplantation: The importance of donor pharmacological management. Transplantation Proceedings. 2010;**42**(3):710-712. DOI: 10.1016/j.transproceed.2010.03.027

[26] Segovia J, Cosio MD, Barcelo JM, et al. RADIAL: A novel primary graft failure risk score in heart transplantation. The Journal of Heart and Lung Transplantation. 2011;**30**(6):644-651. DOI: 10.1016/j.healun.2011.01.721

[27] Gorlitzer M, Ankersmit J, Fiegl N, et al. Is the transpulmonary pressure gradient a predictor for mortality after orthotopic cardiac transplantation? Transplant International. 2005;**18**(4):390-395. DOI: 10.1111/j.1432-2277.2004.00038.x

[28] Patarroyo M, Simbaqueba C, Shrestha K, et al. Pre-operative risk factors and clinical outcomes associated with vasoplegia in recipients of orthotopic heart transplantation in the contemporary era. The Journal of Heart and Lung Transplantation. 2012;**31**(3):282-287. DOI: 10.1016/j.healun.2011.10.010

[29] Butler J, Stankewicz MA, Wu J, et al. Pre-transplant reversible pulmonary hypertension predicts higher risk for mortality after cardiac transplantation. The Journal of Heart and Lung Transplantation. 2005;**24**(2):170-177. DOI: 10.1016/j.healun.2003.09.045

[30] Murali S, Kormos RL, Uretsky BF, et al. Preoperative pulmonary hemodynamics and early mortality after orthotopic cardiac transplantation: The Pittsburgh experience. American Heart Journal. 1993;**126**:896-904. DOI: 10.1016/0002-8703(93)90704-D

[31] Awad M, Czer LS, De Robertis MA, et al. Adult heart transplantation following ventricular assist device implantation: Early and late outcomes. Transplantation Proceedings. 2016;**48**(1):158-166. DOI: 10.1016/j.transproceed.2015.12.007

[32] Young JB, Hauptman PJ, Naftel DC, et al. Determinants of early graft failure following cardiac transplantation, a 10-year, multi-institutional, multivariable analysis. The Journal of Heart and Lung Transplantation. 2001;**20**(2):212. DOI: 10.1016/S1053-2498(00)00460-5

[33] Hong KN, Iribarne A, Worku B, et al. Who is the high-risk recipient? Predicting mortality after heart transplant using pretransplant donor and recipient risk factors. The Annals of Thoracic Surgery. 2011;**92**(2):520-527; discussion 7. DOI: 10.1016/j.athoracsur.2011.02.086

[34] Liu Y, Liu Y, Su L, Jiang SJ. Recipient-related clinical risk factors for primary graft dysfunction after lung transplantation: A systematic review and meta-analysis. PLoS One. 2014;**9**(3):e92773. DOI: 10.1371/journal.pone.0092773

[35] Cosio Carmena MD, Gomez Bueno M, Almenar L, et al. Primary graft failure after heart transplantation: Characteristics in a contemporary cohort and performance of the RADIAL risk score. The Journal of Heart and Lung Transplantation. 2013;**32**(12):1187-1195

[36] Nicoara A, Ruffin D, Cooter M, Patel CB, Thompson A, Schroder JN, et al. Primary graft dysfunction after heart transplantation: Incidence, trends, and associated risk factors. American Journal of Transplantation. 2017 Dec 14;**129**(3):e28-e10. DOI: 10.1111/ajt.14588

[37] Sabatino M, Vitale G, Manfredini V, et al. Clinical relevance of the International Society for Heart and Lung Transplantation consensus classification of primary graft dysfunction after heart transplantation: Epidemiology, risk factors, and outcomes. The Journal of Heart and Lung Transplantation. 2017;**36**:1217-1225. DOI: 10.1016/j.healun.2017.02.014

[38] Opelz G. Success rate and impact of HLA matching on kidney graft survival in highly immunized recipients. Collaborative transplant study. Transplant International. 1992;**5**(Suppl 1):S601-S603

[39] Schaffer JM, Singh SK, Reitz BA, Oyer PE, Robbins RC, Mallidi HR. Heart transplant graft survival is improved after a reduction in panel reactive antibody activity. The Journal of Thoracic and Cardiovascular Surgery. 2013;**145**(2):555-564; discussion 64-5. DOI: 10.1016/j.jtcvs.2012.10.025

[40] de Perrot M, Bonser RS, Dark J, et al. Report of the ISHLT working group on primary lung graft dysfunction part III: Donor-related risk factors and markers. The Journal of Heart and Lung Transplantation. 2005;**24**(10):1460-1467. DOI: 10.1016/j.healun.2005.02.017

[41] Martinez-Selles M, Almenar L, Paniagua-Martin MJ, et al. Donor/recipient sex mismatch and survival after heart transplantation: Only an issue in male recipients? An analysis of the Spanish heart transplantation registry. Transplant International. 2015;**28**(3):305-313. DOI: 10.1111/tri.12488

[42] Squiers JJ, Saracino G, Chamogeorgakis T, et al. Application of the International Society for Heart and Lung Transplantation (ISHLT) criteria for primary graft dysfunction after cardiac transplantation: Outcomes from a high-volume centredagger. European Journal of Cardio-Thoracic Surgery. 2017;**51**(2):263-270. DOI: 10.1093/ejcts/ezw271

[43] Sanchez-Lazaro IJ, Almenar L, Martinez-Dolz L, et al. Does amiodarone influence early mortality in heart transplantation? Transplantation Proceedings. 2006;**38**(8):2537-2538. DOI: 10.1016/j.transproceed.2006.08.022

[44] Blomberg PJ, Feingold AD, Denofrio D, et al. Comparison of survival and other complications after heart transplantation in patients taking amiodarone before surgery versus those not taking amiodarone. The American Journal of Cardiology. 2004;**93**(3):379-381. DOI: 10.1016/j.amjcard.2003.10.027

[45] Chin C, Feindel C, Cheng D. Duration of preoperative amiodarone treatment may be associated with postoperative hospital mortality in patients undergoing heart transplantation. Journal of Cardiothoracic and Vascular Anesthesia. 1999;**13**(5):562-566. DOI: 10.1016/S1053-0770(99)90008-3

[46] Cooper LB, Mentz RJ, Edwards LB, et al. Amiodarone use in patients listed for heart transplant is associated with increased 1-year post-transplant mortality. The Journal of Heart and Lung Transplantation. 2017;**36**:202-210. DOI: 10.1016/j.healun.2016.07.009

[47] Warnes CA, Williams RG, Bashore TM, et al. ACC/AHA 2008 guidelines for the management of adults with congenital heart disease: Executive summary: A report of the American College of Cardiology/American Heart Association task force on practice guidelines. Circulation. 2008;**118**:2395-2451. DOI: 10.1161/CIRCULATIONAHA.108.190811

[48] Hosseinpur AR, Cullen S, Tsang VT. Transplantation in adults with congenital heart disease. European Journal of Cardio-Thoracic Surgery. 2006;**30**:508-514. DOI: 10.1016/j.ejcts.2006.06.007

[49] Karamlou T, Hirsch J, Welke K, et al. A united network for organ sharing analysis of heart transplantation in adults with mortality and retransplantation. The Journal of Thoracic and Cardiovascular Surgery. 2010;**140**:161-168. DOI: 10.1016/j.jtcvs.2010.03.036

[50] Smith JD, Ogino H, Hunt D, et al. Humoral immune response to human aortic valve homograft. The Annals of Thoracic Surgery. 1995;**60**:S127-S130

[51] Hasan A, Au J, Hamilton JR, et al. Orthotopic heart transplantation for congenital heart disease: Technical considerations. European Journal of Cardio-Thoracic Surgery. 1993;**7**:65-70

[52] Irving C, Parry G, O'Sullivan J, et al. Cardiac transplantation in adults with congenital heart disease. Heart. 2010;**96**:1217-1222. DOI: 10.1136/hrt.2009.184713

[53] McGothlin D, De Marco T. Transplantation in adults with congenital heart disease. Progress in Cardiovascular Diseases. 2011;**53**:312-323. DOI: 10.1016/j.pcad.2010.12.002

[54] Shah DK, Deo SV, Althouse AD, Teuteberg JJ, Park SJ, Kormos RL, Burkhart HM, Morell VO. Perioperative mortality is the Achilles heel for cardiac transplantation in adults with congenital heart disease: Evidence from analysis of the UNOS registry. Journal of Cardiac Surgery. 2016:755-764. DOI: 10.1111/jocs.12857

[55] Patel ND, Weiss ES, Allen JG, et al. Heart transplantation for adults with congenital heart disease: Analysis of the united network for organ sharing database. The Annals of Thoracic Surgery. 2009;**88**:814-821. DOI: 10.1016/j.athoracsur.2009.04.071

[56] Kirklin JK, Naftel DC, Kirklin JW, et al. Pulmonary vascular resistance and the risk of heart transplantation. The Journal of Heart Transplantation. 1988;**7**:331-336

[57] Nwakanma LU, Williams JA, Weiss ES, et al. Influence of pretransplant panel-reactive antibody on outcomes in 8,160 heart transplant recipients in recent era. The Annals of Thoracic Surgery. 2007;**84**:1556-1562. (discussion 1562-1563). DOI: 10.1016/j.athoracsur.2007.05.095

[58] Loh E, Bergin JD, Couper GS, Mudge GH Jr. Role of panel-reactive antibody cross-reactivity in predicting survival after orthotopic heart transplantation. The Journal of Heart and Lung Transplantation. 1994;**13**:194-201

[59] Thompson JS, Thacker LR II, Takemoto S. The influence of conventional and cross-reactive group HLA matching on cardiac transplant outcome: An analysis from the united network of organ sharing scientific registry. Transplantation. 2000;**69**:2178-2186

[60] Daebritz SH. Update in adult congenital cardiac surgery. Pediatric Cardiology. 2007;**28**: 96-104. DOI: 10.1007/s00246-006-1446-5

[61] Hulman M, Artemiou P, Ondrusek M, Hudec V, Gasparovic I, Bena M, et al. Short-term mechanical circulatory support for severe primary graft dysfunction following orthotopic heart transplant. Interactive Cardiovascular and Thoracic Surgery. 2018 Mar 5;**27**:943-945. DOI: 10.1093/icvts/ivy050

[62] D'Alessandro C, Aubert S, Golmard JL, et al. Extracorporeal membrane oxygenation temporary support for early graft failure after cardiac transplantation. European Journal of Cardio-Thoracic Surgery. 2010;**37**:343-349. DOI: 10.1016/j.ejcts.2009.05.034

[63] Marasco SF, Esmore DS, Negri J, et al. Early institution of mechanical support improves outcomes in primary cardiac allograft failure. The Journal of Heart and Lung Transplantation. 2005;**24**(12):2037-2042. DOI: 10.1016/j.healun.2005.06.007

[64] Tanaka D, Hirose H, Cavarocchi N, et al. The impact of vascular complications on survival of patients on venoarterial extracorporeal membrane oxygenation. The Annals of Thoracic Surgery. 2016;**101**:1729-1734. DOI: 10.1016/j.athoracsur.2015.10.095

[65] Williams B, Bernstein W. Review of venoarterial extracorporeal membrane oxygenation and development of intracardiac thrombosis in adult cardiothoracic patients. The Journal of Extra-Corporeal Technology. 2016;**48**:162-167

[66] Takeda K, Li B, Garan AR, et al. Improved outcomes from extracorporeal membrane oxygenation versus ventricular assist device temporary support of primary graft dysfunction in heart transplant. The Journal of Heart and Lung Transplantation. 2017;**36**(6):650. DOI: 10.1016/j.healun.2016.12.006

[67] Tran BG, La Cruz DK, Grant S, Meltzer J, Benharash P, Dave R, et al. Temporary venoarterial extracorporeal membrane oxygenation. Journal of Intensive Care Medicine. 2018;**33**(5):288-295. DOI: 10.1177/0885066616654451

[68] Aissaoui N, Luyt CE, Leprince P, Trouillet JL, Léger P, Pavie A, Diebold B, Chastre J, Combes A. Predictors of successful extracorporeal membrane oxygenation (ECMO) weaning after assistance for refractory cardiogenic shock. Intensive Care Medicine. 2011;**37**:1738-1745. DOI: 10.1007/s00134-011-2358-2

[69] Aso S, Matsui H, Fushimi K, Yasunaga H. The effect of intraaortic balloon pumping under venoarterial extracorporeal membrane oxygenation on mortality of cardiogenic patients: An analysis using a nationwide inpatient database. Critical Care Medicine. 2016;**44**(11):1974-1979. DOI: 10.1097/CCM.0000000000001828

[70] Patel SM, Lipinski J, Al-Kindi SG, Patel T, Saric P, Li J, Nadeem F, et al. Simultaneous venoarterial extracorporeal membrane oxygenation and percutaneous left ventricular decompression therapy with impella is associated with improved outcomes in refractory cardiogenic shock. ASAIO Journal. 2018 Feb 27. DOI: 10.1097/MAT.0000000000000767. [Epub ahead of print]

[71] Lima EB, Cunha CRD, Barzilai VS, Ulhoa MB, de Barros MR, Moraes CS, et al. Experience of ECMO in primary graft dysfunction after orthotopic heart transplantation. Arquivos Brasileiros de Cardiologia. 2015 Sep;**105**(3):285-291. DOI: 10.5935/abc.20150082

[72] Kittleson M, Patel J, Moriguchi J, Kawano M, Davis S, Hage A, et al. Heart transplant recipients supported with extracorporeal membrane oxygenation: Outcomes from a single-center experience. The Journal of Heart and Lung Transplantation. 2011;**30**(11):1250-1256. DOI: 10.1016/j.healun.2011.05.006

[73] Listijono D, Watson A, Pye R, Keogh A, Kotlyar E, Spratt P, et al. Usefulness of extracorporeal membrane oxygenation for early cardiac allograft dysfunction. The Journal of Heart and Lung Transplantation. 2011;**30**(7):783-789. DOI: 10.1016/j.healun.2011.01.728

Chapter 8

Extracorporeal Membrane Oxygenation Support for Post-Cardiotomy Cardiogenic Shock

Takashi Murashita

Additional information is available at the end of the chapter

http://dx.doi.org/10.5772/intechopen.76217

Abstract

Cardiogenic shock following cardiac surgery is rare, but a serious complication. Patients who suffer from severe valvular disease, low cardiac function, massive myocardial infarction, and acute aortic dissection have high risk of cardiogenic shock after surgery. Extracorporeal membrane oxygenation (ECMO) is a last resort treatment option for such patients. However, ethical concerns exist regarding whether ECMO is worthwhile for them, because it carries a huge financial burden, and the mortality of ECMO patients following cardiac surgery is reported to be as high as 60–80%. No guideline exists regarding optimal patient selection, duration of mechanical support, and management of ECMO. There are many unanswered questions in this field. This is a comprehensive review regarding the most recent available evidences in the field of ECMO support for post-cardiotomy cardiogenic shock

Keywords: cardiac surgery, cardiogenic shock, extracorporeal membrane oxygenation support

1. Introduction

Post-cardiotomy cardiogenic shock occurs in approximately 1% of adult cardiac surgical patients [1, 2]. For these patients, extracorporeal membrane oxygenation (ECMO) is a device for temporary mechanical circulatory support allowing cardiac and pulmonary recovery or as a bridge to further therapeutic alternatives.

However, the outcomes of ECMO use for post-cardiotomy patients are not satisfactory. Inhospital mortality has been reported to be as high as 60–85%. In addition, ECMO use requires blood products, manpower, and special resources; therefore, it is associated with a significant financial burden to the institution.

No clear guidelines exist regarding the management of ECMO after cardiac surgery. The decision to place a patient on ECMO after cardiac surgery is difficult. Physicians have to make a decision based on individual circumstances, considering the balance between risks and benefits of ECMO.

2. VA-ECMO for post-cardiotomy cardiogenic shock

2.1. Initiation of ECMO

The causes of cardiogenic shock following cardiac surgery are divided into three categories: reversible, potentially reversible, and irreversible [3]. Reversible and potentially reversible causes of inability to wean from cardiopulmonary bypass include myocardial stunning, localized acute myocardial infarction, and acute pulmonary hypertension. Irreversible causes include pre-existing severe ventricular dysfunction, massive acute myocardial infarction, and chronic pulmonary hypertension.

ECMO offers the possibility of providing a bridge for maintaining organ perfusion and oxygenation allowing time for the heart and lung function to recover [4]. Theoretically, ECMO is indicated for reversible or potentially reversible cardiogenic shock; however, it is hard to tell the reversibility of stunned or infarcted myocardium, and how long it would take for recovery.

2.2. ECMO set-up

ECMO following cardiac surgery is often established centrally, i.e., an arterial line through the ascending aorta and a venous line through the right atrium [5, 6]. If the chest is not open, or if there is a concern for leaving the chest open due to the risk of infection or bleeding, ECMO is established peripherally. This consists of a venous cannula in the femoral vein and an arterial cannula in the femoral artery.

If central ECMO is initiated, one can consider tunneling arterial and venous cannulas through the abdomen, so that the chest can be closed to reduce the risk of infection and bleeding [7].

2.3. Management of ECMO

ECMO management should be done in an intensive care unit, and perfusionists, cardiac surgeons, and intensivists should be involved.

Heparinization is a controversial issue in ECMO management. While anticoagulation is necessary to prevent formation of clots in the ECMO circuit, it increases the risk of bleeding from the cannulation sites and surgical fields [8]. Ko et al. suggested avoiding use of heparin for the first 24 hours of ECMO support [9].

http://dx.doi.org/10.5772/intechopen.76217

There is no consensus regarding anticoagulation management. Most centers use activated clotting time (ACT) to monitor the level of anticoagulation. ACT should be kept above 160 seconds during full flow of ECMO; whereas, it should be kept higher (>180 or >200 seconds) if patients have artificial valves or ECMO is in low flow [10]. Blood transfusion is to be expected due to blood loss and coagulopathy. Some centers use thromboelastography to guide what blood products (platelets, fresh frozen plasma, or cryoprecipitate) are necessary during ECMO management [11].

Some centers use bivalirudin instead of heparin for the management of ECMO, and some previous studies showed the superiority of bivalirudin over heparin [12, 13].

2.4. Management of left ventricular distension

Left ventricular distension can happen as a result of inadequate drainage of the right atrium, shunting of blood between the bronchial and pulmonary artery circulation, and inadequate ejection of the left ventricle against the afterload posted by the ECMO. This can result in increased wall stress, increased myocardial oxygen consumption, pulmonary edema, and hemorrhage. There are some strategies to alleviate left ventricular distension [14].

Seib et al. described a technique of left heart decompression with blade and balloon atrial septostomy [15]. They reported that this technique could successfully alleviate left atrial hypertension and pulmonary edema.

Aiyagari et al. described a technique of decompressing the left atrium by placing a transseptal left atrial drainage incorporated into the ECMO circuit [16]. This drainage cannula can be placed via a patent foramen ovale [17]. The left ventricle can be vented directly by placing a catheter percutaneously through the aortic valve into the left ventricle [18, 19].

Alternatively, other type of mechanical circulatory assist devices such as the Impella (Abiomed Inc., Danvers, MA) or the TandemHeart (CardiacAssist Inc., Pittsburgh, PA) can decompress the left ventricle [20].

2.5. Weaning of ECMO

The length of ECMO support ranges between 3 and 14 days [21]. Fiser et al. suggested that consideration of discontinuing ECMO should be given after 48 to 72 hours of ECMO initiation, either by moving to an implantable ventricular assist device or by withdrawal of ECMO [22]. Distelmaier et al. reviewed their experience of ECMO use in 354 patients, and found that prolonged ECMO support was associated with poor outcomes [23]. They suggested reevaluation of therapeutic strategies after 7 days of ECMO, because mortality increases dramatically afterward.

A pulmonary artery catheter and transesophageal echocardiography are essential in weaning ECMO to assess the cardiac function. If a patient can successfully maintain a reasonable cardiac output on a low pump flow, ECMO can be discontinued.

2.6. Outcomes

The surgical outcomes of ECMO support for post-cardiotomy cardiogenic shock in adult patients are summarized in **Table 1**. Overall, about half of the patients could be weaned off ECMO; however, inhospital mortality was around 60–80%. In other words, only a quarter of the patients survived to be discharged home. Pokersnik et al. concluded that advancements in technology improved oxygenator durability, but had little impact on overall survival rates [39].

Study	Number of pts	Successful weaning of ECMO	Survival
Rastan et al. [24]	517	63.3% was successfully weaned from ECMO	Inhospital mortality was 75.2%. Cumulative survivals were 17.6% after 6 months, 16.5% after 1 year, and 13.7% after 5 years.
Muehrcke et al. [25]	23	39.1% was weaned from ECMO, 13.0% underwent LVAD	Inhospital mortality was 69.6%.
Elsharkawy et al. [26]	233	12.0% was converted to implantable LVAD	Inhospital mortality was 64%.
Zhao et al. [27]	24	66.7% was weaned off ECMO	Inhospital mortality was 66.7%.
Ko et al. [9]	76	55.3% was weaned off ECMO, 2.6% underwent LVAD, and 2.6% underwent transplantation	Inhospital mortality was 73.7%.
Biancari et al. [28]	148	4.1% underwent LVAD	Inhospital mortality was 64.2%. One-, 2-, and 3-year survival was 31.0%, 27.9%, and 26.1%, respectively.
Khorsandi et al. [29]	27	15% underwent short-term VAD implantation	Inhospital mortality was 59.3%.
Ariyaratnam et al. [3]	14	50% was weaned off ECMO	Inhospital mortality was 85.7%.
Smedira et al. [30]	202	23.8% underwent transplantation, 35.1% was weaned off ECMO	30-day mortality was 62%. Survival at 5 years was 24%.
Bakhtiary et al. [31]	45	56% had successful weaning of ECMO	Inhospital mortality was 71%. During follow-up period up to 3 years, 22% were alive.
Hsu et al. [32]	51	53% had successful weaning of ECMO	Inhospital mortality was 67%. 29% patients were alive at 1-year postop.
Li et al. [33]	123	56% had successful weaning of ECMO	Inhospital mortality was 65.9%.
Saxena et al. [34]	45	53% were weaned off ECMO	Inhospital mortality was 75.6%.
Papadopoulos et al. [35]	360	58% had successful weaning of ECMO	Inhospital mortality was 70%.
Unosawa et al. [36]	47	62% had successful weaning of ECMO	Inhospital mortality was 32%. The actuarial survival rates were 34.0% at 30 days, 29.8% at 1 year, and 17.6% at 10 years.

http://dx.doi.org/10.5772/intechopen.76217

Study	Number of pts	Successful weaning of ECMO	Survival
Slottosch et al. [37]	77	62% had successful weaning of ECMO	30-day mortality was 70%.
Zhang et al. [38]	32	44% had successful weaning of ECMO	30-day mortality was 68.8%. At a follow-up period of 3.9 years, the overall survival rate was 12.5%.
Doll et al. [2]	219	60% had successful weaning of ECMO	Inhospital mortality was 76%. Among survivors, 74% were alive at 5-year follow-up.
Magovern et al. [10]	55	65% were weaned off ECMO	Inhospital mortality was 64%.
Pokersnik et al. [39]	49	55% were weaned off ECMO	Inhospital mortality was 67%.
Guihaire et al. [40]	92	48% were weaned off ECMO	Inhospital mortality was 63%. Overall 1-month and 6-month survival rates were, 42% and 39%, respectively.

Table 1. Outcomes of ECMO use for post-cardiotomy cardiogenic shock.

Risk factors associated with hospital mortality were age [24, 26, 33, 35, 37, 40], diabetes [24, 26], obesity [24], female gender [33], pulmonary disease [28], atrial fibrillation [34], and chronic kidney disease [24, 28, 30, 34]. It is also suggested that the level of lactate [24, 28, 34, 35, 37, 38, 40], creatine kinase isoenzyme MB [38], longer duration of ECMO support [36, 37], mean lactate concentration [33], and lactate clearance [33] were predictors of inhospital mortality. In terms of surgical procedures, valvular surgery is generally associated with poor outcomes [40], and coronary artery bypass is associated with better outcomes [24].

Not many papers reported long-term outcomes after ECMO use for post-cardiotomy cardiogenic shock. One-year survival rate was around 20–30%. Despite high inhospital mortality, some papers reported the quality of life of survivors were acceptable with New York Heart Association functional class I or II [2, 9].

Biancari et al. performed a meta-analysis of the outcomes of ECMO for post-cardiotomy adult patients [41]. They investigated 31 studies reported on 2986 patients who required post-cardiotomy ECMO. The weaning rate from ECMO was 59.5%, and hospital survival was 36.1%. One-year survival rate was 30.9%. However, there is a criticism for this paper, as it included post-transplant patients [42]. Usually the outcomes of planned ECMO use following heart transplantation are better than those of unplanned non-transplant post-cardiotomy ECMO.

2.7. Complications of ECMO

ECMO is associated with high incidence of complications.

Major hemorrhage is the most commonly reported complication associated with ECMO institution. The reasons for excessive bleeding in ECMO patients are the surgical trauma, thrombocytopenia, activation of leukocytes, and necessity of anticoagulation. Rastan et al.

reported that more than half of the patients required re-exploration of the chest for bleeding [24]. Golding et al. reported that 87.3% required re-exploration for bleeding [43].

Cerebrovascular events also occurred frequently. Smedira et al. reported that 33% of the patients developed neurologic events [30], and Rastan et al. reported that the incidence of cerebrovascular events was 17.4% [24]. The reasons for high incidence of cerebrovascular events include the operative procedure itself, hemodynamic instability, lack of pulsatile flow, retrograde perfusion via peripheral circuit, and anticoagulation-related injuries.

Leg ischemia is a complication specifically associated with peripheral ECMO institution [44]. Rastan et al. reported that about 20% of the patients developed leg ischemia and 9.2% required leg fasciotomy [24]. However, the risk of this complication can be reduced by using a distal leg perfusion cannula [24], or by using a dacron or hemashield prosthetic graft sewn onto the artery to maintain both central arterial blood flow as well as distal limb perfusion [32].

A meta-analysis performed by Biancari et al. reported that the rate of reoperation for bleeding was 42.9%, major neurological event 11.3%, lower limb ischemia 10.8%, deep sternal wound infection 14.7%, and renal replacement therapy 47.1% [41].

2.8. Bridge to alternatives

When patients have difficulty of being weaned from ECMO, physicians need to consider if they have to withdraw ECMO from them, or if they proceed to alternative options. Patients were more likely to be considered for bridging to heart transplantation if they are less than 60 years of age. Smedira et al. reported that 24% were bridged to heart transplantation [30]. However, heart transplantation is not an available option in all countries.

Other options include left ventricular assist device (LVAD) or right ventricular assist device (RVAD). Muehrcke et al. reported that 4 out of 23 patients were transferred to an implantable LVAD from ECMO [25]. Pokersnik et al. reported that 2 out of 49 patients were bridged to long-term devices—bi-ventricular assist devices [39].

2.9. Hospital transfer

Post-cardiotomy shock may happen at institutions which do not have much experience with the management of mechanical circulatory support devices. In addition, not all institutions have options of long-term devices such as LVAD, or transplantation. Therefore, the development of a robust program of tertiary referral is of paramount importance [45]. Javidfar et al. reported no transport-related mortality or morbidity in patients who were transported via an ambulance with ECMO [46].

Teman et al. reported that patients with post-cardiotomy cardiac shock transported to a tertiary care center had a nearly 50% survival [47].

Weaning to recovery, institution of long-term support as a bridge to recovery, transition to transplantation or destination therapy, as well as device withdrawal and palliative care should be discussed in a multidisciplinary team including cardiologists, surgeons, intensivists, psychiatrists, and social workers [21].

3. Conclusions

The surgical mortality after ECMO use for post-cardiotomy cardiogenic shock remains high despite technological advancement. However, ECMO is the last resort to keep a patient alive who would otherwise expire on the operating table. According to the literatures, ECMO can be a salvage treatment in about one-third of these patients. Increased age, chronic kidney disease, and high level of lactate are major risk factors associated with hospital mortality. Also longer duration of ECMO support is associated with poor outcome. There is no guideline regarding optimal patient selection, duration of mechanical support, and management of ECMO.

A careful decision-making is necessary before ECMO is initiated, because ECMO is associated with a significant burden to a facility. As patients who need ECMO are always heterogeneous, the decision should be based on an individual basis.

A transfer to a tertiary center is critically important, because they can provide the transition to further supports, such as heart transplantation and implantable ventricular assist devices for patients who have difficulty of being weaned from ECMO.

Author details

Takashi Murashita

Address all correspondence to: tmurashita@gmail.com

West Virginia University, Heart and Vascular Institute, Morgantown, WV, USA

References

[1] Muehrcke DD, McCarthy PM, Stewart RW, Seshagiri S, Ogella DA, Foster RC, Cosgrove DM. Complications of extracorporeal life support systems using heparin-bound surfaces. The risk of intracardiac clot formation. The Journal of Thoracic and Cardiovascular Surgery. 1995;**110**:843-851

[2] Doll N, Kiaii B, Borger M, Bucerius J, Krämer K, Schmitt DV, Walther T, Mohr FW. Five-year results of 219 consecutive patients treated with extracorporeal membrane oxygenation for refractory postoperative cardiogenic shock. The Annals of Thoracic Surgery. 2004;**77**:151-157

[3] Ariyaratnam P, McLean LA, Cale AR, Loubani M. Extra-corporeal membrane oxygenation for the post-cardiotomy patient. Heart Failure Reviews. 2014;**19**:717-725. DOI: 10.1007/s10741-014-9428-9

[4] Bardia A, Schonberger RB. Postcardiotomy venoarterial extracorporeal membrane oxygenation (VA ECMO) in adult patients - Many questions, few answers, and hard choices. Journal of Cardiothoracic and Vascular Anesthesia. 2017 Oct 31. pii: S1053-0770(17)30821-2. DOI: 10.1053/j.jvca.2017.10.037

[5] Khorsandi M, Dougherty S, Bouamra O, Pai V, Curry P, Tsui S, Clark S, Westaby S, Al-Attar N, Zamvar V. Extra-corporeal membrane oxygenation for refractory cardiogenic shock after adult cardiac surgery: A systematic review and meta-analysis. Journal of Cardiothoracic Surgery. 2017;**12**:55. DOI: 10.1186/s13019-017-0618-0

[6] Khorsandi M, Shaikhrezai K, Prasad S, Pessotto R, Walker W, Berg G, Zamvar V. Advanced mechanical circulatory support for post-cardiotomy cardiogenic shock: A 20-year outcome analysis in a non-transplant unit. Journal of Cardiothoracic Surgery. 2016;**11**:29. DOI: 10.1186/s13019-016-0430-2

[7] Kohler K, Valchanov K, Nias G, Vuylsteke A. ECMO cannula review. Perfusion. 2013;**28**:114-124. DOI: 10.1177/0267659112468014

[8] Muntean W. Coagulation and anticoagulation in extracorporeal membrane oxygenation. Artificial Organs. 1999;**23**:979-983

[9] Ko WJ, Lin CY, Chen RJ, Wang SS, Lin FY, Chen YS. Extracorporeal membrane oxygenation support for adult postcardiotomy cardiogenic shock. The Annals of Thoracic Surgery. 2002;**73**:538-545

[10] Magovern GJ Jr, Simpson KA. Extracorporeal membrane oxygenation for adult cardiac support: The Allegheny experience. The Annals of Thoracic Surgery. 1999;**68**:655-661

[11] Panigada M, Iapichino EG, Brioni M, Panarello G, Protti A, Grasselli G, Occhipinti G, Novembrino C, Consonni D, Arcadipane A, Gattinoni L, Pesenti A. Thromboelastography-based anticoagulation management during extracorporeal membrane oxygenation: A safety and feasibility pilot study. Annals of Intensive Care. 2018;**8**:7. DOI: 10.1186/s13613-017-0352-8

[12] Ranucci M, Ballotta A, Kandil H, Isgrò G, Carlucci C, Baryshnikova E, Pistuddi V. Surgical and clinical outcome research group. Bivalirudin-based versus conventional heparin anticoagulation for postcardiotomy extracorporeal membrane oxygenation. Critical Care. 2011;**15**:275. DOI: 10.1186/cc10556

[13] Pieri M, Agracheva N, Bonaveglio E, Greco T, De Bonis M, Covello RD, Zangrillo A, Pappalardo F. Bivalirudin versus heparin as an anticoagulant during extracorporeal membrane oxygenation: A case-control study. Journal of Cardiothoracic and Vascular Anesthesia. 2013; **27**:30-34. DOI:10.1053/j.jvca.2012.07.019

[14] Soleimani B, Pae WE. Management of left ventricular distension during peripheral extracorporeal membrane oxygenation for cardiogenic shock. Perfusion. 2012;**27**:326-331. DOI: 10.1177/0267659112443722

[15] Seib PM, Faulkner SC, Erickson CC, Van Devanter SH, Harrell JE, Fasules JW, Frazier EA, Morrow WR. Blade and balloon atrial septostomy for left heart decompression in patients with severe ventricular dysfunction on extracorporeal membrane oxygenation. Catheterization and Cardiovascular Interventions 1999;**46**:179-186

[16] Aiyagari RM, Rocchini AP, Remenapp RT, Graziano JN. Decompression of the left atrium during extracorporeal membrane oxygenation using a transseptal cannula incorporated into the circuit. Critical Care Medicine. 2006;**34**:2603-2606

[17] Madershahian N, Salehi-Gilani S, Naraghi H, Stoeger E, Wahlers T. Biventricular decompression by trans-septal positioning of venous ECMO cannula through patent foramen ovale. The Journal of Cardiovascular Surgery. 2011;**52**:900

[18] Fumagalli R, Bombino M, Borelli M, Rossi F, Colombo V, Osculati G, Ferrazzi P, Pesenti A, Gattinoni L. Percutaneous bridge to heart transplantation by venoarterial ECMO and transaortic left ventricular venting. The International Journal of Artificial Organs. 2004;**27**:410-413

[19] Barbone A, Malvindi PG, Ferrara P, Tarelli G. Left ventricle unloading by percutaneous pigtail during extracorporeal membrane oxygenation. Interactive Cardiovascular and Thoracic Surgery. 2011;**13**:293-295. DOI: 10.1510/icvts.2011.269795

[20] Cheng A, Swartz MF, Massey HT. Impella to unload the left ventricle during peripheral extracorporeal membrane oxygenation. ASAIO Journal. 2013;**59**:533-536. DOI: 10.1097/MAT.0b013e31829f0e52

[21] Sylvin EA, Stern DR, Goldstein DJ. Mechanical support for postcardiotomy cardiogenic shock: Has progress been made? Journal of Cardiac Surgery. 2010;**25**:442-454. DOI: 10.1111/j.1540-8191.2010.01045.x

[22] Fiser SM, Tribble CG, Kaza AK, Long SM, Zacour RK, Kern JA, Kron IL. When to discontinue extracorporeal membrane oxygenation for postcardiotomy support. The Annals of Thoracic Surgery. 2001;**71**:210-214

[23] Distelmaier K, Wiedemann D, Binder C, Haberl T, Zimpfer D, Heinz G, Koinig H, Felli A, Steinlechner B, Niessner A, Laufer G, Lang I, Goliasch G. Duration of extracorporeal membrane oxygenation support and survival in cardiovascular surgery patients. The Journal of Thoracic and Cardiovascular Surgery. 2017. pii: S0022-5223 (17)33057-X. DOI: 10.1016/j.jtcvs. 2017.12.079

[24] Rastan AJ, Dege A, Mohr M, Doll N, Falk V, Walther T, Mohr FW. Early and late outcomes of 517 consecutive adult patients treated with extracorporeal membrane oxygenation for refractory postcardiotomy cardiogenic shock. The Journal of Thoracic and Cardiovascular Surgery. 2010;**139**:302-311. DOI: 10.1016/j.jtcvs.2009.10.043

[25] Muehrcke DD, McCarthy PM, Stewart RW, Foster RC, Ogella DA, Borsh JA, Cosgrove DM 3rd. Extracorporeal membrane oxygenation for postcardiotomy cardiogenic shock. The Annals of Thoracic Surgery 1996;**61**:684-691

[26] Elsharkawy HA, Li L, Esa WA, Sessler DI, Bashour CA. Outcome in patients who require venoarterial extracorporeal membrane oxygenation support after cardiac surgery. Journal of Cardiothoracic and Vascular Anesthesia. 2010;**24**:946-951. DOI: 10.1053/j.jvca.2010.03.020

[27] Zhao Y, Xing J, Du Z, Liu F, Jia M, Hou X. Extracorporeal cardiopulmonary resuscitation for adult patients who underwent post-cardiac surgery. European Journal of Medical Research. 2015;**20**:83. DOI: 10.1186/s40001-015-0179-4

[28] Biancari F, Dalén M, Perrotti A, Fiore A, Reichart D, Khodabandeh S, Gulbins H, Zipfel S, Al Shakaki M, Welp H, Vezzani A, Gherli T, Lommi J, Juvonen T, Svenarud P, Chocron S,

Verhoye JP, Bounader K, Gatti G, Gabrielli M, Saccocci M, Kinnunen EM, Onorati F, Santarpino G, Alkhamees K, Ruggieri VG, Dell'Aquila AM. Venoarterial extracorporeal membrane oxygenation after coronary artery bypass grafting: Results of a multicenter study. International Journal of Cardiology. 2017;**241**:109-114. DOI: 10.1016/j.ijcard.2017.03.120

[29] Khorsandi M, Dougherty S, Sinclair A, Buchan K, MacLennan F, Bouamra O, Curry P, Zamvar V, Berg G, Al-Attar N. A 20-year multicentre outcome analysis of salvage mechanical circulatory support for refractory cardiogenic shock after cardiac surgery. Journal of Cardiothoracic Surgery. 2016;**11**:151. DOI: 10.1186/s13019-016-0545-5

[30] Smedira NG, Moazami N, Golding CM, McCarthy PM, Apperson-Hansen C, Blackstone EH, Cosgrove DM 3rd. Clinical experience with 202 adults receiving extracorporeal membrane oxygenation for cardiac failure: Survival at five years. The Journal of Thoracic and Cardiovascular Surgery 2001;**122**:92-102

[31] Bakhtiary F, Keller H, Dogan S, Dzemali O, Oezaslan F, Meininger D, Ackermann H, Zwissler B, Kleine P, Moritz A. Venoarterial extracorporeal membrane oxygenation for treatment of cardiogenic shock: Clinical experiences in 45 adult patients. The Journal of Thoracic and Cardiovascular Surgery. 2008;**135**:382-388. DOI: 10.1016/j.jtcvs.2007.08.007

[32] Hsu PS, Chen JL, Hong GJ, Tsai YT, Lin CY, Lee CY, Chen YG, Tsai CS. Extracorporeal membrane oxygenation for refractory cardiogenic shock after cardiac surgery: Predictors of early mortality and outcome from 51 adult patients. European Journal of Cardio-Thoracic Surgery. 2010;**37**:328-333. DOI: 10.1016/j.ejcts.2009.07.033

[33] Li CL, Wang H, Jia M, Ma N, Meng X, Hou XT. The early dynamic behavior of lactate is linked to mortality in postcardiotomy patients with extracorporeal membrane oxygenation support: A retrospective observational study. The Journal of Thoracic and Cardiovascular Surgery. 2015;**149**:1445-1450. DOI: 10.1016/j.jtcvs.2014.11.052

[34] Saxena P, Neal J, Joyce LD, Greason KL, Schaff HV, Guru P, Shi WY, Burkhart H, Li Z, Oliver WC, Pike RB, Haile DT, Schears GJ. Extracorporeal membrane oxygenation support in postcardiotomy elderly patients: The Mayo clinic experience. The Annals of Thoracic Surgery. 2015;**99**:2053-2060. DOI: 10.1016/j.athoracsur.2014.11.075

[35] Papadopoulos N, Marinos S, El-Sayed Ahmad A, Keller H, Meybohm P, Zacharowski K, Moritz A, Zierer A. Risk factors associated with adverse outcome following extracorporeal life support: Analysis from 360 consecutive patients. Perfusion. 2015;**30**:284-290. DOI: 10.1177/0267659114542458

[36] Unosawa S, Sezai A, Hata M, Nakata K, Yoshitake I, Wakui S, Kimura H, Takahashi K, Hata H, Shiono M. Long-term outcomes of patients undergoing extracorporeal membrane oxygenation for refractory postcardiotomy cardiogenic shock. Surgery Today. 2013;**43**:264-270. DOI: 10.1007/s00595-012-0322-6

[37] Slottosch I, Liakopoulos O, Kuhn E, Deppe AC, Scherner M, Madershahian N, Choi YH, Wahlers T. Outcomes after peripheral extracorporeal membrane oxygenation therapy for postcardiotomy cardiogenic shock: A single-center experience. The Journal of Surgical Research. 2013;**181**:47-55. DOI: 10.1016/j.jss.2012.07.030

[38] Zhang R, Kofidis T, Kamiya H, Shrestha M, Tessmann R, Haverich A, Klima U. Creatine kinase isoenzyme MB relative index as predictor of mortality on extracorporeal membrane oxygenation support for postcardiotomy cardiogenic shock in adult patients. European Journal of Cardio-Thoracic Surgery. 2006;**30**:617-620

[39] Pokersnik JA, Buda T, Bashour CA, Gonzalez-Stawinski GV. Have changes in ECMO technology impacted outcomes in adult patients developing postcardiotomy cardiogenic shock? Journal of Cardiac Surgery. 2012;**27**:246-252. DOI: 10.1111/j.1540-8191.2011.01409.x

[40] Guihaire J, Dang Van S, Rouze S, Rosier S, Roisne A, Langanay T, Corbineau H, Verhoye JP, Flécher E. Clinical outcomes in patients after extracorporeal membrane oxygenation support for post-cardiotomy cardiogenic shock: A single-centre experience of 92 cases. Interactive Cardiovascular and Thoracic Surgery. 2017;**25**:363-369. DOI: 10.1093/icvts/ivx155

[41] Biancari F, Perrotti A, Dalén M, Guerrieri M, Fiore A, Reichart D, Dell'Aquila AM, Gatti G, Ala-Kokko T, Kinnunen EM, Tauriainen T, Chocron S, Airaksinen JKE, Ruggieri VG, Brascia D. Meta-analysis of the outcome after postcardiotomy venoarterial extracorporeal membrane oxygenation in adult patients. Journal of Cardiothoracic and Vascular Anesthesia. 2017. pii: S1053-0770(17)30730-9. DOI: 10.1053/j.jvca.2017.08.048

[42] Charlesworth M, Venkateswaran R, Barker JM, Feddy L. Postcardiotomy VA-ECMO for refractory cardiogenic shock. Journal of Cardiothoracic Surgery. 2017;**12**:116. DOI: 10.1186/s13019-017-0674-5

[43] Golding LA, Crouch RD, Stewart RW, Novoa R, Lytle BW, McCarthy PM, Taylor PC, Loop FD, Cosgrove DM 3rd. Postcardiotomy centrifugal mechanical ventricular support. The Annals of Thoracic Surgery 1992;**54**:1059-1063

[44] Bisdas T, Beutel G, Warnecke G, Hoeper MM, Kuehn C, Haverich A, Teebken OE. Vascular complications in patients undergoing femoral cannulation for extracorporeal membrane oxygenation support. The Annals of Thoracic Surgery. 2011;**92**:626-631. DOI: 10.1016/j.athoracsur.2011.02.018

[45] Fukuhara S, Takeda K, Garan AR, Kurlansky P, Hastie J, Naka Y, Takayama H. Contemporary mechanical circulatory support therapy for postcardiotomy shock. General Thoracic and Cardiovascular Surgery. 2016;**64**:183-191. DOI: 10.1007/s11748-016-0625-4

[46] Javidfar J, Brodie D, Takayama H, Mongero L, Zwischenberger J, Sonett J, Bacchetta M. Safe transport of critically ill adult patients on extracorporeal membrane oxygenation support to a regional extracorporeal membrane oxygenation center. ASAIO Journal. 2011;**57**:421-425. DOI: 10.1097/MAT.0b013e3182238b55

[47] Teman NR, Demos DS, Reames BN, Pagani FD, Haft JW. Outcomes after transfer to a tertiary center for postcardiotomy cardiopulmonary failure. The Annals of Thoracic Surgery. 2014;**98**:84-89. DOI: 10.1016/j.athoracsur.2013.12.091

Chapter 9

Use of ECMO in Sepsis and Septic Shock

Koen De Decker

Additional information is available at the end of the chapter

http://dx.doi.org/10.5772/intechopen.77120

Abstract

The use of extracorporeal membrane oxygenation (ECMO) has always been controversial in the past. Evidence was mainly build up in neonates and much controversy remained in adults. The main adult indications were mechanical support (e.g., in cardiogenic shock) or respiratory support (e.g., in the field of acute respiratory distress syndrome (ARDS)). Sepsis was historically often considered as a contraindication. As a consequence of several worldwide flu outbreaks, the use of ECMO in infectious diseases increased. Besides in these viral infections, there was also growing interest for its use in bacterial septicemia, although often as escape therapy. In the recent years, other techniques gained increasing interest like for example, immunoadsorption, implemented in dialysis or ECMO circuits. In this chapter, we resume the available literature on the use of ECMO in septic shock including the use of immunoadsorption techniques.

Keywords: ECMO, sepsis, septic shock, immunoadsorption

1. Introduction

Since the publication in the early 1970s of the first successful use of extracorporeal membrane oxygenation (ECMO) in a post-traumatic adult respiratory distress (ARDS) patient [1], ECMO has been used tremendously. The approach can be either by veno-venous cannulation, which is mainly used in hypoxic respiratory failure, or by veno-arterial cannulation, which is the preferred modality for cardiac (or combined) support. This implements that most indications are in the field of ARDS and cardiogenic shock states.

Septic shock is a serious disorder that, despite progress in treatment over the last decades, still has a high mortality (between 20 and 30%) [2]. The ECMO survival in septic neonates [3, 4] and children [5] has improved to ~90 and 75%, respectively. There is however far more controversy on its use in adult refractory septic shock, although successful salvage cases have been published [6, 7]. In parallel with the reports on its effectiveness during the influenza A (H1N1) outbreaks [8, 9], the interest for using ECMO in noninfluenza-induced sepsis has grown.

This chapter mainly focuses on indications, the difference between children and adults, causative pathogens, outcome and outcome prediction. It will not go into further detail on the technical aspects (cannulation, oxygenators and pumps).

2. Study population

2.1. Adults

2.1.1. Case report

A typical case of refractory septic shock is the following, unpublished, case out of our own ICU. A 42-year-old (type I) diabetic female was found unconscious by her husband and was brought to the emergency department after she was intubated at home by a medical team. She was diagnosed with diabetic ketoacidosis (initial pH 6.96) and was in of severe shock signs, requiring high doses of norepinephrine (0.5 μg/kg/′) in the emergency department. The patient was transferred to the ICU and after sampling (respiratory and hemocultures) empirical amoxicillin-clavulanate was started.

Because of refractory shock despite aggressive fluid resuscitation, vasopressin was added as well as low doses of hydrocortisone (3 × 100 mg daily). This led to normalization of blood pressures and pH, but the patient remained oliguric and overnight oxygenation deteriorated despite increasing PEEP and FiO2. Early continuous renal replacement therapy (CRRT) was started.

Approximately 14 h after ICU admission, she suffered cardiac arrest due to sudden onset of ventricular fibrillation. After initial successful resuscitation (after cardiac massage and defibrillation), her oxygenation and hemodynamic status deteriorated further, necessitating peripheral cannulation of the femoral vein and artery and afterward the initiation of veno-arterial ECMO.

Antibiotic therapy was empirically switched to a combination of meropenem and vancomycin and (single shot) amikacin. The initial hemocultures were positive for Gram-positive cocci, later identified as *Enterococcus faecalis*.

Over the following days, the patient suffered no further complications. Hemodynamics and oxygenation stabilized, inflammatory parameters slowly resolved. Seven days after starting mechanical support, ECMO support could be weaned and stopped.

Four days later, she suffered a new bacteremic episode with ***E. coli*** due to the development of empyema of the left hemithorax with. ***E. coli***. This time, however, without the need for mechanical support. After thoracospic drainage and antibiotic switch to cefepime, based on culture results, inflammation went down. After repeat empyema, urokinase in loco was administered with finally complete resolution of the empyema. The patient was extubated 30 days after hospital admission after 6 weeks she was discharged to the ward.

2.1.2. ICU case series

The available literature on ECMO use in adult septic shock patients consists mainly of case reports or (usually single-centered) retrospective case series. In a recent multicenter study [10], the data from 42 Japanese intensive care units were retrospectively collected and propensity score analysis was performed. Out of 3195 patients included in the JSEPTIC DIC study [11], 570 patients suffered from severe respiratory failure and in 285 of them respiratory failure was induced by lung infection. Overall 40 patients were supported with ECMO and these were matched with 150 patients in the control group. Sepsis-related organ failure (SOFA) scores were comparable (12 vs. 13).

A second propensity analysis was performed between the 25 ECMO patients with lung infection-induced respiratory failure and 89 patients in the control group. Overall no marked differences were found in 28-day mortality (47.2% in the control group vs. 32% in the ECMO group, p 0.168) and the in-hospital mortality (60.7% in control group vs. 40% in the ECMO group, p 0.07). However, in the second analysis comparing 89 controls with 25 ECMO patients with lung infection-induced respiratory failure, the survival time in the ECMO group was significantly longer (hazard ratio (HR), 0.498; 95% confidence interval (CI), 0.279–0.889; p 0.018). The numbers of renal replacement therapy and vasopressor-free days were also significantly higher in the ECMO group.

These results are similar with those reported by Nesseler et al. [12], who questioned the use of ECMO in patients with intra-abdominal sepsis-induced ARDS. Although the overall ECMO group (n = 40) received more red blood cell transfusions, there was no significant difference in the rate of severe bleeding complications. The numbers of renal replacement therapy and vasopressor-free days were significantly higher in the ECMO group.

Another retrospective study [13] describes 32 ECMO patients with refractory septic shock. Fourteen patients had undergone cardiopulmonary resuscitation (CPR) in which ECMO was started during CPR (ECPR). The most frequently infected site was the lung and 20 patients had bacteremia. Thirteen patients (40.6%) were successfully weaned of ECMO but only seven (21.9%) survived to discharge. Interestingly, none of the patients in whom ECMO was initiated more than 30 h after the onset of septic shock survived. CPR appeared to be an independent predictor of in-hospital mortality (adjusted HR, 4.61; 95% CI, 1.55–13.69; p 0.006). On the other hand, patients with myocardial injury (higher peak troponin I > 15 ng/ml) had a lower risk of in-hospital mortality (adjusted HR, 0.34; 95% CI, 0.12–0.97; P = 0.04).

The low survival rate was partially due to the ECPR cases, of who only 2 out of 14 survived and they both had return of spontaneous circulation within minutes. One of the conclusions of this trial was evidently that ECMO should be avoided in patients who have received CPR. The fact that patients with signs of myocardial injury had better survival rates could be explained by the reversibility of septic cardiomyopathy. There are two patterns of early death in septic shock: distributive shock or a cardiogenic form of septic shock [14]. ECMO may be a valuable support in patients with the latter form that is unresponsive to highly dosed cathecholamines [15]. Finally, survivors appeared to have lower SOFA score at day 3 compared with the nonsurvivors (15 vs. 18, p = 0.01).

In another case series [16], 14 patients received ECMO support as salvage therapy for refractory septic shock, 24 h (3–108) after shock onset. Mean simplified acute physiology score (SAPS) III was 84 (75–106) SOFA score was 18 (8–21). Twelve patients (86%) could be weaned off and 10 patients (71%) were discharged home and were alive after a median follow-up of 13 months (3–43) with normalized ejection fraction and a good quality of life.

During a 6-year period, 52 septic shock patients had undergone ECMO support in a South Korean ICU [17]. Almost half of them (n = 21) was receiving CPR at the time of ECMO implantation. Not surprisingly overall outcome data were poor with only 15% survival to discharge. The nonsurvivors were significantly older than survivors (59.3 vs. 43.8 years, P = 0.009) and all patients aged 60 or older died.

2.1.3. *Specific populations*

2.1.3.1. *Obstetrical cases*

Maternal sepsis is a predominant cause of maternal death in low-income countries, but also in Western countries maternal mortality from sepsis has increased [18]. In 15 years, the incidence in the UK almost doubled from 0.65 to 1.12 per 100,000 cases [19]. Twenty-one deliveries per 100,000 develop sepsis with a case fatality rate of 7–8%. In the presence of septic shock, mortality goes up to 60%. Pregnant women are not only vulnerable to sepsis because of changes in the immune system, predisposition to pyelonephritis due to ureteral compression and increased invasive interventions. They also tend to decompensate quickly in case of sepsis due to the physiological changes (cardiovascular, respiratory, and metabolic) of pregnancy. These changes can finally also mask the early recognition of sepsis.

Sharma et al. [20] examined 31 published reports (with a total of 67 patients) of ECMO use in pregnancy. Fetal survival was 70% and maternal survival 80% which was comparable to nonpregnant patients requiring ECMO support. Fifteen reports of V-V ECMO, 16 reports of V-A ECMO, and 1 report of a lung assist device. But, indications for ECLS use included mainly severe ARDS, postpartum cardiogenic shock and amniotic fluid embolism. Besides a lot of H1N1 infected patients, only one patient with staphylococcal-induced ARDS and septic shock was included. There was no consensus on an optimal anticoagulation strategy in these patients, though most preferred to keep anticoagulation at lower therapeutic levels. A few cases of vaginal bleeding were reported, but occurrence of catastrophic bleeding was rare.

After this review, several case reports on bacterial septic shock were published [21, 22]. A 24-year-old multiparous woman was admitted with multiple organ failure in the third trimester of pregnancy [21], after suffering from high fever and diarrhea since 1 day. Cesarean section was performed due to fetal distress but the patient remained in refractory circulatory failure with consequent, progressive multiple organ failure. Cateacholamines were increased after ICU admission and low doses hydrocortisone were given.

Continuous hemodiafiltration was initiated 4 h after ICU admission. Piperacillin/tazobactam was started at hospital admission but after the identification of Streptococcus pyogenes, the diagnosis of Streptococcal toxic shock syndrome was made. Antibiotics were switched to penicillin, and clindamycin and intravenous immunoglobulins were added. Despite the abovementioned therapy and the increase of the hemofilter membrane area, multiple organ failure continued to progress. Repeated echocardiography showed left ventricular ejection fraction (LVEF) of 10%. Therefore, veno-arterial ECMO was initiated from the right atrium to the right femoral artery. With blood and oxygen flows of both 3.0 L/min lactate levels decreased from 20 to 8.9 mmol/l after 24 h of ECMO support. On day 7, she was weaned from ECMO; on day 8, vasopressors were stopped; on day 10, ventilation could be stopped and renal function recovered. The patient was discharged after 53 days and cardiac function recovered after 4 months. The patient suffered no bleeding complications.

In a very recent case report [22], another 24-year-old was readmitted to the hospital 2 days after a normal vaginal delivery following an uneventful pregnancy. Despite starting vasopressors and broad-spectrum antibiotics, she continued to decline with intubation 14 h after admission. An echocardiogram revealed an LVEF of 20%. Blood cultures grew Gram-positive cocci (group a streptococcus). The patient was transferred to a tertiary center where the diagnosis of endometritis was made and emergent total abdominal hysterectomy was performed after starting VA ECMO support. The fascia was left open and wound vacuum system was left in place. Vasopressors could be weaned on postoperative day (POD) 1, but she returned to the operating room (OR) for intra-abdominal bleeding. Afterward she suffered no more adverse events until decannulation, which was done on POD 5 in the OR. She was extubated on POD 7 and by POD 12 LVEF had normalized.

Finally, a third case of an 18-year-old nulliparous woman was reported [23]. She was admitted after 26 weeks of pregnancy with high fever, nausea, headache and increasing inflammatory parameters. After blood cultures were taken, empirical cefuroxime (750 mg every hours intravenously). On the second day of hospitalization, contractions started and a preterm low birth weight premature girl was born after urgent C-section. Surgery was uncomplicated but suddenly tachycardia developed and diffuse intravascular coagulation (DIC) with consecutive bleeding problems from wounds and catheter insertion sites started after about an hour after the procedure. Sepsis was supposed to be the cause of the DIC and antibiotics were switched to vancomycin and meropenem after new hemocultures were obtained. The patient was transferred to the ICU because of pulmonary edema, which started 4 h after the bleeding problems.

She was intubated and vasopressors were started. Blood cultures grew positive for ***Staphylococcus aureus*** and ***Enterobacter cloacae***. As septic shock and cardiorespiratory failure deteriorated, hysterectomy was performed 4 days after the C-section. Afterward the patient recovered slightly, but respiratory failure further deteriorated and 3 days after the hysterectomy VA ECMO was started between the femoral vein and subclavian artery. She suffered from a hematoma at the arterial insertion point which encapsulated and infected, resulting in a thoracotomy. This had to be repeated several times because of bleeding complications, but finally the ECMO could be weaned 3 weeks after it had been initiated. Respiratory failure regressed and in the end she was discharged home after 105 days.

2.1.3.2. The immunocompromised patient

Several publications [24–27] report on the use of ECMO in immunocompromised patients, mainly kidney and liver transplanted patients. Infections are the leading cause of critical illness and mortality in liver transplant patients. More than half of the patients develop an infection during the first year, almost always ending in ICU admission. Bacteremia associated from 10 to 52%. Mortality is higher in recipients with bacteremia due to 'ESKAPE' pathogens, which stands for *Enterococcus faecium*, ***Staphylococcus aureus***, ***Klebsiella pneumoniae***, *Acinetobacter baumannii*, *Pseudomonas aeruginosa* and *Enterobacter* species [28]. Over a 7-year period, a South Korean university center [24] used ECMO in 8 (of in total 854) liver transplanted patients with refractory septic shock. Primary liver disease in these patients was hepatocellular carcinoma (n = 3), liver cirrhosis due to hepatitis B infection (n = 3), alcoholic liver cirrhosis (n = 1) and toxic hepatitis (n = 1). These patients suffered mainly from intra-abdominal and lung infections. They were infected by a variety of pathogens, but in five out of eight, *Acinetobacter baumannii* was cultured.

ECMO was initiated after a median of 6, 5 h under vasoactive drugs were started and six patients received cardiopulmonary resuscitation (CPR) with initiation of ECMO after a median of 41, 5 min (range, 20–154 min) after onset of CPR. The interval between the transplantation and the onset of infection was not mentioned. Three patients (37.5%) were successfully weaned from ECMO but only 2 (25%) survived until hospital discharge. Illness severity scores at onset were not different between survivors and nonsurvivors. Lactate levels and SOFA scores tended to decrease over the course of treatment in survivors while in nonsurvivors total bilirubin and CRP levels tended to increase.

Another successful use of ECMO support was reported in a 49-year-old male liver transplant [25] suffering from alcoholic liver cirrhosis-induced acute-on-chronic liver failure. Immediately before the emergent liver transplantation, he developed pulmonary tuberculosis and tuberculosis peritonitis. The latter caused intermittent small-bowel obstruction and subsequent ischemia and led to emergency adhesiolysis on POD 114. In the postoperative phase, the patient developed aspiration pneumonia leading to septic shock and ARDS. After 11 days of ECMO support, the patient could be weaned and finally was discharged on day 204.

The largest available series of ECMO in adult liver transplant patients was published by Park et al. [26]. Over a 3-year period, 18 out of 1076 liver transplanted patients required VV ECMO. The main indication, however, was refractory respiratory failure, not necessarily with concomitant septic shock. Eight patients could be weaned.

The electronic medical records of kidney transplanted (KT) patients that received ECMO support were reviewed [27]. Between December 2010 and December 2014, 12 KT patients required ECMO management. In half of them, this was due to bacterial sepsis only or combined viral/bacterial pneumonia or sepsis. The others suffered from viral pneumonia or in 1 case fulminant myocarditis secondary to fungemia. The mean period between the KT and the ECMO support was 44.4 months (range, 1.2–184.3 months) and in three patients ECMO was started during the admission for the transplant.

The mean duration of ECMO support was 9.1 days (range, 3.5–15.1 days) and six patients were successfully weaned from ECMO. However, two of them died after being weaned from ECMO. During ECMO support, all patients needed renal replacement therapy (RRT). Among the six survivors, five could be weaned after a mean period of 53 + 37.5 days (range, 16–97 days). The pH just before the beginning of ECMO appeared to be significantly lower in the nonsurvivors than in the survivors (P = 0.046).

2.2. Children

In contrast with the adult population, there is far more acceptance for using ECMO in pediatric cases of septic shock. In a French study [29], the use of VA ECMO in 14 neonates and 9 children with refractory septic shock was reported. The mean age of the pediatric population was 30 months. Overall, in more than half of the cases septic shock was due to streptococcal or ***E. coli*** bacteremia. Fifty-seven percent of the neonates suffered from Streptococcus B infection. All patients were ventilated and received vasopressors before ECMO initiation.

In two patients, cannulation was performed during chest compressions because of cardiac arrest. The mean duration of support was 7.43 days (range, 1–17) and 5.9 days (range, 3–10) in neonates and children, respectively. Six neonates (42%) and three children (37%) had mechanical (mainly clotting) complications with the ECMO circuit. One neonate and three children required renal replacement therapy.

The overall survival rate was 59.1%, with 64.% of the newborns (n = 9) surviving to discharge and 50% (n = 4) of the pediatric population. So survival was significantly higher in the newborns (p = 0.02), although ECMO weaning rates were comparable (64 and 66% respectively).

These results are somewhat lower than those reported in older trials [3, 4, 30, 31], with survival rates up to 80% in neonates and 74% in older children. But in the French cohort [29], the patients seemed to have more severe cardiovascular failure with higher inotropic scores and lower pH. The authors conclude that ECMO can be safely used to resuscitate children with refractory shock and propose to transfer infants to an ECMO referral center in case of persisting oliguria and without decrease of lactate levels within 6 h after the initiation of maximum drug therapy.

In some of the older trials [5], central cannulated ECMO (atrio-aortal cannulaton) was used in 23 children, almost all (96%) having at least three organ failures and eight (35%) suffered cardiac arrest and required massage during ECMO placement. All had microbiological evidence of infection and meningococcemia was the most common causative pathogen. Despite the severe setting at onset, 18 patients (78%) could be weaned of ECMO and 17 (74%) survived to hospital discharge.

More recently, several case reports of pediatric ECMO use were published in specific indications [32] like liver transplanted infants or with more rare pathogens [33] like community-acquired Legionella infection.

Finally, a Taiwanese group [34] recently published their retrospective single center review of 55 pediatric septic shock patients. In this cohort, overall survival to discharge was 31%. However, 25 patients were immunocompromised, in whom mortality was 75%. Mean ECMO duration was 9 days (range, 0–103) with a duration in survivors that doubled the one in non-survivors (14 vs. 7 days, $p = 0.09$). In 17 of them, causal pathogens could be identified of which 7 were bacterial and 1 was an invasive fungal infection. In the previously healthy kids, in 18 cases with an identified pathogen 10 were bacteremic (mainly pneumococcal).

3. Adjunctive therapies

The mainstay of etiological treatment in septic shock remains source control and the administration of anti-infective agents. Especially with regard to the latter, dosing issues are extremely important. Finally, there is also some emerging literature, unfortunately mainly anecdotal, on the use of immunoadsorptive strategies.

3.1. Source control

Resection or drainage of an infectious inoculum is important. Due the necessity of anticoagulating ECMO treated patients, this is not without risk of bleeding during or after (at restart of anticoagulation) the procedure. However, as mentioned in previous sections of this chapter, performing surgical procedures in ECMO patients is feasible [22, 23].

3.2. Dosing of anti-infective agents

In the last decade, the interest in pharmacodynamics and therapeutic drug monitoring (especially for antibiotics) has grown tremendously. With regard to prescribing antibiotics, several reports have dealt with therapeutic drug monitoring in ICU patients in the absence [35] or in the presence [36] of concomitant use of renal replacement therapy.

However, there are no clear guidelines for dosing antibiotics in ECMO-treated patients. Therefore, the interest on the matter increased in the latest years and several publications investigated this topic [37–39], mainly in the class of beta-lactam antibiotics.

In ECMO patients, the volume of distribution increases tremendously, but clearance is usually lower than controls [37]. Although pharmacokinetic variability is high, decreased meropenem clearance usually compensates for ECMO and critical illness-related increases in the volume of distribution. With standard 1 g IV dosing 8-hourly, target concentrations of >2 mg/L are usually met, but an increase in dose may be appropriate in patients with elevated creatinine clearance or when higher concentrations are needed for less susceptible microorganisms.

The use of continuous infusions of carbapenems might be useful in this regard [38]. In a pediatric ECMO case, a bolus of 40 mg/kg meropenem followed by a continuous infusion of 200 mg/kg/day resulted in target attainment of 100% for serum and lung concentrations above the MIC.

http://dx.doi.org/10.5772/intechopen.77120

Also, other beta-lactam antibiotics [39] were investigated. For piperacillin/tazobactam insufficient concentrations were more frequent than with meropenem therapy in the treatment of *Pseudomonas aeruginosa* infections.

Also while prescribing antifungal agents, caution is warranted for subtherapeutic exposure. In pediatric ECMO case [40], insufficient plasma levels were measured despite the administration of normal to high doses of caspofungin.

3.3. Immunoadsorption

In the last decade, several publications report on the use of cytokine adsorption techniques [41–46]. In several case reports [41–43], the Cytosorb hemoadsorption column (Linc Medical, Leicestershire, United Kingdom) was installed either in the ECMO circuit or in the CRRT circuit in order to stabilize septic shock patients more rapidly and to improve their outcome. Cytosorb removes the proinflammatory cytokines and has been shown to reduce vasopressor doses and serum inflammatory markers in septic patients. A similar device is the polymethylmethacrylate membrane hemofilter is also available for clinical use and a report on its use has been published [46]. Although promising, the addition of these immunabsorption techniques is costly and still under investigation.

4. Outcome prediction

Giving the debatable indication (at least in adults), the high cost and the invasive nature of ECMO treatment and the consequent complications, outcome prediction before treatment initiation is important. In **Table 1**, the outcome predictors of the previously cited publications

Predictor	cut off	impact on survival	Reference
ADULTS			
SAPS II	< 80	increased	50
ECPR at implementation		decreased	13
Pneumonia induced septic shock		increased	51
Gram-positive vs. Gram-negative septicemia		increased	51
Door-to ECMO time	< 96 hours	increased	51
	> 30 hours	decreased	24
Age	> 60	decreased	10, 24
Troponin I levels	> 15 ng/ml	increased	13
lower SOFA score at day 3 of support		increased	15
CHILDREN			
Arterial blood gas pH	< 7,2	decreased	37
Arterial blood gas CO2	> 56,9 mm Hg	decreased	37
Glasgow Coma Scale	<9	decreased	37
SOFA	< 15	increased	37
Central cannulation		increased	34

Table 1. Outcome predictors for ECMO use in septic shock.

are listed and a few other publications [47–49], that have investigated survival predictors for septic shock patients under mechanical support, were added.

In a Korean case series [47], 28 patients were treated with ECMO, of whom 21 with VA ECMO. The overall survival to discharge rate was 35.7% and predictors of survival appeared to be: a simplified acute physiology score II (SAP II) of 80 or less and pre-ECMO albumin levels.

In another report [48], better outcomes were seen if door-to ECMO times were < 96 h. Furthermore, survival was better in case of Gram-positive infections rather than Gram-negative septic shock. Finally, outcome was better for pneumonia rather than primary bloodstream infections.

The same group [49] also published that the implementation of ECMO during CPR is not beneficial for septic shock patients.

5. Conclusions

Although the use of VA ECMO has been controversial in adults with septic shock, it is commonly used in the pediatric population, with good results. Despite the ongoing controversy, VA ECMO has seen increased use in septic adults with SICM, with survival and complete cardiac recovery in as high as 70% of patients. However, outcomes vary enormously and VA ECMO seems especially beneficial in certain subsets, like, for example, lung infection-induced septic shock. On the other hand, survival rates are poor when ECMO is initiated in a CPR setting. Other currently reported, negative predictors (at ECMO onset) are SAPS II scores >80, Gram-negative septicemia, age > 60 years, SOFA scores >15. Also in immunocompromised patients, mortality rates are high and ECMO, which does not exclude its use in escape therapy (e.g., after liver transplantation). The use of ECMO does not prohibit other surgical interventions, with the aim of infectious source control. Procedures like hysterectomy, laparotomy, all have been performed under or immediately before ECMO therapy.

Conflict of interest

The author has no conflicts of interest to be declared.

Author details

Koen De Decker

Address all correspondence to: koen.de.decker@olvz-aalst.be

Onze Lieve Vrouw Hospital, Aalst, Belgium

References

[1] Hill JD, O'Brien TG, Murray JJ, Dontigny L, Bramson ML, Osborn JJ, Gerbode F. Prolonged extracorporeal oxygenation for acute post-traumatic respiratory failure (shock-lung syndrome). Use of the Bramson membrane lung. New England Journal of Medicine. 1972; 23;**286**(12):629-634

[2] Martin GS, Mannino DM, Eaton S, Moss M. The epidemiology of sepsis in the United States from 1979 through 2000. The New England Journal of Medicine. 2003;**348**:1546-1554

[3] McCune S, Short BL, Miller MK, Lotze A, Anderson KD. Extracorporeal membrane oxygenation therapy in neonates with septic shock. Journal of Pediatric Surgery. 1990; **25**:479-482

[4] Hocker JR, Simpson PM, Rabalais GP, Stewart DL, Cook LN. Extracorporeal membrane oxygenation and early-onset group B streptococcal sepsis. Pediatrics. 1992;**89**:1-4

[5] MacLaren G, Butt W, Best D, Donath S. Central extracorporeal membrane oxygenation for refractory pediatric septic shock. Pediatric Critical Care Medicine. 2011;**12**:133-136

[6] Firstenberg MS, Abel E, Blais D, Louis LB, Steinberg S, Sai-Sudhakar C, et al. The use of extracorporeal membrane oxygenation in severe necrotizing soft tissue infections complicated by septic shock. American Surgeon. 2010;**76**:1287-1289

[7] MacLaren G, Pellegrino V, Butt W, Preovolos A, Salamonsen R. Successful use of ECMO in adults with life-threatening infections. Anaesthesia and Intensive Care. 2004;**32**:707-710

[8] Noah MA, Peek GJ, Finney SJ, et al. Referral to an extracorporeal membrane oxygenation center and mortality among patients with severe 2009 influenza a (H1N1). JAMA. 2011;**306**:1659-1668

[9] Munshi L, Telesnicki T, Walkey A, et al. Extracorporeal life support for acute respiratory failure a systematic review and metaanalysis. Annals of the American Thoracic Society. 2014;**11**:802-810

[10] Takauji S, Hayakawa M, Ono K, Makise H. Respiratory extracorporeal membrane oxygenation for severe sepsis and septic shock in adults: A propensity score analysis in a multicenter retrospective observational study. Acute Medicine & Surgery. 2017;**4**:408-417

[11] Hayakawa M, Kudo D, Saito S, et al. Recombinant human soluble thrombomodulin and mortality in sepsis-induced disseminated intravascular coagulation. A multicenter retrospective study. Thrombosis and Haemostasis. 2016;**115**:1157-1166

[12] Nesseler N, Launey Y, Isslame S, et al. Is extracorporeal membrane oxygenation for severe acute respiratory distress syndrome related to intra-abdominal sepsis beneficial? Intensive Care Medicine. 2015;**41**(5):943

[13] Park TK, Yang JH, Jon K, et al. Extracorporeal membrane oxygenation for refractory septic shock in adults. European Journal of Cardio-Thoracic Surgery. 2015;**47**:e68-e74

[14] Court O, Kumar A, Parrillo JE, Kumar A. Clinical review: Myocardial depression in sepsis and septic shock. Critical Care. 2002;**6**:500-508

[15] Maclaren G, Butt W. Extracorporeal membrane oxygenation and sepsis. Critical Care and Resuscitation. 2007;**9**:76-80

[16] Brechot N, Luyt CE, Schmidt M, et al. Venoarterial extracorporeal membrane oxygenation support for refractory cardiovascular dysfunction during severe bacterial septic shock. Critical Care Medicine. 2013;**41**:1616-1626

[17] Huang CT, Tsai YJ, Tsai PR, Ko WJ. Extracorporeal membrane oxygenation resuscitation in adult patients with refractory septic shock. The Journal of Thoracic and Cardiovascular Surgery. 2013;**146**:1041-1046

[18] Say L, Chou D, Gemmill A, et al. Global causes of maternal death: A WHO systematic analysis. The Lancet Global Health. 2014;**2**:e323-e333

[19] Acosta CD, Kurinczuk JJ, Lucas DN, et al. Severe maternal sepsis in the UK, 2011-2012: A national case-control study. PLoS Medicine. 2014;**370**:2211-2218

[20] Sharma NS, Wille KM, Bellot SC, et al. Modern use of extracorporeal life support in pregnancy and postpartum. ASAIO Journal. 2015;**61**:110-114

[21] Imaeda T, Nakada T, Abe R, Tateishi Y, Oda S. Ven-arterial extracorporeal membrane oxygenation for streptococcus pyogenes toxic shock syndrome in pregnancy. Journal of Artificial Organs. 2016;**19**:200-203

[22] Perdue SM, Poore BJ, Babu AN, Stribling WK. Successful use of extracorporeal membrane oxygenation support in severe septic shock with associated acute cardiomyopathy. Journal of Cardiac Surgery. 2018;**33**:50-52

[23] Benetis R, Nadisauskiene R, Sirvinskas E, et al. Successfully treated severe obstetric sepsis and acute respiratory distress syndrome with extracorporeal membrane oxygenation. Perfusion. 2016;**31**(4):343-346

[24] Lee KW, Cho CW, et al. Extracorporeal membrane oxygenation support for refractory septic shock in liver tranplantation recipients. Annals of Surgical Treatment Research. 2017;**93**(3):152-158

[25] Park JI, Jung BH, Lee SG. Veno-arterial-venous hybrid mode of extracorporeal membrane oxygenation for acute respiratory distress syndrome combined with septic shock in a liver transplant patient: A case report. Transplantation Proceedings. 2017 Jun; **49**(5):1192-1195

[26] Baeka JK, Leaa JS, Kima TH, et al. Four-year experience with extracorporeal membrane oxygenation for kidney transplant patients with severe refractory cardiopulmonary insufficiency. Transplantation Proceedings. 2016;**48**:2080-2083

[27] Park YH, Hwang S, Park HW, et al. Effect of pulmonary support using extracorporeal membrane oxygenation for adult liver transplant recipients with respiratory failure. Transplantation Proceedings. 2012;**44**:757-761

[28] Ye QF, Zhao J, Wan QQ, et al. Frequency and clinical outcomes of ESKAPE bacteremia in solid organ transplantation and the risk factors for mortality. Transplant Infectious Disease. 2014;**16**:767-774

[29] Rambaud J, Guellec I, Léger PL, Renolieau S, Guilbert J. Venoarterial extracorporeal membrane oxygenation support for neonatal and pediatric refractory septic shock. Indian Journal of Critical Care Medicine. 2015;**19**(10):600-605

[30] Bartlett RH. Extracorporeal support for septic shock. Pediatric Critical Care Medicine. 2007;**8**:498-499

[31] Maclaren G, Butt W, Best D, Donath S, Taylor A. Extracorporeal membrane oxygenation for refractory septic shock in children : One institution's experience. Pediatric Critical Care Medicine. 2007;**8**:447-451

[32] Abe M, Ide K, Nishimura N et al. Successful venoarterial extracorporeal membrane oxygenation for postoperative septic shock in a child with liver transplantation : A case report. Pediatric Transplantation. 2017;**21**(8): doi: 10.1111/petr.13063. Epub 2017 Sep 12

[33] Leruste A, Rambaud J, Picard C, et al. Successful pediatric ECMO in a rare case of septic shock due to a community-acquired legionella infection. Médecine et Maladies Infectieuses. 2017;**47**:68-70

[34] Chang TH, Wu ET, Lu CY, et al. Pathogens and outcomes in pediatric septic shock patients supported by extracorporeal membrane oxygenation. Journal of Microbiology, Immunology, and Infection. 2017;**4**:S1684-S1182

[35] Wong G, Brinkman A, Benefield RJ, et al. An international, multicenter survey of B-lactam antibiotic therapeutic drug monitoring practice in intensive care units. The Journal of Antimicrobial Chemotherapy. 2014;**69**:1416-1423

[36] Economou CJ, Wong G, McWhinney B, et al. Impact of B-lactam antibiotic therapeutic drug monitoring on dose adjustments in critically ill patients undergoing continuous renal replacement therapy. International Journal of Antimicrobial Agents. 2017; **49**:589-594

[37] Shekar K, Fraser JF, Taccone FS, et al. The combined effects of extracorporeal membrane oxygenation and renal replacement therapy on meropenem pharmacokinetics : A matched cohort study. Critical Care. 2014;**18**:565-573

[38] Cies JJ, Moore WS, Dickerman MJ, et al. Pharmacokinetics of continuous-infusion meropenem in a pediatric patient receiving extracorporeal life support. Pharmacotherapy. 2014;**34**:e175-e179

[39] Donadello K, Antonucci E, Cristallini S, et al. Beta-lactam pharmacokinetics during extracorporeal membrane oxygenation therapy : A case-control study. International Journal of Antimicrobial Agents. 2015;**45**:278-282

[40] Koch BC, Wildschut ED, de Goede AL, de Hoog M, Brüggemann RJ. Insufficient serum caspofungin levels in a paediatric patient on ECMO. Medical Mycology Case Reports. 2013;**2**:23-24

[41] Lees NJ, Rosenberg AJ, Hurtado-Doce AI et al. Combination of ECMO and cytokine adsorption therapy for severe sepsis with cardiogenic shock and ARDS due to Panton-valentine leukocidin-positive *Staphylococcus aureus* pneumonia and H1N. Journal of Artificial Organs. 2016;**19**:399-402

[42] Bruenger F, Kizner L, Weile J, Morshuis M, Gummert JF. First successful combination of ECMO with cytokine removal therapy in cardiogenic septic shock: A case report. The International Journal of Artificial Organs. 2015;**38**:113-116

[43] Bracht H, Schneider EM, Weiss M, Hohmann H, Georgieff M, Barth E. Pattern of cytokine removal using an adsorption column Cytosorb during severe candida albicans induced septic shock. Infection. 2013;**41**:S1-S9

[44] Morris C, Gray L, Giovannelli M. Early report: The use of Cytosorb haemoabsorption column as an adjunct in managing severe sepsis: Initial experiences, review and recommendation. Journal of the Intensive Care Society. 2015;**16**:257-264

[45] Nakada TA, Oda S, Matsuda K, et al. Continuous hemodiafiltration with PMMA hemofilter in the treatment of patients with septic shock. Molecular Medicine. 2008;**14**:257-263

[46] Song M, Winchester J, Albright RL, et al. Cytokine removal with a novel adsorbent polymer. Blood Purification. 2004;**22**:428-434

[47] Choi MJ, Ha SO, Kim HS, et al. The simplified acute physiology score II as a predictor of mortality in patients who underwent extracorporeal membrane oxygenation for septic shock. The Annals of Thoracic Surgery. 2017;**103**:1246-1253

[48] Cheng A, Sun HY, Tsai MS, et al. Predictors of survival in adults undergoing extracorporeal membrane oxygenation with severe infections. The Journal of Thoracic and Cardiovascular Surgery. 2016 Dec;**152**:1526-1536

[49] Cheng A, Sun HY, Lee CW, et al. Survival of septic adults compared with no septic adults receiving extracorporeal membrane oxygenation for cardiopulmonary failure: A propensity-matched analysis. Journal of Critical Care. 2013;**28**:532 e1-532 10

Section 2

Technology

Chapter 10

Education Curriculum on Extracorporeal Membrane Oxygenation: The Evolving Role of Simulation Training

Simon Sin Wai Ching, Pauline Yeung Ng,
Wallace Ngai Chun Wai, Peter Lai Chi Keung,
Ricky Chan Wai Kit and Andy Mok Yuen Tin

Additional information is available at the end of the chapter

http://dx.doi.org/10.5772/intechopen.76656

Abstract

Continuing education is essential for the success and safety of an extracorporeal membrane oxygenation (ECMO) programme. However, it is challenging due to the intrinsic characteristic of ECMO—a complex, high-risk, low-volume clinical activity which require teamwork, inter-professional communication, critical decision and rapid response especially in emergency. Thus, simulation is a rapidly evolving teaching methodology in ECMO education to address those training needs that cannot be entirely addressed by traditional teaching modalities. The development of a simulation programme requires commitment on resources for equipment, environment setup and training of personnel. Knowledge on ECMO management, education science and debriefing technique forms the cornerstone of successful ECMO simulation facilitators and hence the simulation programme. Currently, researches have already shown that ECMO simulation can improve individual and team performance despite that its impact on patient outcome is still unknown. In the future, the role of simulation will increase importantly in multicentre research, certifying specialists and credentialing if standardization of training curriculum can be achieved.

Keywords: extracorporeal membrane oxygenation, human learning, high-fidelity simulation, debriefing, credentialing

1. Introduction

Extracorporeal membrane oxygenation (ECMO) is well known to be a highly complex but low-volume clinical activity. Complications may arise at many stages of ECMO care—from cannulation to during the ECMO run, to weaning and decannulation. Most complications are low occurrence but potentially life-threatening events. As a result, continuing education is essential to ensure the success and safety of an ECMO programme. Due to the inherent characteristics of ECMO service provision, the implementation of such educational activities is not straightforward. Firstly, professionals who undergo training for ECMO are usually experienced health-care providers. The learning processes of experienced adults are more complex, requiring assimilation of newly acquired knowledge with past experiences and roles. In these instances, learning will be more effective when the teaching is learner-centred and the learner is actively engaged. Secondly, the low-volume nature of severe ECMO complications renders training by apprenticeship difficult. Thirdly, while most ECMO runs are uneventful, in situation when crises occur, ECMO care providers have to respond emergently and proficiently under a stressful environment and often in a team-based approach. Fourthly, the provision of ECMO care often requires critical decision-making across specialties and professions.

Traditional ECMO teaching modalities like reading, didactic lectures, water drills (referring to deliberate practice in a closed-loop ECMO circuit model, e.g. changing the oxygenator or using the hand crank) and practices in the animal laboratory (where a living animal is cannulated to simulate human responses) primarily focus on cognitive and technical skills, with little emphasis on behavioural skills like communication and leadership that are fundamental during training for ECMO. ECMO simulation has rapidly evolved as an effective learning methodology that supplements traditional teaching modalities. It creates a standardized, controlled, safe and repeatable environment that aims to mimic the realistic clinical environments, so that new skills can be learnt and practised without doing harm to patients and learners.

In this chapter, we discuss simulation training in ECMO from the perspectives of human learning theory, simulation programme setup (including scenario design, equipment and resources), debriefing, current evidence and future challenges.

2. Human learning models and simulation-based education

Simulation is often considered simply as an exercise where learners perform actions in an environment simulated to resemble reality, and facilitators are present to ensure its smooth running and to lead a discussion afterwards. As a relatively new method of teaching in medical education, there are often misunderstandings about simulation training and inadequate knowledge of its execution. High-quality simulation is backed by evidence-based educational theories and includes purposefully designed scenarios and well-trained facilitators.

Kolb's theory on experiential learning forms the foundation of simulation-based education. In his theory, learners enter the learning cycle through experiencing an event—either a real patient experience or simulated activities ('concrete experience'). Afterwards, through self-reflection or reflection assisted by facilitator ('reflection'), a new insight of the event is created ('abstract conceptualization'). Finally, this new insight is applied in a similar simulated or real-life event ('active experimentation') [1].

Neil Flemming's VARK model describes four modalities in an individual's preferred method of learning—Visual, Auditory, Reading and Kinesthetic [2]. Different individuals learn more effectively when they receive specific types of stimulation. Simulation, through active engagement with hands-on action, produces better training effect in kinesthetic learners.

Simulation experiences can trigger learner emotions and it is known that a highly activated core affect can positively influence the uptake and retention of knowledge and skills. The Change Theory proposed by Lewin/Schein highlights the relationship between affect and learning. It theorized a three-stage model of change, namely unfreezing, transition and refreezing. 'Unfreezing' refers to the motivation to change by adding new force or removing existing concepts that are influencing behaviour. It unavoidably leads to emotional stress, largely a sense of dissatisfaction with oneself as a result of disconfirmation of the present condition. Moreover, it creates a survival anxiety as the pre-existing belief is rejected and a learning anxiety in which the previously learnt knowledge has to be unlearnt. 'Unfreezing' is followed by 'transition', a process of moving onto a new state, which requires reconstruction of one's thoughts, feelings and behaviours. 'Refreezing' is the final stage in which the newly acquired knowledge, concepts and behaviours are adopted and assimilated [3].

The principles underlying simulation scenario design, together with the debriefing process, are largely developed based on one of these educational theories. Simulation training aims to facilitate acquisition of knowledge and skills and to change one's perceptions and behaviour. The following sections further elaborate on scenario design and debriefing in ECMO simulation.

3. Scenario design in ECMO simulation

Scenario design is one of the key elements in simulation education. On designing a scenario, thorough understanding of the background, training needs and experience of learners is essential. In particular, meticulous attention must be paid to tailor the learning goals and objectives to the target learner. The goal of a scenario refers to the overall educational mission the learners are expected to achieve. Detailed objectives may be made up of cognitive, psychomotor, behavioural or affective component [4]. As an example, the goals and objectives for novice ECMO learners would be different from experienced ECMO learners in a scenario of ECMO blood pump failure. For the novice, the goal would be 'to switch to a standby machine in emergency setting', with objectives including 'recognize blood pump failure and its related physiological changes' (cognitive) and 'acquire the technical skill of using hand crank' (psychomotor). For the experienced learner, the goal may be more advanced, such as 'demonstration of teamwork in managing blood pump failure crisis', achieved through the objective of 'demonstrating effective communication and leadership skills' (behavioural), in addition to the cognitive and psychomotor skills. **Table 1** lists examples of common scenarios used in an Asia-Pacific ELSO Adult ECMO Training Course and **Table 2** illustrates the goals and objectives of some of these scenarios.

Some deviation of simulation scenarios from the real-world practice is acceptable. Especially for novice ECMO learners, they are expected to adopt the role of the ECMO specialist during simulation learning, regardless of their current position as senior consultants, junior doctors, nurses or perfusionists. This is to ensure competency in the various aspects of troubleshooting and response to ECMO emergencies after they undergo training. This training concept reflects the reality that

Scenario Topic	Examples
Routine ECMO circuit management	External compression on return tubing
	Heater failure with hypothermia
	Oxygenator failure
Emergencies in ECMO care	Blood pump failure
	Oxygen supply failure
	Circuit air embolism
Patient management	Venous insufficiency
	Recirculation
	Permissive hypoxaemia in VV ECMO
	Tension pneumothorax
	Ventricular fibrillation in VA ECMO
	Differential hypoxaemia in VA ECMO

Table 1. Examples of scenarios in adult ECMO simulation training (adopted from Asia-Pacific ELSO Adult ECMO Training Course, Queen Mary Hospital).

Scenarios	Goals and learning objectives
External compression on return tubing	Goal:
	Understand the change in circuit pressure related to preload and afterload conditions.
	Objectives:
	(C) Recognize high return pressure with drop in ECMO blood flow signifying post-pump obstruction.
	(P) Systematic circuit check.
Oxygenator failure	Goal:
	Diagnosis of oxygenator failure.
	Objectives:
	(C) Recognize features of oxygenator failure – elevated transmembrane pressure, decrease oxygenator function, clot in oxygenator, disseminated intravascular coagulopathy blood picture.
	(P) Circuit check for clot in oxygenator.
Blood pump failure	Goal:
	Management of blood pump failure.
	Objectives:
	(C) Recognize presentation of blood pump failure—loss of ECMO blood flow, change of patient's hemodynamic and physiological parameters.
	(P) Technique of using hand crank.
	(B) Communication to call for help for resuscitation and patient stabilization.

Scenarios	Goals and learning objectives
Oxygen supply failure	Goal:
	Understand the importance of complete circuit check in ECMO emergency.
	Objectives:
	(C) Recognize patient desaturation, loss of color difference in ECMO limbs.
	(P) Systematic circuit check and potential sites of oxygenation supply disconnection.
Circuit air entrainment	Goal:
	Diagnose and manage circuit air entrainment.
	Objectives:
	(C) Recognize presentation of circuit air entrainment—abnormal noise from ECMO circuit, decrease ECMO blood flow with corresponding change in patient's hemodynamic and physiological parameters.
	(C) Recognize potential source of air entrainment—negative pressure side.
	(P) Complete circuit check to identify source of air and stop further entrainment. Technical skill for circuit de-airing or technical skill to change to new circuit.
	(B) Teamwork and communication skills during circuit de-airing, changing ECMO circuit, and patient resuscitation.
Venous insufficiency	Goal:
	Understand the cause of venous insufficiency and its management.
	Objectives:
	(C) Recognize presentation of venous insufficiency—drainage limb chattering, more negative venous pressure, decrease ECMO blood flow.
	(C) Recognize the cause of venous insufficiency—hypovolaemia, excessive pump speed, inappropriate drainage catheter position; and their respective management.
Recirculation	Goal:
	Understand the physiology of recirculation and its management.
	Objectives:
	(C) Recognize the presentation of recirculation—desaturation without problems in ECMO blood flow and oxygen supply, loss of color differential in drainage and return limb, elevated SvO2.
	(C) Recognize the causes of recirculation—close proximity of drainage and return cannula, excessive pump speed.

Table 2. Examples of goals and learning objectives of common ECMO simulation scenarios (C = cognitive, P = psychomotor, B = behavioural) (adopted from Asia-Pacific ELSO Adult ECMO Training Course, Queen Mary Hospital).

many ECMO centres nowadays adopt a mixed ECMO care model, with the ECMO team consisting of physicians, nurses, perfusionists and respiratory therapists [5, 6]. The other advantage of including mixed roles in simulation is the possibility of modifying the focus of training as the team matures, to aspects such as leadership, communication and teamwork during emergencies.

Furthermore, simulation scenarios can be adjusted according to the characteristics of the respective ECMO team and health-care institution. The scenario design for institutions using a bedside nurse ECMO care model will be different from that using a perfusionist care model.

By fine-tuning the expected roles of participants, flexibility in meeting the training needs of individual centres can be met, although possibly at the expense of lack of standardization and generalizability across centres.

4. Setup of a high-fidelity and immersive simulation

High-fidelity simulation usually involves full-body manikins set up in environments made to simulate real-life situations. The presentation of changing patient physiology data and machine or physiological parameter alarms is used to mimic realistic health-care settings and elicits desired responses from learners. This is in contrast to water drills, considered low-fidelity simulation, which runs in the form of deliberate practice in a static and alarm-free environment. High-fidelity simulation is an immersive experience for the participant and offers the opportunity to introduce knowledge through challenging and reflecting upon learners' individual responses. It is also a useful tool to introduce concepts related to team-based care.

4.1. Simulation environment

A variety of clinical environments involving ECMO care may be simulated, for example, ICU, operating theatre and emergency room. In institutions without dedicated simulation facilities, one can consider setting up the simulation model in an unoccupied cubicle in the ICU or the emergency room to achieve contextual reality.

Typical equipment for veno-venous ECMO simulation will include an intubated manikin (e.g. megacode Kelly) attached to a mechanical ventilator. Arterial lines, drug infusion devices and Foley catheters may be added as necessary. Essential physiological parameters, for example, arterial blood pressure, pulse rate, ECG rhythm, SpO2 and central venous pressure should be clearly displayed (**Figure 1**), and these should be controlled remotely by a compatible computer programme (e.g. Laerdal SimMan).

4.2. Manikin modification and incorporation of an ECMO circuit

A commonly used method in ECMO simulation is to connect the access and return cannulae of the ECMO circuit to a volume reservoir hidden inside the manikin (**Figure 2**, left upper panel). Access ports on the volume reservoir are mandatory (**Figure 2**, left lower panel) to allow manipulation of volume and hence pressure status within the ECMO circuit in different simulation scenarios. For example, access insufficiency is simulated by withdrawal of fluid from the reservoir, causing collapse of the reservoir, a decreased ECMO flow, and a negative access pressure. Circuit air entrainment may be simulated by the controlled introduction of air into the circuit. Additional modification may be required for the display of pressure changes, depending on the ECMO machine used—the Medos Deltastream and Maquet Cardiohelp systems display the operating pressures directly on the screen of the ECMO consoles, whereas older ECMO systems like the Maquet Rotaflow require connection of pressure transducers to different parts of the ECMO circuit (**Figure 2**, right panel). Lansdowne et al.

http://dx.doi.org/10.5772/intechopen.76656

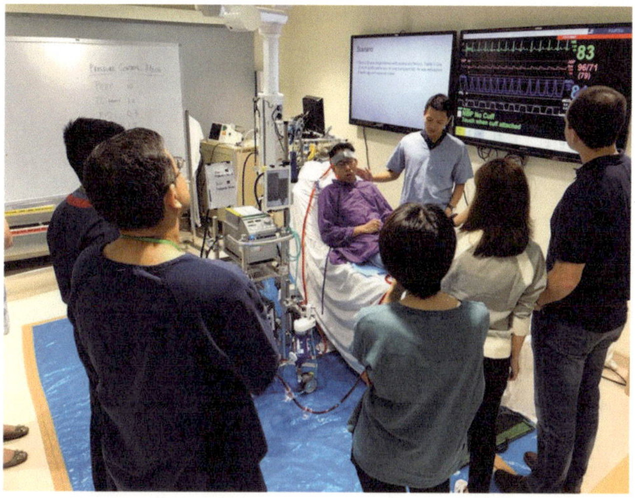

Figure 1. Basic setup of a high-fidelity ECMO simulation environment. A confederate (dressed in blue scrubs) participated in this scenario (adopted from Asia-Pacific Adult ECMO Course, Queen Mary Hospital).

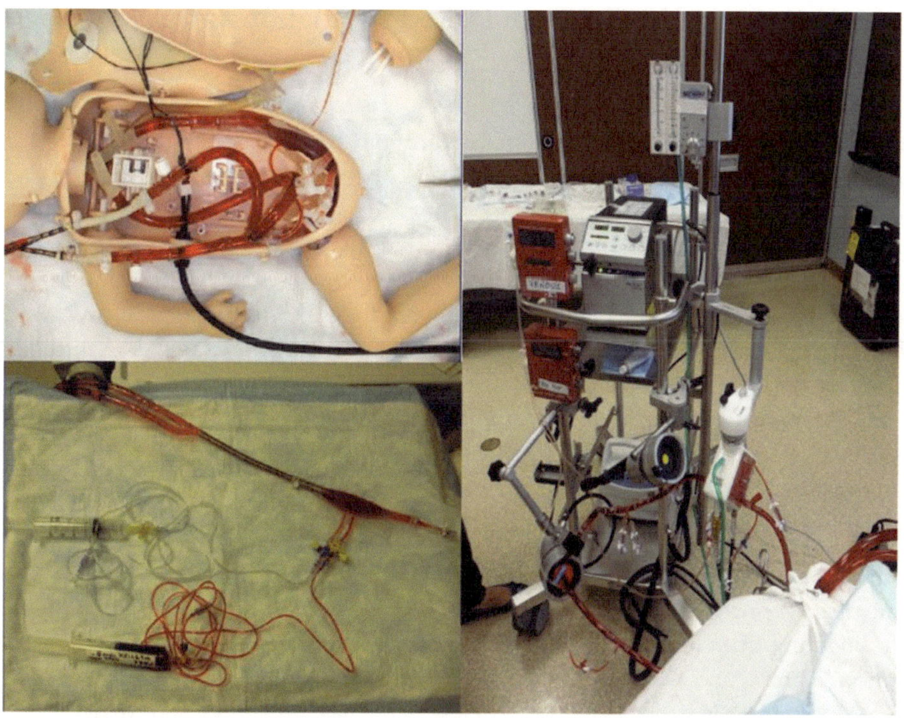

Figure 2. Left upper and lower panels—hidden volume reservoir and tubings inside a pediatric manikin; and the setup of a volume reservoir (photos courtesy of Dr. Mark Ogino). Right panel—ECMO circuit setup with additional pressure transducers (in red) for circuit pressure display.

described a model that incorporates a modified manikin, an ECMO circuit and the hydraulic module of the Orpheus Perfusion Simulator to produce a realistic simulation [7].

4.3. Limitations

A major limitation in ECMO simulation is the cost of medical devices and ECMO consumables. The abovementioned simulation models all require a functioning ECMO machine and a complete ECMO circuit, including the oxygenator, that are subject to wear and tear. The availability of equipment and the costs of replacement are real economical concerns, especially for newly developed centres. The advent of 3-D printing technologies may hold promise for the construct of economical oxygenators [8].

Other limitations arise from the technological parts of the simulation. For instance, it is difficult to simulate the difference in colour of oxygenated and deoxygenated blood, which is important in scenarios related to recirculation and oxygen supply failure. Other technical difficulties include simulating blood clots in the oxygenator and access line chattering. Ongoing research to overcome these challenges is underway, such as the use of thermochromic fluid to simulate colour changes of the circuit blood [8].

5. Special role of the facilitator in ECMO simulation and the debriefing process

The important role of facilitators in simulation education cannot be underscored. Firstly, facilitators should have a thorough understanding of ECMO physiology, patient physiology and their interaction. This forms the prerequisite for facilitators to react swiftly and accurately in real time according to the actions of learners, by manipulating the ECMO flow and pressure (through volume manipulation of the reservoir) and the physiological parameters (through the computer software). For example, when learners increase the ECMO pump speed excessively, the facilitator should make a series of changes to the circuit and patient parameters, which includes withdrawing volume from the reservoir to create a state of venous insufficiency, dropping the SpO2 and SvO2, creating mild tachycardia, and so on. More importantly, during the simulation exercise, facilitators have to denote key actions and behaviours that will be valuable for discussion in the subsequent debriefing session. As a result of the many roles and actions required of facilitators in ECMO simulation, most scenarios require the presence of at least two facilitators.

The other role of the facilitator is the debriefer. Debriefing, the reflective process in Kolb's learning theory provides an opportunity for learners to reflect upon their performance, resolve lingering questions and reinforce learning objectives. It is the most crucial part of simulation learning and was described as the 'heart and soul' of the simulation experience. The aim of debriefing is to constructively review 'what has happened' and 'why it happened' in the simulated event. In the 'frame-action-result' model described by Rudolph, learners have their own 'frames'—their assumption, knowledge and feelings that drive their 'actions', which in turn end up with different 'results' [9]. While actions and results are easily observable, frames are often invisible. A successful debriefer needs to act as a 'cognitive detector', to uncover the 'frame of mind' of the learners and to help them gain better insight of their own frames, so that behavioural change may follow.

The detailed techniques to achieve an effective debriefing are out of the scope of this chapter. Nonetheless, it is worthwhile to mention some of the main principles. As a rule of thumb, confidentiality with regard to learners' performance should be strictly complied, so that they feel safe to express themselves, especially after difficult, stressful, or poorly performed scenarios.

Mutual respect and trust among learners and debriefers are essential to encourage free communication. Debriefers should positively acknowledge the contribution and motivation of the learners. Even when faced with an apparently 'poor' performance, debriefers should remain curious and explore the reasons behind the behaviour [10]. The 'advocacy-inquiry' conversation technique has been described to facilitate this process.

Simulation educators have developed frameworks to facilitate the debriefing process. Scholars from the Center for Medical Simulation at Harvard Medical School advocate a three-step model (reaction, understanding and summary), while those from the Winter Institute for Simulation Education and Research (WISER) of University of Pittsburgh use the 'gather, analyze, and summarize' (GAS) debriefing tool. Debriefers should familiarize themselves with different tools and adopt a systematic approach during debriefing.

Heading forward, efforts are underway to enhance the quality of debriefing by developing assessment tools. In The Debriefing Assessment for Simulation in Healthcare (DASH), the following aspects are considered the key elements of a good debriefer:

1. establishes an engaging learning environment;
2. maintains an engaging learning environment;
3. structures debriefing in an organized way;
4. provokes engaging discussions;
5. identifies and explores performance gaps; and
6. assists trainee achieve or sustain good future performance.

6. Current evidence and status of ECMO simulation

In a recent survey from the United States, lectures (99%), water drills (99%) and bedside training (99%) remain the chief training modalities for new ECMO specialists. Forty-six per cent of ECMO centres had an ECMO simulation programme. ECMO centres with access to a simulation centre, those with higher case numbers and pediatric cardiothoracic ICU are more likely to have an ECMO simulation programme [11].

Simulation-based ECMO education is a growing research area with increasing evidence to support its effectiveness. Earlier publications were mainly descriptive and focused on the setup and content of simulation courses and the evaluation of the learner [12, 13]. Some studies reported an improvement in confidence and performance after ECMO simulation training. Su et al. reported a faster deployment time to ECPR initiation after simulation training [14], and Allan et al. reported a decrease in cannulation time for ECPR in pediatric cardiac surgery trainees [15].

Recently, Zakhary et al. published the first randomized controlled trial comparing the performance after conventional water-drill training and simulation training. In this study, the simulation training group had a higher scenario score and a shorter time to critical action in certain scenarios. More importantly, this superior performance was sustained over 1 year [16]. However, it must be noted that despite the ongoing research and implementation of simulation training, there is yet evidence of association with better patient outcomes.

7. Challenge and future directions

Percutaneous cannulation for ECMO is increasingly performed by intensivists, cardiologists and emergency physicians. Despite infrequent occurrences, complications of cannulation may be associated with significant morbidity and mortality [17]. Existing simulation models mainly focus on ECMO circuit management, with less emphasis on percutaneous cannulation, and there are yet publications related to percutaneous cannulation model. Collaborative international endeavours targeted to improve cannulation safety are in progress. We have developed a simulation model for fluoroscopic-assisted dual-lumen cannulation (https://www.youtube.com/watch?v=dr02RAMRk1A) and two-cannula cannulation in veno-venous ECMO.

Despite the increasing use of simulation in many ECMO education programmes, the role of simulation remains unclear in currently available guidelines and international recommendations. The latest Extracorporeal Life Support Organization (ELSO) guideline on ECMO specialist training published in 2010 only included didactic lectures, water drills, animal laboratory sessions and bedside training as the main training modalities. Moreover, it only targeted 'ECMO specialists' (i.e. nurses, respiratory therapists, perfusionists and medical professions providing care under the guidance of ECMO physicians) and not ECMO physicians.

In a United States survey published in 2015, simulation has been adopted as part of the institutional ECMO credentialing programme for ECMO physicians in 73% of the centres, highlighting its increasing importance [18]. The EuroELSO guidelines for training and continuing education of ECMO physicians published in 2017 have incorporated high-fidelity simulation training as an alternative training modality to supplement bedside clinical hours. More importantly, its significance in teamwork and communication skills training has been acknowledged [19]. It is expected that the role of simulation will be further expanded in future versions of the ELSO guideline.

As mentioned earlier, ECMO training curriculum and thus simulation programmes are institutional specific and may be modified according to the characteristics and training needs of the institution. As a result, significant variances exist among different institutions, imposing difficulties in standardization and validation of the assessment tools. Currently, there are no validated assessment tools to assess the learning efficacy of common and essential ECMO scenarios. Joint efforts are ongoing among international ECMO educators to develop

http://dx.doi.org/10.5772/intechopen.76656

a standardized curriculum. Only through the implementation of a uniform ECMO simulation programme can multi-centred studies be carried out to provide a better understanding of the best approach in ECMO education.

8. Conclusion

ECMO is a low-volume but highly complex technology. The management of ECMO patients often requires an integration of cognitive, psychomotor and behavioural skills that can be addressed by simulation training. As a result, simulation is increasingly acknowledged as one of the essential learning tools in ECMO education. Further researches in simulation technology, medical science pedagogy and clinical trials are warranted to delineate its impact on patient outcomes.

Acknowledgements

The authors would like to acknowledge all the members of the ECMO team, Dr. Chan Wai Ming, the Chief of Service of the Department of Adult Intensive Care, Queen Mary Hospital, Dr. Mark Ogino, Director, Critical Care Services Nemours/Alfred I duPont Hospital for Children and Mr. Kenneth KY Yu, Department Operation Manager of the Department of Adult Intensive Care, Queen Mary Hospital, for their zealous support of the ECMO simulation programme.

Author details

Simon Sin Wai Ching[1,2]*, Pauline Yeung Ng[1], Wallace Ngai Chun Wai[1], Peter Lai Chi Keung[1], Ricky Chan Wai Kit[1] and Andy Mok Yuen Tin[1]

*Address all correspondence to: drwcsin@gmail.com

1 Department of Adult Intensive Care, Queen Mary Hospital, Hong Kong, China

2 Li Ka Shing Department of Medicine, The University of Hong Kong, Hong Kong, China

References

[1] Kolb DA. Experiential Learning: Experience as the Source of Learning and Development. Englewood Cliffs, NJ: Prentice Hall; 1984

[2] Fleming ND. The ADRK modalities. Available from: vark-learn.com [Accessed: March 17, 2018]

[3] Edgar S. Kurt Lewin's change theory in the field and in the classroom: Notes toward a model of managed learning. Systemic Practice and Action Research: 1996;**9**(1):27-47

[4] Johnston L, Williams SB, Ades A. Education for ECMO providers: Using education science to bridge the gap between clinical and educational expertise. Seminars in Perinatology. 2018;**42**(2):138-146

[5] Cavarocchi NC, Wallace S, Hong EY, Tropea A, Byrne J, Pitcher HT, et al. A cost-reducing extracorporeal membrane oxygenation (ECMO) program model: A single institution experience. Perfusion. 2015;**30**(2):148-153

[6] Daly KJ, Camporota L, Barrett NA. An international survey: The role of specialist nurses in adult respiratory extracorporeal membrane oxygenation. Nursing in Critical Care. 2017;**22**(5):305-311

[7] Lansdowne W, Machin D, Grant DJ. Development of the orpheus perfusion simulator for use in high-fidelity extracorporeal membrane oxygenation simulation. The Journal of Extra-Corporeal Technology. 2012;**44**(4):250-255

[8] Al Disi M, Alsalemi A, Alhomsi Y, Bensaali F, Amira A, Alinier G. Revolutionizing ECMO simulation with affordable yet high-Fidelity technology. The American Journal of Emergency Medicine. 2017

[9] Rudolph JW, Simon R, Raemer DB, Eppich WJ. Debriefing as formative assessment: Closing performance gaps in medical education. Academic Emergency Medicine. 2008;**15**(11):1010-1016

[10] Gardner R. Introduction to debriefing. Seminars in Perinatology. 2013;**37**(3):166-174

[11] Weems MF, Friedlich PS, Nelson LP, Rake AJ, Klee L, Stein JE, et al. The role of extracorporeal membrane oxygenation simulation training at extracorporeal life support organization centers in the United States. Simulation in Healthcare. 2017;**12**(4):233-239

[12] Endo T, Kagaya Y, Arata Y, Imai H. Long-term efficacy of an extracorporeal membrane oxygenation simulation with a novel, low-cost vascular model "endo-circuit". Acute Medicine & Surgery. 2017;**4**(1):79-88

[13] Thompson JL, Grisham LM, Scott J, Mogan C, Prescher H, Biffar D, et al. Construction of a reusable, high-fidelity model to enhance extracorporeal membrane oxygenation training through simulation. Advances in Neonatal Care. 2014;**14**(2):103-109

[14] Su L, Spaeder MC, Jones MB, Sinha P, Nath DS, Jain PN, et al. Implementation of an extracorporeal cardiopulmonary resuscitation simulation program reduces extracorporeal cardiopulmonary resuscitation times in real patients. Pediatric Critical Care Medicine. 2014;**15**(9):856-860

[15] Allan CK, Pigula F, Bacha EA, Emani S, Fynn-Thompson F, Thiagarajan RR, et al. An extracorporeal membrane oxygenation cannulation curriculum featuring a novel integrated skills trainer leads to improved performance among pediatric cardiac surgery trainees. Simulation in Healthcare. 2013;**8**(4):221-228

[16] Zakhary BM, Kam LM, Kaufman BS, Felner KJ. The utility of high-fidelity simulation for training critical care fellows in the management of extracorporeal membrane

oxygenation emergencies: A randomized controlled trial. Critical Care Medicine. 2017;**45**(8):1367-1373

[17] Conrad SA, Grier LR, Scott LK, Green R, Jordan M. Percutaneous cannulation for extracorporeal membrane oxygenation by intensivists: A retrospective single-institution case series. Critical Care Medicine. 2015;**43**(5):1010-1015

[18] Muratore S, Beilman G, John R, Brunsvold M. Extracorporeal membrane oxygenation credentialing: Where do we stand? The American Journal of Surgery. 2015;**210**(4):655-660; (e2)

[19] EuroELSO guideline for training and continuing education on ECMO physicians. Jan 2017. www.euroelso.net/PhysiciansGuidelines.pdf

Chapter 11

Holder System for External Pumps Positioned Remote from the CPB Console: 23 Years' Experience

Umberto Borrelli, Marc Detroux, Remi Nottin,
Stephane Nikis and Pierre Nakers

Additional information is available at the end of the chapter

http://dx.doi.org/10.5772/intechopen.77121

Abstract

Since 1995, our objective is to set up the extracorporeal circulation (ECC) in a manner that is both safe and versatile with a holder system which makes possible to install the oxygenator and vacuum-assisted venous drainage (VAVD) hard-shell venous reservoir (HSVR) together with the external pumps, at a distance from the cardiopulmonary bypass (CPB) console but at the same height as the patient's shoulder. The aim is to reduce the effects of ECC by reducing surface of air/blood, blood/materials contact, the dead space of the system and priming volume of the circuit. Our ECC systems have a biocompatible surface treatment, the oxygenator and HSVR are adapted to the patient (body surface area, pathologies, etc.) and circuit includes short 3/8 in arterial and venous line (adult patients). We introduced into routine VAVD, retrograde autologous priming (RAP), including arterial line, arterial filter and antegrade autologous priming of the venous line (VAP) before the start of ECC. To confirm this development strategy of the ECC, we conducted a series of studies that have permitted to demonstrate the positive impact on postoperative outcomes of patients. Since September 2007, our objective was attained through the creation of a holder system (System U. Borrelli).

Keywords: extracorporeal circulation, holder system, external pumps, reducing surface, vacuum-assisted venous drainage

1. Introduction

The extracorporeal circulation (ECC) is associated with a systemic inflammatory response (SIRS), with an activation of different biological pathways such as the coagulation and the fibrinolysis [1]. The ECC creates many hemostatic disturbances that may lead to major bleeding risks, and eventually to thrombotic, myocardial, renal or pulmonary complications and neurological dysfunctions [2–4]. During the last decade, several improvements have been made on the ECC used within cardiac surgery, especially with the arrival of many systems in the market, such as the mini-ECC and the optimised conventional ECC which are closer to the patient's physiology and having surface treatments capable of improving the hemocompatibility of ECC [5]. These new systems have allowed to reduce the aggressiveness of the ECC on the patients, allowing as a consequence a reduction of the SIRS and its negative effects on them; the final result is a decrease of morbidity and mortality of patients postoperatively.

2. Miniaturised conventional extracorporeal circulation system

In 1995, our project was to set up a new concept of a miniaturised conventional extracorporeal circulation (McECC) system that is both safe and versatile, which allows to reduce to the maximum console and the circuit of the ECC. A brand-new console of CPB with a holder system that permits the installation of oxygenator and HSVR at the height of the patient's shoulder, together with the five external pumps (**Figures 1** and **2**).

When I realise the drawing of **Figure 1**, the CPB console of that type did not exist yet, and it was absolutely unthinkable and impossible to place the holder system on the CPB consoles which would have been launched on the market in 1995. For this reason, we put the project regarding the holder system on hold.

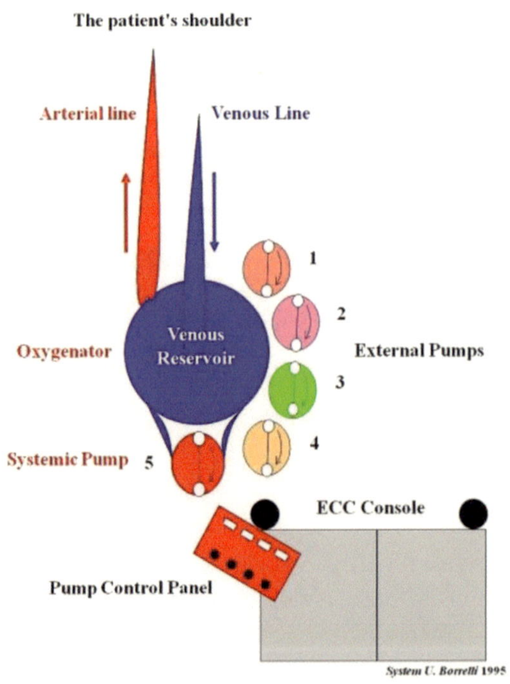

Figure 1. Top view.

http://dx.doi.org/10.5772/intechopen.77121

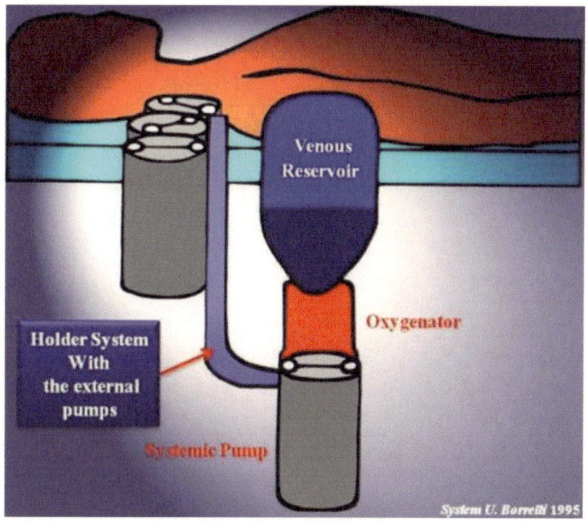

Figure 2. Profile view.

2.1. Study on the ECC surface reduction

In order to be able to confirm the hypothesis stating that the decrease of the ECC system can enhance the postoperative period on patients that have undergone a cardiac surgery, in 1997 we asked the technician of the society (Stöckert®, Müchen, Germany) to carry out some modifications on our CPB console "CAPS "of that time (**Figures 3** and **4**). This action has allowed the positioning of the systemic pump near the oxygenator, and the introduction of a set consisted of the console, oxygenator and the HSVR as close as possible to the patient.

The outcome has been a drastic reduction of the length of the lines, dead space and the ECC priming volume. We gave it the name of "Compact ECC" (**Figures 3** and **4**). Regarding the" Compact ECC", we have conducted many studies and research that we have published [6, 7].

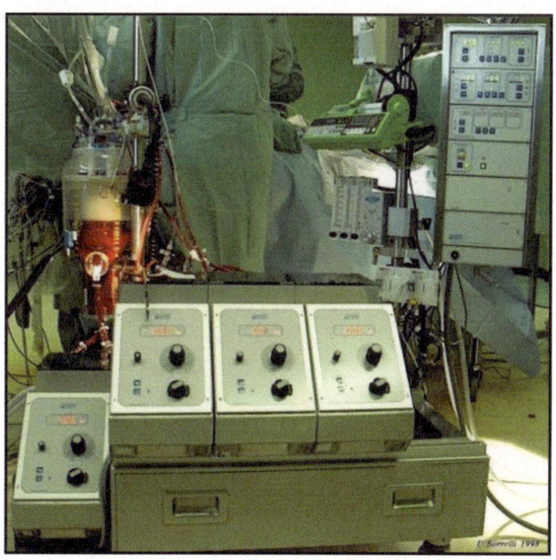

Figure 3. Modified CPB "CAPS"console 1998.

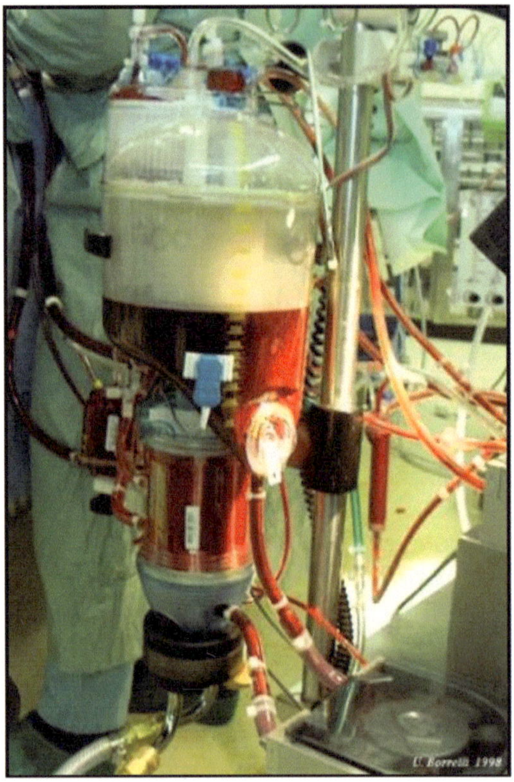

Figure 4. Systemic pump near the oxygenator.

In summary, this study has been conducted on three groups of patients which have undergone a coronary artery bypass grafting (CABG), from 1999 to 2004. A total of 50 patients have been analysed for the first group, from 1999 to 2001, and 25 patients in 2001 for the second group, and 25 patients for the third group from 2003 to 2004.

A significant difference among the groups concerning the patient's age, the Parsonnet score, the number of anastomoses performed, the haemoglobin before ECC, the ECC time and the systemic flow of the ECC have not been found. The systemic flow (L/min) has been measured using a flow index of 2.4 $l/min/m^2$ for each group.

All groups were operated with an open circuit McECC. We have reduced from group [1] up to group [3] the surface of air/blood contact, blood/materials contact, the dead space of the system and the priming.

After the distribution of the new systems (oxygenator and HSVR) and knowing that the surface of contact of oxygenators is the most important of the ECC circuit set, the reduction of the membrane surface area of the oxygenator adapted to the patient (e.g., body surface area, pathologies, etc.) from the group [1] up to the group [3] has been fundamental (**Figure 5**).

For each group, we have used the oxygenator, HSVR and the ECC circuit of the same company (Dideco®, Mirandola, Italy).

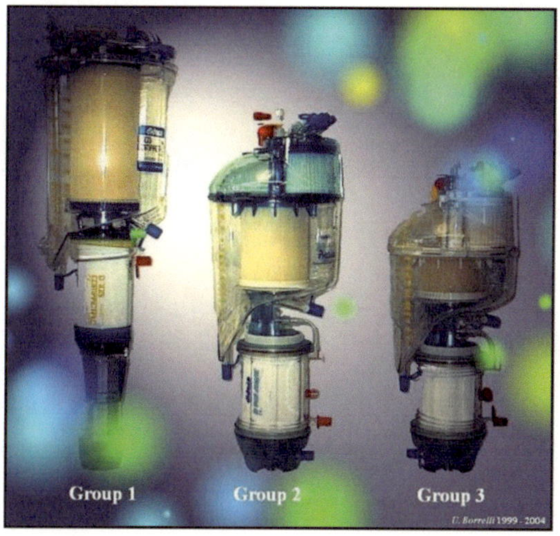

Figure 5. Group [1] oxygenator Compact Flow D703; group [2] oxygenator Avant D903; group [3] oxygenator Eos D905 and compatible HSVR with VAVD (Dideco®, Mirandola, Italy).

We introduced into routine retrograde autologous priming (RAP), including arterial line, arterial filter and antegrade autologous priming of the venous line (VAP) before the start of CPB. This action has allowed a precise control of the hemodilution of patients.

In interventions like CABG, during the aortic cross-clamping (closed-heart surgery), discharge of the left heart by aortic root vent is performed for the group [1–2] by gravity and for the group [3] by vacuum-assisted venous drainage (VAVD); the depression exerted in the aortic root is equal to that applied in the venous reservoir by the VAVD system (**Figures 6** and **7**).

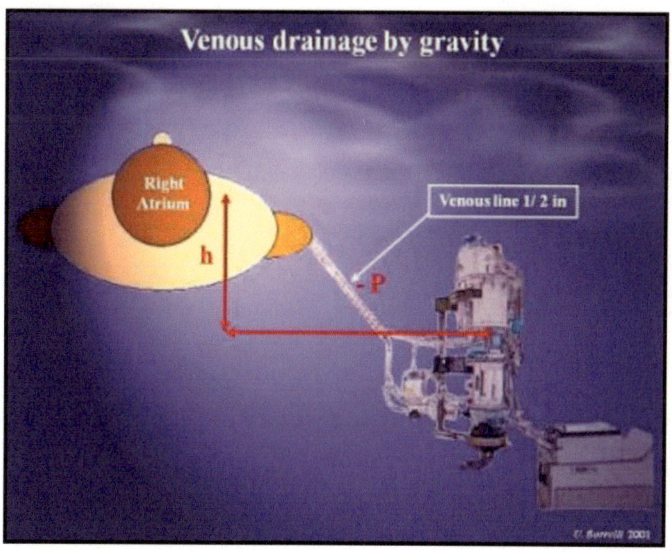

Figure 6. Group [1] and group [2].

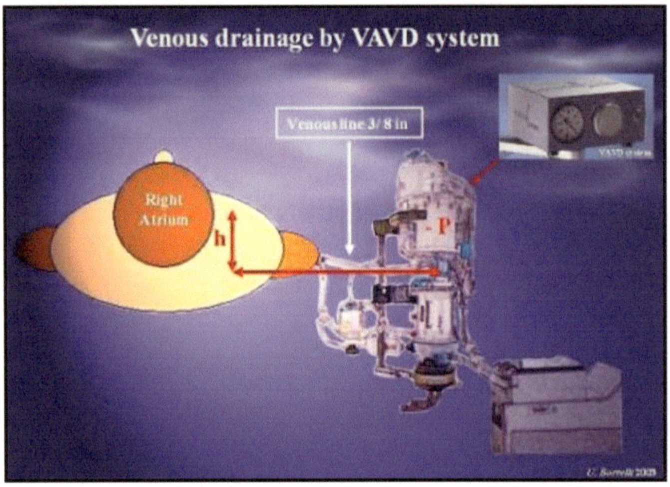

Figure 7. Group [3].

In all three groups, ECC was conducted under normothermia with warm intermittent blood cardioplegia based on potassium and magnesium. In order to verify the quality of our cardioplegia protocol, we have realised a series of studies in which one of these has been published in 2003 with the title *Comparison of the troponin i levels during coronary artery bypass graft in cardiac surgery procedures, realised with and without extracorporeal circulation* [8].

The auto transfusion system Electa (Dideco®, Mirandola, Italy) was employed for all the three groups. The volume of red blood cell concentrate re-injected for the three groups at the end of surgery did not exceed 320 ml. In order to optimise the management of the auto transfusion system, in 1998 we realised a study: *Improving the quality of red blood cells recovered with the Stat, perioperative autotransfusion system: Study of residues* [9].

2.1.1. Group [1]

- The ECC was performed with an oxygenator Compact Flow D703 (Dideco®, Mirandola, Italy)
- Membrane surface area of the oxygenator 2 m^2
- Maximum blood flow rate of the oxygenator 7 l/min
- Flow index: 2.4 $l/min/m^2$
- Mean systemic flow of ECC 4.5 l/min
- Drainage by gravity and venous line ½ in
- Arterial line 3/8 in
- Residual priming or hemodilution of the patient at the start of ECC = 900 ml
- Level detector on the venous reservoir

2.1.2. Group [2]

- The ECC was performed with an oxygenator Avant D903 (Dideco®, Mirandola, Italy)
- Membrane surface area of the oxygenator 1.7 m^2
- Maximum blood flow rate of the oxygenator 7.5 l/min
- Flow index: 2.4 l/min/m^2
- Mean systemic flow of ECC 4.4 l/min
- Drainage by gravity and venous line ½ in
- Arterial line 3/8 in
- Residual priming or hemodilution of the patient at the start of ECC = 500 ml
- Level detector on the venous reservoir
- Surface coating" Phosphorylcholine"(Dideco®, Mirandola, Italy)

2.1.3. Group [3]

We have positioned the set of oxygenator and compatible HSVR with VAVD as close as possible to the patient's shoulder, replacing the gravity venous drainage with a ½ in vein line through a 3/8 in vein line and routinely introduced the vacuum-assisted venous drainage, VAVD, system (Maquet® Cardiopulmonary GmbH, Germany) (**Figures 6** and **7**).

The ECC was performed with an oxygenator EOS D905 (Dideco®, Mirandola, Italy)

- Membrane surface area of the oxygenator 1.1 m^2
- Maximum blood flow rate of the oxygenator 5 l/min
- Flow index: 2.4 l/min/m^2
- Mean systemic flow of ECC 4.3 l/min
- VAVD system with the arterial/venous line 3/8 in and the HSVR
- Residual priming or hemodilution of the patient at the start of ECC = 250 ml
- Level detector on the HSVR
- Surface coating" Phosphorylcholine"(Dideco®, Mirandola, Italy) (**Figures 3–5**)

The result of this study shows a reduction of postoperative ventilation time from the group [1] to group [3] (mean 508 ± 325 vs. 194.6 ± 39.2 min), blood loss (mean 489.2 ± 196.4 vs236 ± 39.6 ml), duration of stay in intensive care unit (mean 3.6 vs. 1.9 days) and need for blood transfusion (mean 0.4 ± 0.7 vs. 0.1 ± 0.3 units/patient).

The study also highlights that the systems used in the first two groups were very big in relation to the patients (BSA, pathologies, physiological needs), and the postoperative impact of these systems on the patients can be compared to an artificial increase in ECC time [10–17].

3. Development of ECC with a holder system for five external pumps

In parallel with this study, we have continued to develop the McECC concept because it was not possible to set up a new CPB console.

In 2006, we decided to test an Heart Lung console: HL30 machine (Maquet® Cardiopulmonary GmbH, Germany), which was marketed only in the late 1990s. The circular base of the CPB HL30 console consists of the housing of emergency batteries, a large part of electronics and five wheels. This particular configuration has allowed to lower the centre of gravity and, therefore, it has permitted to provide a CPB console with greater stability.

The HL30 has very lightweight modular roller pumps because they consist largely of alloy.

From the initial test, it was clear that this concept console could progress into an CPB capable of housing a holder system that authorises the remote placement of oxygenator and HSVR at the height of the patient's shoulder, together with the external pumps.

Therefore, I have created a prototype that has been submitted to Maquet® Cardiopulmonary GmbH, Germany. This society has produced this prototype without making any modifications. Furthermore, the Maquet® society has made several resistance tests of the materials in order to homologate it by giving it the name of Holder System U.Borrelli (**Figures 8–10**).

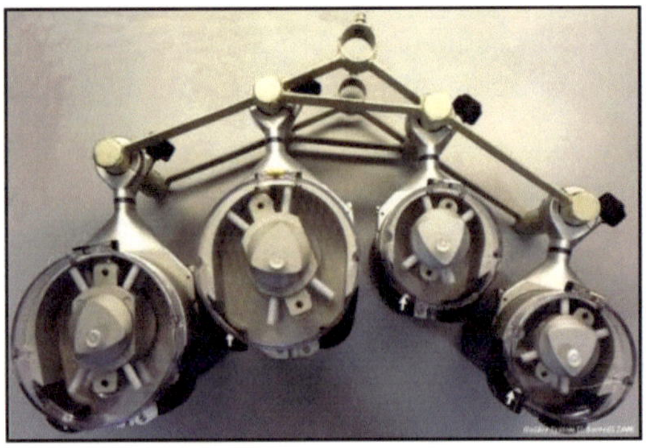

Figure 8. Prototype of the holder system, top view.

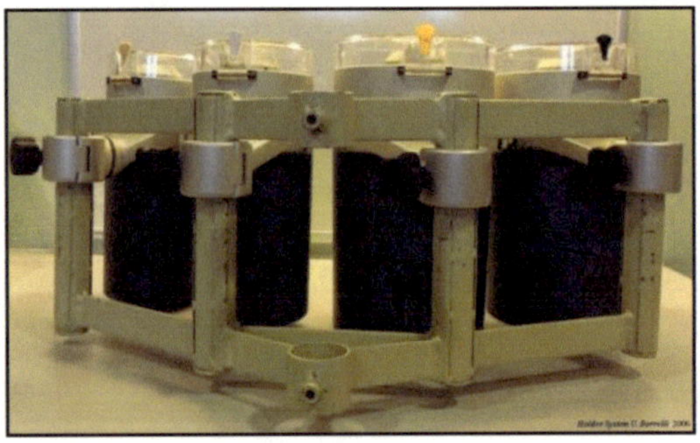

Figure 9. Prototype of the holder system, profile view.

http://dx.doi.org/10.5772/intechopen.77121

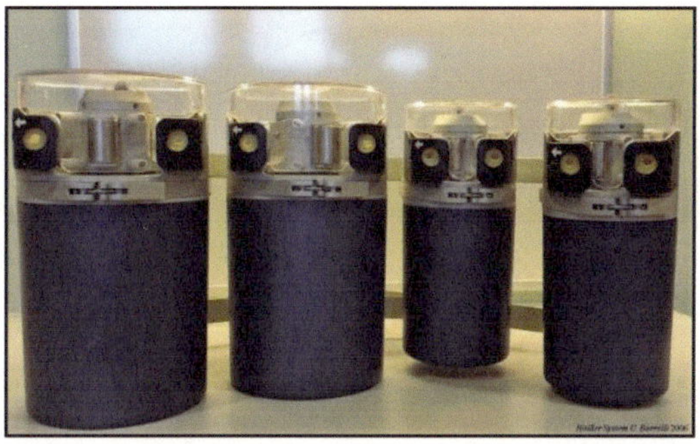

Figure 10. Prototype the holder system, front view.

In September 2007, our goal was achieved by placing on the CPB HL30 console the definitive Holder System. It was positioned using an additional mast and a four-point attachment system. The set is very stable and flexible, the weight of the overall holder system equipped with four roller pumps is 33 kg.

We placed a light at the top of the CPB console to ensure a good observation of the inner area of the heads of the roller pumps that are grey in colour. A second light at the bottom is oriented toward the oxygenator and HSVR (**Figures 11** and **12**).

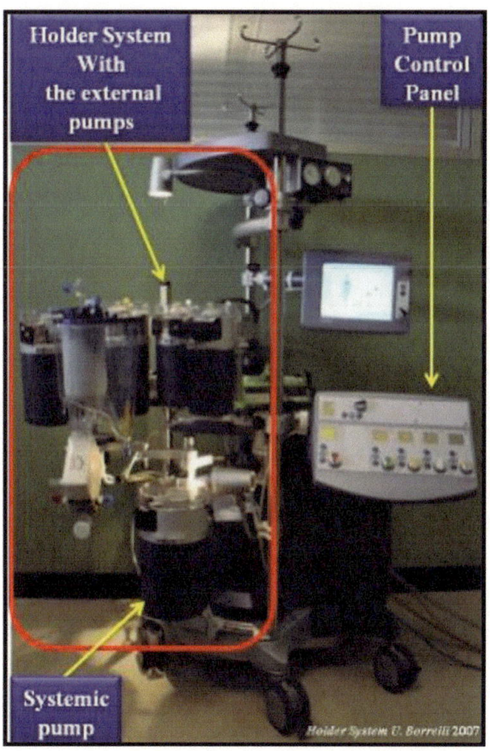

Figure 11. CPB console with the holder system, profile view.

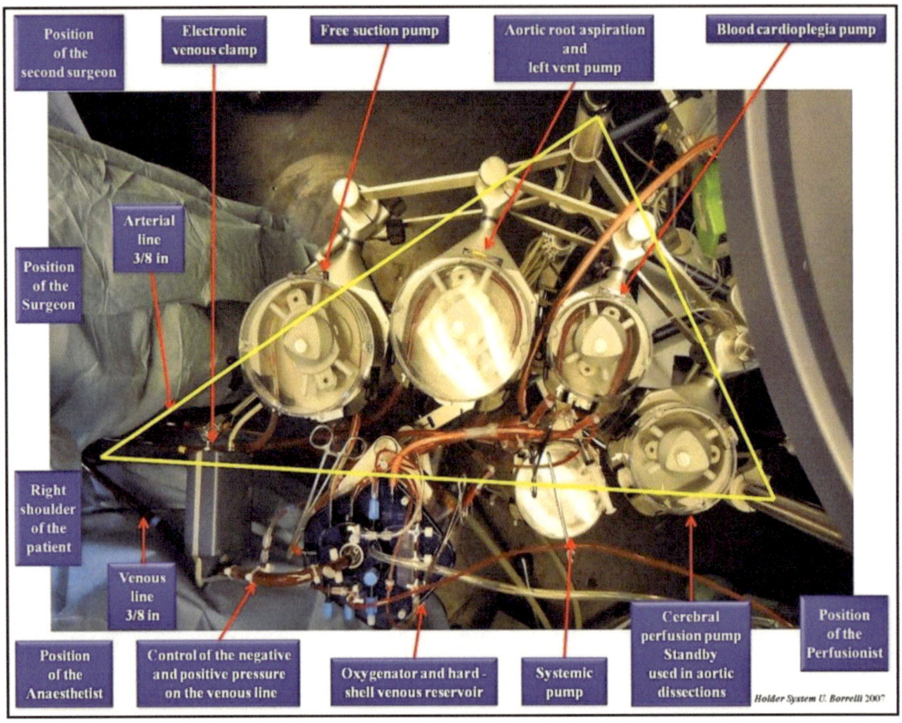

Figure 12. CPB console with the holder system, top view.

4. Optimisation of the circuit and the CPB console with a holder system

The holder system calibrates the CPB console against the ECC circuit to optimise its performance. The triangular shape of the holder system allows its remote placement of the CPB console, its distal end is near the surgeon's left hip. This has the effect of freeing up space for the different operators who are around the patient (**Figures 12** and **13**).

The concept of the CPB console with a holder system, has given us the possibility of reducing the lengths of lines of aspirations of +/−50%. The length of the arterial line of 3/8 in is +/− 100 cm (from the output of the arterial filter of the oxygenator up to the connection of the arterial cannula). Furthermore, the length of the venous line of 3/8 in is also +/− 100 cm (from the venous cannula up to the connection of the HSVR inlet). Therefore, there is a massive reduction of the air/blood surface, blood/contact materials, the dead space of the system and the priming volume (as a reminder: 100 cm of tubing 3/8 in contains 68 ml of liquid). All the dead spaces of the circuit are reduced to a minimum and it is very easy to perform an autologous priming retrograde (RAP) without any significant variation in the patient's volemia, including arterial line, arterial filter and antegrade autologous priming of the venous line (VAP) before the start of CPB [11] (**Figures 12–14**).

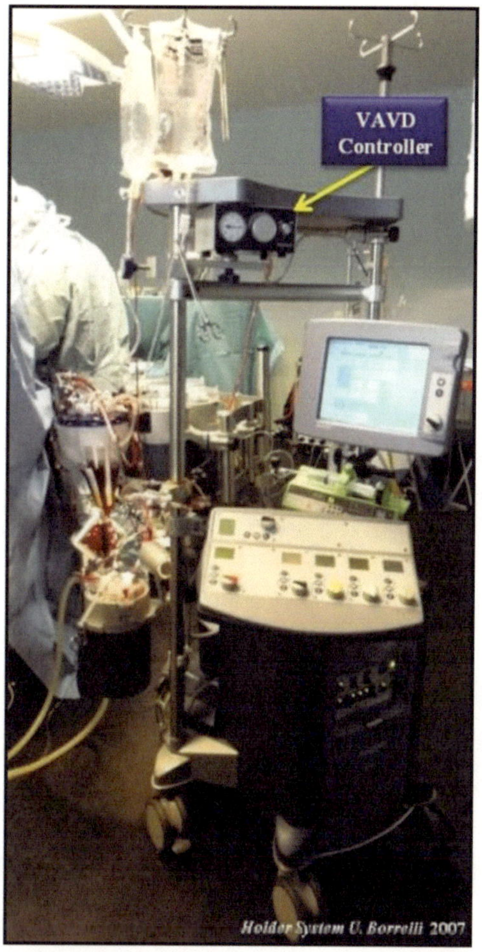

Figure 13. Position of the CPB console in the operating room.

4.1. Example of the circuit and the oxygenator and HSVR used

Alternative 1

- For a patient whose body surface is inferior or equal to 1.9 m^2
- Flow index: 2.4/min/m^2
- Oxygenator Quadrox—I Small Adult (Maquet® Cardiopulmonary GmbH, Germany)
- Membrane surface area of the oxygenator 1.3 m^2
- Maximum blood flow rate of the oxygenator 5 l/min
- Surface coating Bioline the oxygenator of the circuit of the ECC and the compatible HSVR with VAVD (Maquet® Cardiopulmonary GmbH, Germany)

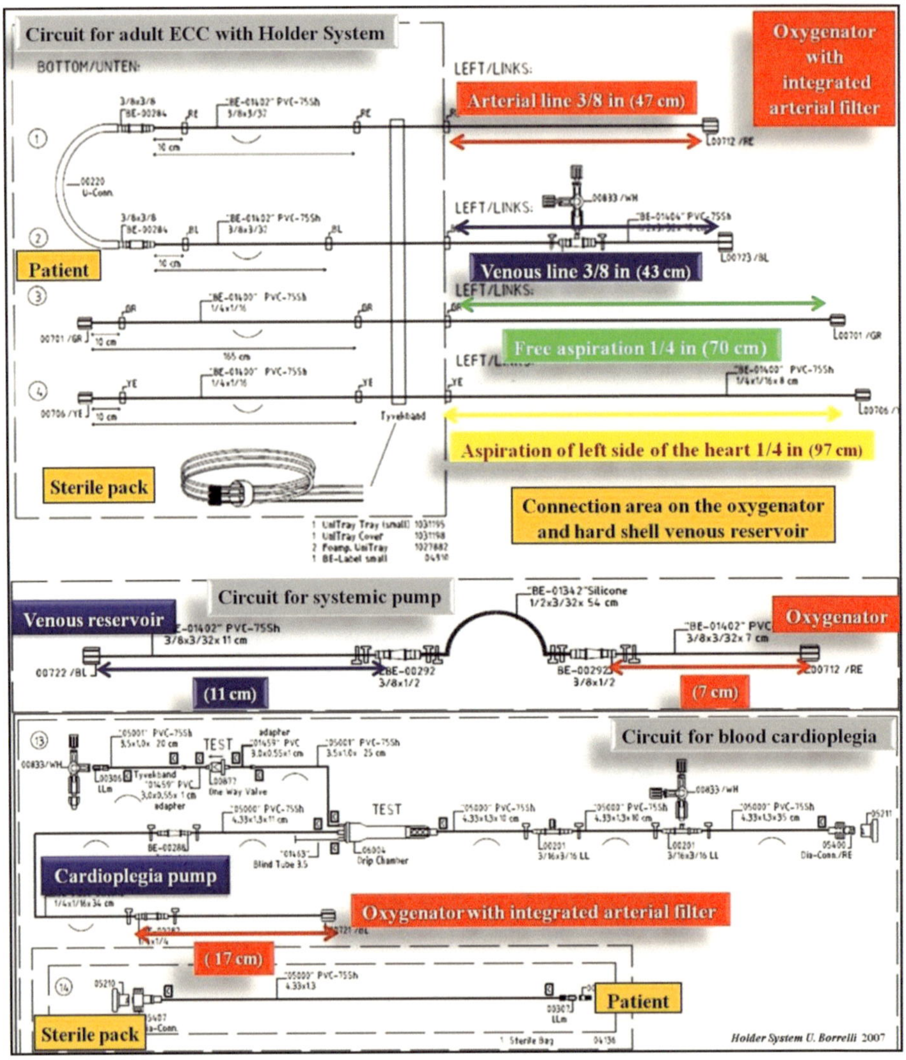

Figure 14. ECC circuit for adult patients with the holder system.

- VAVD system and arterial /venous line 3/8 in
- Level detector on the HSVR
- Retrograde autologous priming (RAP), including arterial line, arterial filter and antegrade autologous priming of the venous line (VAP)
- Residual priming or hemodilution of the patient at the start of ECC = 250 ml

Alternative 2

- For a patient whose body surface is superior to 1.9 m^2

http://dx.doi.org/10.5772/intechopen.77121

- Flow index: 2.4 l/min/m^2
- Oxygenator INSPIRE 6 FM (LivaNova® Mirandola, Italy)
- Membrane surface area of the oxygenator 1.4 m^2
- Maximum blood flow rate of the oxygenator 6 l/min
- Surface coating Phosphorylcholine the oxygenator of the circuit of the ECC and the compatible HSVR with VAVD (LivaNova® Mirandola, Italy)
- VAVD system and arterial/venous line 3/8 in
- Level detector on the HSVR
- Retrograde autologous priming (RAP), including arterial line, arterial filter and antegrade autologous priming of the venous line (VAP)
- Residual priming or hemodilution of the patient at the start of ECC = 300 ml

Alternative 3

- For a patient whose body surface is superior to 2.5 m^2
- Flow index: 2.4 l/min/m^2
- Oxygenator Quadrox—I Adult (Maquet® Cardiopulmonary GmbH, Germany)
- Membrane surface area of the oxygenator 1.8 m^2
- Maximum blood flow rate of the oxygenator 7 l/min
- Surface coating Bioline the oxygenator of the circuit of the ECC and the compatible HSVR with VAVD (Maquet® Cardiopulmonary GmbH, Germany)
- VAVD system and arterial/venous line 3/8 in
- Level detector on the HSVR
- Retrograde autologous priming (RAP), including arterial line, arterial filter and antegrade autologous priming of the venous line (VAP)
- Residual priming or hemodilution of the patient at the start of ECC = 300 ml

We routinely use the VAVD system with venous cannulas that are chosen according to their hemodynamic characteristics (design, size, internal-external diameter, pressure drop, etc.). The atrio-caval venous cannulae of reduced diameter have the disadvantage of slipping into the inferior vena cava during the surgical intervention and necessitate a greater negative pressure in the HSVR by the VAVD system. It is important to choose an armed venous cannula in a diameter adapted to the right atrium and a central cage that eliminates the phenomenon of massive suction of the right atrial wall. Venous cannulae with orifices of the central cage of sufficiently large size offset each other considerably reduce the incidence of this phenomenon of chattering (**Figure 15**).

With an appropriate venous cannula and a venous line of 3/8 in diameter, the vacuum required in the HSVR achieved by the VAVD system needs to simply replace the vacuum generated by venous drainage by gravity in a venous line of 1/2 in diameter, taking into account the internal pre-gravity of the HSVR from the right atrium of the patient to the lower part of the HSVR.

For example, for a systemic flow of 4.5–5 l/min with a venous cannula of 33–43 Fr (TF33430 Edwards®, USA) and a venous line of 3/8 in diameter, the vacuum necessary by the VAVD system is −20 to −25 mmHg (**Figure 15**).

In order to have a precise control of the VAVD system, we placed on the venous line of 3/8 in a monitoring of the negative and positive pressure. This triggers an alarm if the values reach −40 mmHg or + 3 mmHg. The VAVD system (Maquet® Cardiopulmonary GmbH, Germany) has internal safeguards that protects the HSVR from pressures above +3 mmHg and below −100 mmHg. Before each ECC intervention, we check the correct calibration of our roller pumps (**Figures 12**, **13**, and **15**).

The optimisation of venous return with VAVD is conditioned by the optimal choice of the venous cannula and its positioning; it improves the hemodynamics of the ECC and the

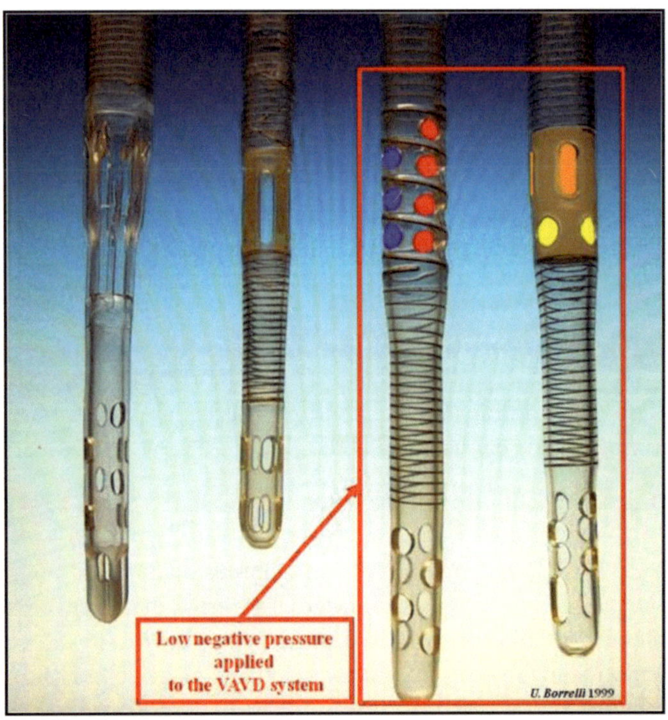

Figure 15. Venous cannulae.

patient. As the ECC becomes an arteriovenous extension of the patient's vascular network, the arterial flow and venous flow of the ECC must be in equilibrium. This constant ensures an adequate arteriovenous systemic flow capable of satisfying the patient's physiological needs during ECC [18–22].

Reducing the surface area contact of air/blood, blood/materials, the dead space of the system and the balance of arteriovenous flow results in a reduction of the risk of abdominal stasis and its repercussions on tissue perfusion. This ensures stability of the patient's blood volume that is in the HSVR. This optimisation of the hemodynamic equilibrium gives the possibility to widen the range of the strategies which are used during the management of the patients who undergo surgery under ECC (reduction of hemodilution, transfusions, etc.).

In order to limit the area contact of air/blood, blood/materials during ECC, the excess blood volume in the HSVR is isolated in biocompatible transfer bags. If necessary, it is re-infused to the patient during or at the end of the ECC. In general, the hematic volume in our HSVR during ECC is 350 to 400 ml.

The shape of the lower part of the HSVR that we use is conical or cylindrical, this has the consequence of limiting the free contact surface of the blood with the air and the biomaterials which constitute the base part of the HSVR (wall, filters, etc.) [23] (**Figures 15**).

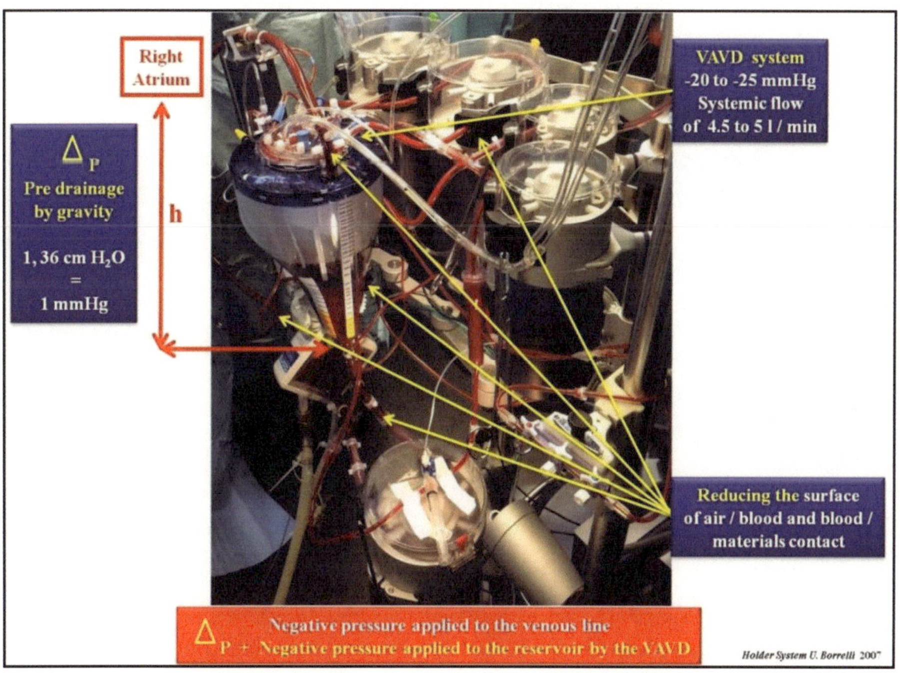

Figure 16. CPB console with the holder system, top view.

5. Conclusions

The optimisation of ECC management through:

- Used techniques (cardioplegia, autotransfusion system, etc.)
- Optimal choice of material (VAVD system, HSVR, surface coating, cannulas, design, hemodynamic, safe and accurate monitoring, security, etc.)
- The reduction of contact area surface of air/blood, blood/materials, dead space of the circuit and priming volume
- Hemodynamic equilibrium of the patient and ECC (arterial and venous flow)
- Accurate control of the patient's hemodilution

It has a direct impact on postoperative patients who have undergone surgical intervention under ECC; it could be comparable to an artificial reduction of ECC time.

For 23 years, this strategy of developing the McECC and the CPB console with the Holder System, the circuit, the various components that constitute the ECC allowed us to operate all types of patients with various pathologies with a safe and versatile system that is adapted to each patient. It gave us the possibility of a different approach for fragile patients or having to undergo paediatric, valvular or minimally invasive heart surgery.

The CPB HL30 console is very stable; thanks to its concept with its center of gravity which is low, it allowed us to place the Holder system away from the CPB console without having any technical problems. The assembly is very safe and flexible, the weight of the overall holder system provided with four roller pumps is 33 kg.

For 11 years, we have realised more than 3600 cardio-thoracic surgeries in our hospital with this concept of McECC and holder system.

This holder system was placed in 2009 on two CPB consoles at the Azienda Ospedaliera Universitaria "Ospedali Riuniti In Trieste, Italy, where more than 4300 cardio-vascular surgery were carried out with this ECC concept.

6. Future goals

Create a VAVD system with a servo controller to monitor the different pressures in HSVR (positive and negative) with respect to the hemodynamics of the patient and the ECC (arterial flow and venous flow).

Reduce the contact surface of the blood with air and biomaterials caused by HSVR, by creation of a safe and versatile VAVD HSVR that can be used as a closed or open system according to the needs of the users.

http://dx.doi.org/10.5772/intechopen.77121

Conflict of interest

The authors declare that they have no conflicts of interest.

Notes/Thanks/Other declarations

The author wishes to thank the people who made this project possible:
G. Baert MD and B. Trifan MD from Department of Cardiovascular Surgery, Grand Hôpital de Charleroi, Gilly, Belgium;
A.M. Calafiore MD from Department of Cardiac Surgery, Prince Sultan Cardiac Center, Riyadh, Saudi Arabia;
N. Al-Attar MD from Department of Cardiac Surgery, Golden Jubilee Hospital, Glasgow, UK;
A. Silvestri ECCP and S. Mercurio ECCP from Department of Cardiovascular Perfusion, Grand Hôspital de Charleroi, Gilly, Belgium;
A. Pappalardo MD, M. Gabrielli MD, C. Gripari CCP, G. Gustin CCP, D. Fasolo CCP, and A. Scala CCP from Department of Cardiac Surgery, Ospedali Riuniti, Trieste, Italy;
F. Perron CCP from Department of Cardiovascular Perfusion, Kelowna General Hospital, BC, Canada;
Mr. Dominique Bourgeois, professional welder.

Author details

Umberto Borrelli[1]*, Marc Detroux[2], Remi Nottin[3], Stephane Nikis[2] and Pierre Nakers[2]

*Address all correspondence to: umberto.borrelli@hotmail.com

1 Department of Cardiovascular Perfusion, Grand Hôspital de Charleroi, Gilly, Belgium

2 Department of Cardiovascular Surgery, Grand Hôpital de Charleroi, Gilly, Belgium

3 Department of Cardiac Surgery, Center Surgical Marie Lannelongue, Paris, France

References

[1] Butler J, Rocker GM, Westaby S. Inflammatory response to cardiopulmonary bypass. The Annals of Thoracic Surgery. 1993;**55**:552-559

[2] Bracey AW, Radovancevic R. The hematologic effects of cardiopulmonary bypass and the use of hemotherapy in coronary artery bypass grafting. Arch Pathol Lab Med 93;**118**: 411-416

[3] Williamson LM, Lowe S, Love EM, Cohen H, Soldan K, McClelland DBL, Skacel P, Barbara JAJ. Serious hazards of transfusion (SHOT) initiative: Analysis of the first two annual reports. British Medical Journal. 1999;**319**:16-19

[4] Moulton MJ, Creswell LL, Mackey ME, Cox JL, Rosembloom M. Reexploration for bleeding is a risk factor for adverse outcomes after cardiac operations. The Journal of Thoracic and Cardiovascular Surgery. 1996;**111**:1037-1046

[5] Fromes Y, Gaillard D, Ponzio O, Chauffert M, Gerhardt MF, Deleuze P, Bical OM. Reduction of the inflammatory response following coronary bypass grafting with total minimal extracorporeal circulation. European Journal of Cardio-Thoracic Surgery. 2002;**22**:527-533

[6] Borrelli U, Detroux M, Nackers P, Nikis S, et al. Impact on the inflammatory reaction by optimization of the extracorporeal circulation in cardiac surgery. Biomedical Journal, Innovation and Technology in Biology and Medicine; Editions Scientific and Medical. 2003 November;**24**(Suppl 1):80

[7] Borrelli U, Al-Attar N, Detroux M, Nottin R, Nikis S, et al. Compact extracorporeal circulation: Reducing of cardiopulmonary bypass to improve outcomes. Surgical Technology International. 2007;**16**:159-166

[8] Borrelli U, Detroux M, Nackers P, Nikis S, et al. Comparison of the troponin I levels during coronary artery bypass graft in cardiac surgery procedures, realised with and without extracorporeal circulation. Biomedical Journal. Innovation and Technology in Biology and Medicine; Editions Scientific and Medical Elsevier. 2003 November;**24**(Suppl. 1) 79 p

[9] Borrelli U, Detroux M, Nackers P, Nikis S, et al. Amélioration de la qualité des globules rouges récupérés avec le Stat, système d'autotransfusion périopératoire: Étude des résidus. Biomedical Journal, Innovation and Technology in Biology and Medicine; Editions Scientific and Medical Elsevier. 1998 October;**20**(Suppl 1)

[10] Bronson SL, Riley JB, Blessing JP, Ereth MH, Dearani JA. Prescriptive patient extracorporeal circuit and oxygenator sizing reduces Hemodilution and allogeneic blood product transfusion during adult cardiac surgery. The Journal of ExtraCorporeal Technology. 2013;**45**:167-117

[11] Ariyaratnam P, Bennett RT, McLean LA, Jagannadham KK, Turner E, Griffin S, Chaudhry MA, Loubani M. Antegrade rapid prime displacement in elective coronary artery surgery is associated with lower perioperative blood transfusions and a shorter hospital stay. Interactive Cardiovascular and Thoracic Surgery. 2013 Sep;**17**(3):485-491

[12] DeFoe GR, Ross CS, Olmstead EM, et al. Lowest hematocrit on bypass and adverse outcomes associated with coronary artery bypass grafting. Northern New England cardiovascular disease study group. The Annals of Thoracic Surgery. 2001;**71**:769-776

[13] Engoren MC, Habib RH, Zacharias A, et al. Effect of blood transfusion on long-term survival after cardiac operation. The Annals of Thoracic Surgery. 2002;**74**:1180-1186

[14] Karkouti K, Djaiani G, Borger MA, et al. Low hematocrit during cardiopulmomary bypass is associated with increased risk of perioperative stroke in cardiac surgery. The Annals of Thoracic Surgery. 2005;**80**:1381-1387

[15] Yavari M, Becker RC. Coagulation and fibrinolytic protein kinetics in cardiopulmonary bypass. Journal of Thrombosis and Thrombolysis. 2009 Jan;**27**(1):95-104

[16] Society of Thoracic Surgeons Blood Conservation Guideline Task Force, Ferraris VA, Brown JR, Despotis GJ, Hammon JW, Reece TB, Saha SP, Song HK, Clough ER, Society of Cardiovascular Anesthesiologists Special Task Force on Blood Transfusion, Shore-Lesserson LJ, Goodnough LT, Mazer CD, Shander A, Stafford-Smith M, Waters J, International Consortium for Evidence Based Perfusion, Baker RA, Dickinson TA, FitzGerald DJ, Likosky DS, Shann KG. 2011 update to the Society of Thoracic Surgeons and the Society of Cardiovascular Anesthesiologists blood conservation clinical practice guidelines. The Annals of Thoracic Surgery. 2011 Mar;**91**(3):944-982

[17] Anesthetic Techniques Fluid Management "Literature Abstracts". Society for Advancement of Blood Management; 2007 April;**5**(4)

[18] Nia Y-m, Leskosekb B, Shia L-p. Optimization of venous return tubing diameter for cardiopulmonary bypass. European Journal of Cardio-Thoracic Surgery. 2001;**20**:614-620

[19] Chalegre ST, Salerno PR, Salerno LM, Melo AR, Pinheiro AC, Frazão Cda S, Barros Filho PB, Lima Rde C. Vacuum-assisted venous drainage in cardiopulmonary bypass and need of blood transfusion: Experience of service. Revista Brasileira de Chirurgia Cardiovascular. 2011 Jan-Mar;**26**(1):122-127

[20] Goksedef D, Omeroglu SN, Balkanay OO, Denli Yalvac ES, Talas Z, Albayrak A, Ipek G. Hemolysis at different vacuum levels during vacuum-assisted venous drainage. The Thoracic and Cardiovascular Surgeon. 2012 Jun;**60**(4):262-268

[21] Simons AP, Ganushchak Y, Wortel P, Van Der Nagel T, Van Der Veen FH. Laboratory performance testing of venous Cannulae during inlet obstruction. Artificial Organs. Jul 1, 2008;**32**(7)

[22] Shinde SB, Golam KK, Kumar P, Patil ND. Blood lactate levels during cardiopulmonary bypass for valvular heart surgery. Annals of Cardiac Anaesthesia. 2005 Jan;**8**(1):39-44

[23] Zimmermann AK, Weber N, Aebert H, Ziemer G, Wendel HP. Effect of biopassive and bioactive surface-coatings on the hemocompatibility of membrane oxygenators. Journal of Biomedical Materials Research. Part B, Applied Biomaterials. 2007;**80**(2):433-439

Chapter 12

Utility of Modified Ultrafiltration in Congenital Heart Disease Patients Operated with Cardiopulmonary Bypass

Pedro José Curi-Curi, Juan Calderón-Colmenero,
Samuel Ramírez-Marroquín and
Jorge Luis Cervantes-Salazar

Additional information is available at the end of the chapter

http://dx.doi.org/10.5772/intechopen.77122

Abstract

Modified ultrafiltration is used in cardiac surgery with cardiopulmonary bypass in order to diminish systemic inflammatory response syndrome. We aimed to show its utility for removing pro-inflammatory agents in operated pediatric patients with congenital heart disease and its impact at operative care. A clinical case-control trial was designed, including patients with simple congenital heart disease operated on with cardiopulmonary bypass in a 1-year period. We randomized them to a problem group (with modified ultrafiltration, n = 15) and a control group (without it, n = 16), and blood samples to measure interleukins (6 and 10); 3d and 4d complement fraction concentrations were taken at the following times: baseline, before cardiopulmonary bypass, after it, after modified ultrafiltration, and from the ultrafiltration concentrate. Operative clinical end points of success were defined as hemodynamic stability, absence of morbidity, and lack of mortality. We observed a higher significant interleukin 6 concentration in the problem group patients at baseline, as well as a higher removal of this pro-inflammatory agent at the ultrafiltration concentrate. Modified ultrafiltration has a positive impact over simple congenital heart disease surgery with cardiopulmonary bypass because of removing interleukin 6. We recommend its routine use when hemodynamic conditions are favorable.

Keywords: cardiopulmonary bypass, congenital heart disease, interleukin

1. Introduction

Cardiopulmonary bypass (CPB) allowed the correction of several congenital heart diseases such as intracardiac malformations, but it is well-known that this is not a harmless procedure because it can lead to a systemic inflammatory response syndrome (SIRS), with activation of complement, cytokines, coagulation, and fibrinolysis pathways. Factors that contribute to the development of SIRS include blood contact with the synthetic surface of cardiopulmonary bypass components, as well as leukocyte and endothelial activation after tissue ischemia and reperfusion [1–5]. If there is a severe inflammatory response, it could also develop a multiorganic dysfunction syndrome that increases morbidity and mortality of the patients at pediatric intensive care units (PICUs). Some of the methods used to quantify the magnitude of SRIS due to the use of CPB include measurement of blood cytokine concentrations (interleukins 1 and 6), complement activation products (C3d and C4d), and also coagulation activated factors (Von Willebrand, fibrinogen and factor VIII) [6].

There are several operative strategies for diminishing SRIS and its clinical repercussion, such as the use of steroids, modified tubular surfaces for CPB, and ultrafiltration. Despite the single or combined use of these strategies [7–12], ultrafiltration is the one that probably removes a larger amount of pro-inflammatory agents, as well as water (volume) [13]. The two ultrafiltration technique modalities widely accepted for pediatric cardiac surgery are conventional ultrafiltration (CUF) and modified ultrafiltration (MUF). CUF is applied in CPB during the heart re-warming period and MUF right after ending CPB.

Currently, there is no enough evidence that favor the routine use of MUF [14–19], and we can still find some controversies regarding the benefits of this technique [20–22]. In addition, most reports of the study are focalized in adult cohorts of patients, and there is few information provided for pediatric population that show the real impact of MUF in the re-motion of pro-inflammatory agents due to CPB use. Therefore, we aimed to study the real utility of MUF for re-motion of pro-inflammatory agents induced by CPB in operated pediatric patients with simple congenital heart disease. We made a special emphasis in hemodynamic variables, morbidity, and mortality at the operative period.

2. Materials and methods

2.1. Study design

A prospective, randomized, analytic, and clinical case-control trial was designed at the Department of Pediatric Cardiac and Congenital Heart Surgery of a single center during a 1-year period of time. Inclusion criteria were age ≤ 18 years, and simple congenital heart disease that required elective surgical treatment with CPB use for at least 30 min. Exclusion criteria were preoperative renal failure, preoperative cardiogenic shock requiring the use of inotropics, preoperative sepsis, and preoperative mechanical ventilatory support of ≤48 h, preoperative lactate seric levels of ≥3 mmol/l, and cardiac reoperation. Patients were randomized into two study groups: problem group (with MUF) and control group (without MUF). With the use of an electronic URNA software, a statistical person randomized the patients and told the perfussionist, which was the only surgical team person informed about the results of randomization. All patients included in this study were operated on with informed consent signed by their parents or tutors. The study was also approved by our institutional research and ethics committee.

2.2. Modified ultrafiltration technique

Patients randomized to problem group (with MUF), when informed to the perfussionist, were prepared for CPB with an additional MUF set. Once CPB was ended and hemodynamic stability of the patient was provided, the surgeon was told not to remove the venous canula, and the venous line was clamped just before its connection to the reservoir. Arterial and venous line pathways were released in order to begin MUF with a 10–20-ml/kg/min flow. MUF continuous flow was achieved, pumping the venous residual reservoir volume by means of the arterial line to the patient. A 150–200-mmHg venous vacuum was applied when needed. MUF lasted 10–20 min in order to reach a desired hematocrit level and obtain also a suitable volume and electrolyte balance. MUF was stopped in case of hemodynamic instability. Once ended, MUF volume was restored to the patient from the hemofilter and venous canula, allowing the surgeon for decanulation of the patient.

2.3. Biochemical and clinical operative analysis

Biochemical and clinical results were compared between the two study groups at the operative period. Biochemical results were the concentration of cytokine (interleukins 6 and 10) and complement activated products (C3d and C4d). These concentrations were measured from blood samples at the following times: T0 (baseline, at the beginning of anesthesia induction), T1 (before CPB), T2 (immediately after CPB), and T3 (immediately after MUF, in the problem group). The same agents were measured in the MUF fluid concentrate of the problem group after the procedure (T4). Clinical operative results were evaluated in terms of hemodynamic instability (>20% post CPB variation with respect to previous CPB values of at least three of the following five hemodynamic variables: heart rate, systolic, diastolic and mean blood pressure, and central venous pressure), operative morbidity and mortality. Operative clinical end points of success were defined as hemodynamic stability, absence of morbidity, and lack of mortality.

2.4. Laboratory analysis of the fluid samples

All patient samples were obtained from central or peripheral blood and collected in tubes without heparin (vacutainer, Beckton Dickinson). A 3-ml blood sample was obtained for each of the study times (T0, T1, T2, and T3). The same volume of T4 samples was obtained from the ultrafiltration fluid concentrate. All of the samples were centrifugated at 3000 rpm for 15 min, 4°C, and cryopreserved in aliquots of 15 ml at −75°C. Interleukin concentrations (IL-6 and IL-10) were measured by means of an ELISA-Sandwich technique with the use of monoclonal antibodies (Peprotech, NJ, EUA). Complement activation products (C3d and C4d) were measured with the same technique, using commercial kits (Bachem, San Carlos, CA, EUA). Optical density was determined at 450 nm in the ELISA lector. Concentrations of IL-6, IL-10 (pg/ml), as well as C3d and C4d (ng/ml) were calculated by means of a GraphPad Software v. 4.2.

2.5. Statistical analysis

Information was registered in evaluation sheets, stored in an electronic Excel page and analyzed by means of a Prisma Graphics v3.1 statistical software. Continuous variables are presented as a mean, standard deviation, and variability ranges (minimum and maximum). Categorical data are presented by means of frequency and percentages in relation to the population at risk. Comparison between the two study groups was made by means of a Student's *t*-test for continuous variables. A chi-squared (X^2) test was used for comparing categorical variables with a 95% confidence interval (CI). A p-value <0.05 was considered as statistically significant.

3. Results

A total of 31 patients were enrolled and randomized to this trial: 15 to the problem group (with MUF) and 16 to the control group (without MUF).

3.1. Preoperative characteristics

Table 1 shows the type of congenital diseases that were operated by means of CPB in both groups of study. There are no differences in the total number of congenital heart disease in the studied groups, but control group (without MUF) showed more patients with AV channel than the problem group (with MUF).

Congenital heart disease type	Total series (n = 31) n (%)	Problem group (with MUF) (n = 15) n (%)	Control group (without MUF) (n = 16) n (%)	p
Ventricular septal defect	13 (42%)	8 (52%)	5 (31%)	NS
Balanced AV channel	8 (26%)	1 (7%)	7 (44%)	0.04
Congenital mitral valve disease	4 (13%)	3 (20%)	1 (6%)	NS
Subaortic membrane	3 (10%)	1 (7%)	2 (13%)	NS
Right ventricular outflow tract obstruction	1 (3%)	1 (7%)	0 (0%)	NS
Double chamber right ventricle	1 (3%)	1 (7%)	0 (0%)	NS
Atrial septal defect	1 (3%)	0 (0%)	1 (6%)	NS
Total	31 (100%)	15 (100%)	16 (100%)	NS

Table 1. Congenital heart disease type in the studied groups.

http://dx.doi.org/10.5772/intechopen.77122

Variable	Total series n (%) or mean ± SD (range)	Problem group (with MUF) n (%) or mean ± SD (range)	Control group (without MUF) n (%) or mean ± SD (range)	
Age (years)	4.26 ± 4.11 (0.38–17.18)	37 ± 14 (18–76)	31 ± 11 (18–56)	NS
Gender				
Male	12 (39%)	8 (53%)	4 (25%)	NS
Female	19 (61%)	7 (47%)	12 (75%)	NS
Anthropometric data				
Weight (kg)	14.9 ± 10.8 (4–47)	14.1 ± 10.4 (4–38.3)	15.9 ± 11.6 (5.3–47)	NS
Height (cm)	90 ± 31.1 (12–159)	94.2 ± 31.2 (55–158)	86 ± 31.5 (12–159)	NS
Body surface area (m^2)	0.56 ± 0.27 (0.25–1.32)	0.58 ± 0.31 (0.25–1.32)	0.53 ± 0.18 (0.28–0.78)	NS
Circulating blood volume (ml)	1032 ± 627 (343–2660)	1164 ± 756 (343–2660)	867 ± 385 (452–1560)	NS
Cardiovascular background				
Previous surgery	0 (0%)	0 (0%)	0 (0%)	NS
Previous catheterization	2 (6%)	0 (0%)	2 (6%)	NS
Pathologic background				
Preoperative infection	1 (3%)	0 (0%)	1 (6%)	NS
Pulmonary artery hypertension	4 (13%)	0 (0%)	4 (25%)	NS
None	26 (84%)	15 (100%)	11 (69%)	NS
Syndromes				
Down	3 (10%)	0 (0%)	3 (19%)	NS
None	28 (90%)	15 (100%)	13 (81%)	NS
NYHA/Ross pre-operative functional class				
I	8 (26%)	4 (27%)	4 (25%)	NS
II	21 (68%)	9 (60%)	12 (75%)	NS
III	2 (6%)	2 (13%)	0 (0%)	NS
Operative risk				
RACHS-1 score	2.4 ± 0.5 (1–3)	2.4 ± 0.5 (2–3)	2.4 ± 0.6 (1–3)	NS
Basic aristoteles	7.2 ± 1.5 (3–9)	7 ± 1.2 (6–9)	7.4 ± 1.9 (3–9)	NS
Complete aristoteles	8.1 ± 1.8 (4–11)	7.8 ± 1.5 (6–10)	8.4 ± 2.1 (4–11)	NS
Preoperative morbidity				
Mechanic ventilation	0 (0%)	0 (0%)	0 (0%)	NS
Preoperative inotropic support	0 (0%)	0 (0%)	0 (0%)	NS
Preoperative infection	1 (3%)	0 (0%)	1(6%)	NS
None	30 (97%)	15 (100%)	15 (94%)	NS
Preoperative laboratory exams				
Lactate	1.2 ± 0.3 (0.6–1.7)	1.2 ± 0.3 (0.7–1.7)	1.1 ± 0.3 (0.6–1.5)	NS

Variable	Total series n (%) or mean ± SD (range)	Problem group (with MUF) n (%) or mean ± SD (range)	Control group (without MUF) n (%) or mean ± SD (range)	
Creatinine	0.4 ± 0.1 (0.2–0.7)	0.4 ± 0.1 (0.2–0.7)	0.4 ± 0.1 (0.3–0.5)	NS
Perfusion variables				
Oxigenator type				
Baby Rx	14 (52%)	7 (47%)	7 (58%)	NS
Terumo SX10	6 (22%)	4 (27%)	2 (17%)	NS
Terumo SX18	1 (4%)	1 (7%)	0 (0%)	NS
Mini max	5 (19%)	2 (13%)	3 (25%)	NS
Safe Mini	1 (4%)	1 (7%)	0 (0%)	NS
Arterial filter use	18 (67%)	12 (80%)	6 (50%)	NS
Surgical variables				
CPB time (min)	81.9 ± 26.9 (40–131)	76.5 ± 23.7 (40–122)	87 ± 29.4 (41–131)	NS
Aortic cross clamp time (min)	53.7 ± 23.6 (12–96)	49.5 ± 21.8 (18–90)	57.6 ± 25.2 (12–96)	NS
Temperature (°C)	27 ± 1.6 (24–30)	27 ± 1.5 (24–29)	27.3 ± 1.8 (24–30)	NS
Anterograde cardioplegia	29 (94%)	14 (93%)	15 (94%)	NS
Blood cardioplegia	29 (94%)	14 (93%)	15 (94%)	NS

Table 2. Preoperative characteristics of the studied groups.

Table 2 shows the rest of preoperative characteristics in both studied groups. Note that there are no statistical differences in all variables analyzed between the two groups.

Although more random patients with AV channel in the control group, the rest of the preoperative data showed that both groups are absolutely comparable.

3.2. Biochemical operative results

Table 3 compares the concentration of pro-inflammatory agents between groups before surgical correction (T0). Note a baseline elevated concentration of IL-6 in the problem group (with

Pro-inflammatory agent	T0 Problem group (with MUF) n = 15 Mean ± DE	T0 Control group (without MUF) n = 16 Mean ± DE	p
C3d (ng/ml)	368.66 ± 331.87	413.248 ± 316.804	NS
C4d (ng/ml)	199.57 ± 201.56	213.89 ± 116.72	NS
IL-6 (pg/ml)	**672.249 ± 433.186**	**246.874 ± 365.69**	**0.0061**
IL-10 (pg/ml)	239.698 ± 381.517	299.618 ± 370.148	NS

The words and numbers in "bold" highlight the variables that have a statistical significance ($p<0.005$).

Table 3. Comparison between concentrations of pro-inflammatory agents in both groups of study (with and without MUF) at baseline (T0).

MUF), without differences in both groups for the rest of pro-inflammatory agents (IL-10, C3d, and C4d).

On the other hand, **Table 4** shows a lack of statistically significant difference in the concentrations of pro-inflammatory agents at the control group before surgical correction (T0) and after CPB (T2).

Finally, **Table 5** shows the comparison between the concentration of pro-inflammatory agents in the problem group before surgical correction (T0) and after MUF (T4). There is a statistically significant removal of IL-6, but no difference in the concentrations of the rest of pro-inflammatory agents analyzed (IL-10, C3d, and C4d).

3.3. Clinical operative results

Table 6 summarizes the comparison of clinical end point variables in both groups of study (with and without MUF). There is a statistically significant decrease of hemoglobin (Hb) in the problem group after MUF compared with the baseline level, which is not observed in the control group.

Both groups show an increase in lactate levels and heart rate after surgery when comparing these values with the baseline ones before CPB. Control group (without MUF) showed a statistically significant increase in the central venous pressure after CPB compared with the ones before CPB. There were no differences before and after CPB in the other hemodynamic variables (systolic, diastolic, and mean blood pressures), nor in operative morbidity and mortality. Successful clinical operative endpoints were achieved in both groups of study.

Pro-inflammatory agent	T0 Group control (sin UFM) n = 16 Media ± SD	T2 Control group (without MUF) n = 16 Media ± DE	p
C3d (ng/ml)	413.248 ± 316.804	264.33 ± 198.12	NS
C4d (ng/ml)	213.89 ± 116.72	210.65 ± 141.13	NS
IL-6 (pg/ml)	246.874 ± 365.69	289.499 ± 301.913	NS
IL-10 (pg/ml)	299.618 ± 370.148	387.26 ± 306.07	NS

Table 4. Comparison between concentrations of pro-inflammatory agents at T0 (baseline) and T2 (after CPB) for the control group (without MUF).

Pro-inflammatory agent	T0 Grupo problema (con UFM) n = 15 Media ± SD	T4 Problem group (with MUF) n = 15 Media ± DE	p
C3d (ng/ml)	368.66 ± 331.87	379.99 ± 264.64	NS
C4d (ng/ml)	199.57 ± 201.56	172.89 ± 139.64	NS
IL-6 (pg/ml)	**672.249 ± 433.186**	**366.31 ± 280.25**	**0.0293**
IL-10 (pg/ml)	239.698 ± 381.517	230.453 ± 352.27	NS

The words and numbers in "bold" highlight the variables that have a statistical significance ($p<0.005$).

Table 5. Comparison between concentrations of pro-inflammatory agents at baseline (T0) and after MUF (T4) for the problem group (with MUF).

	Problem group (with MUF)			Control group (without MUF)			Problem versus control groups (with vs. without MUF)		
Operative clinical end point variable	**Control group**	**Problem group**	**p**	**Control group**	**Problem group**	**p**	**Problem group**	**Control group**	**p**
	Before CPB	**After MUF**		**Before CPB**	**After MUF**		**After MUF**	**After CPB**	
	n/total n (%) or	**n/total n (%) or**		**n/total n (%) or**	**n/total n (%) or**		**n/total n (%) or**	**n/total n (%) or**	
	Mean ± SD	**Mean ± SD**		**Mean ± SD**	**Mean ± SD**		**Mean ± SD**	**Mean ± SD**	
Laboratory examinations									
Hematocrit (%)	38 ± 7	34 ± 6	NS	37 ± 5	34 ± 7	NS	34 ± 6	34 ± 7	NS
Hemoglobin (g/dl)	**14 ± 5**	**11 ± 2**	**0.0344**	12 ± 2	11 ± 2	NS	11 ± 2	11 ± 2	NS
CPB hematocrit (%)						26 ± 5*	24 ± 4*	NS	
Lactate (mmol/l)	**1.2 ± 0.3**	**3.5 ± 1.4**	**0.0001**	**1.1 ± 0.3**	**3.3 ± 1.2**	**0.0001**	3.5 ± 1.4	3.3 ± 1.2	NS
Hemodynamic variables									
Heart rate (beats per minute)	**97 ± 15**	**113 ± 18**	**0.012**	**97 ± 16**	**112 ± 15**	**0.0116**	113 ± 18	112 ± 15	NS
Systolic blood pressure (mmHg)	85 ± 16	89 ± 12	NS	83 ± 10	90 ± 20	NS	89 ± 12	90 ± 20	NS
Diastolic blood pressure (mmHg)	53 ± 15	52 ± 12	NS	49 ± 7	49 ± 12	NS	52 ± 12	49 ± 12	NS
Mean blood pressure (mmHg)	64 ± 18	61 ± 12	NS	64 ± 13	64 ± 17	NS	61 ± 12	64 ± 17	NS
Central venous pressure (mmHg)	10 ± 8	12 ± 7	NS	**8 ± 1**	**10 ± 3**	**0.0203**	12 ± 7	10 ± 3	NS
Operative morbidity and mortality									
Morbidity						3 (20%)	1 (6%)		NS
Mortality						0 (0%)	0 (0%)		NS

*CPB measured values (due to hemodilution).
Shades: The words and numbers in "bold" highlight the variables that have a statistical significance (p<0.005).

Table 6. Comparison between operative clinical end point variables in both groups of study (with and without MUF).

4. Discussion

Cardiopulmonary bypass (CPB) is able to trigger a systemic inflammatory response syndrome (SRIS) due to several factors that include (1) cell activation secondary to contact with CPB synthetic surfaces, (2) mechanic stress, (3) tissue ischemia and reperfusion, (4) hypotension, (5) non-pulsatile flow, (6) hemodilution relative anemia, (7) blood and blood products transfusion, (8) heparin and protamine administration, and (9) hypothermic effects. CPB activates the vessels endothelium and releases pro-inflammatory agents such as tumoral necrosis factor α (TNF-α), interleukins, and endotoxins. These agents activate the intracellular transcription factor as well, which increases endothelial pro-inflammatory cytokines and the molecular expression of leukocyte adhesion.

It is a well-known fact that younger age increases the inflammatory effects of CPB even more. Some reasons include an increased metabolic demand in these patients, hyperactivity of their pulmonary vessels, immaturity of their organs/systems, and altered homeostasis. Risk is particularly high in neonates and young infants due to a mismatch between CPB and patient's size, with CPB circuit volume usually 200–300% higher than that of the patient. In addition, an increased metabolic demand requires elevated pump flow up to 200 ml/kg/min in neonates. Combining a relative major size of CPB with an increased perfusion rate leads to a greater blood exposure to synthetic surfaces of the circuit components [23]. In our series, there was no age difference between the studied groups, and it is important to highlight that none of the groups included neonate patients for the reasons already discussed.

One of the most involved cytokines in SRIS development is, indeed, IL-6. Increased concentrations of IL-6 have been reported in patients with postoperative complications and a correlation with the posterior left ventricular wall dyskinesia detected by means of transesophageal echocardiography has been established. IL-6 is also an endogenous pyrogen agent that activates acute phase reactant proteins. Concentration of IL-6 increases independently of the oxygenator type, degree of hypothermia, or heparin use in the CPB circuit surfaces [24, 25]. Although in our study IL-6 concentrations were significantly higher before surgery in the problem group than in the control group, this agent is also the one that is significantly more removed by MUF. This is probably the most relevant fact of our study because it shows that the benefit of MUF in congenital heart disease surgery is the removal of IL-6, an important pro-inflammatory agent, particularly in patients that SRIS is enhanced because of the immaturity of their immune system. Another effect that is important to discuss is the fact that if MUF benefits patients with simple congenital heart disease surgery as were the ones included in our study, it would indeed improve operative outcomes in those operated on for complex congenital heart disease [26]. This single fact justifies the routine use of MUF in all patients with congenital heart disease that are operated on with CPB.

There are several additional methods, despite ultrafiltration, that had been developed in order to diminish SRIS secondary to CPB at surgical correction of congenital heart disease in pediatric population. Some of them are steroids (e.g., dexamethasone 10–30 mg/kg, 6–12 h before CPB), and modified tubular synthetic surfaces in the CPB circuit. However, none of these methods are as useful for this purpose as MUF, which is established right after ending the CPB and before decanulation of the patient [27]. Since 1973, different types of hemofilters have been developed in order to remove priming volume (water) following the principle of pressure gradient, particularly those made of polycarbonate. These filters have been replaced by the ones made out of poliarileter-sulfonate in 1986, and later by the current generation of polyamide hemofilters. These are the most practical ones because of its greater biocompatibility, reduced surface, and more ultrafiltration effectiveness due to a less than physiological pressure.

The effectiveness of ultrafiltration for removing pro-inflammatory agents depends also on the type of hemofilter and on the modality of ultrafiltration procedure used. Berdat et al. studied the effectiveness of poliariletersulfonate filters versus polyamide ones in the two ultrafiltration modalities for the removal of pro-inflammatory agents such as IL-6, IL-10, and TNFα [10]. They prove that IL-6 was better removed by conventional ultrafiltration (CUF) with poliarileter-sulfonate filter, while TNFα was better removed by modified ultrafiltration (MUF) and poliariletersulfonate filter. The rest of the pro-inflammatory agents were not modified neither for the ultrafiltration modality nor for the hemofilter type. Therefore, it seems that MUF with poliariletersulfonate hemofilter is the better strategy for removing pro-inflammatory agents in pediatric patients with congenital heart surgery. Our results are based on the ultrafiltration modality rather than the type of filter, since the material of hemofilters that we used was variable.

It has been reported that MUF is not only useful for removing extracellular fluid excess but also cytokines and other inflammatory agents triggered by CPB and surgical trauma. There is some controversy in the study regarding the efficacy of filters in the removal of cytokines, as well as in the differences between the two ultrafiltration modalities [28]. In addition, the comparative results between both ultrafiltration modalities are difficult to interpret due to variations in the ultrafiltration technique, equipment, definitions and objectives, and measurements of cytokines. Finally, it is still not known if the clinical benefits of MUF are due to the removal of cytokines and other inflammatory agents, or to the isolated reduction of tissue edema [29–33].

5. Conclusion

Based on the results of this study [34], we can say that although the baseline concentrations of IL-6 in the patients of the problem group were higher in relation to those of the control group, the removal of this pro-inflammatory agent by MUF was statistically significant. This indicates that MUF is a procedure that can benefit pediatric patients with congenital heart disease undergoing CPB because it is able to decrease the concentration of IL-6. Therefore, we consider that the use of MUF in pediatric patients should be routinely recommended as long as hemodynamic conditions allow it.

Acknowledgements

We thank the Cardio Slim Foundation for the financial support provided to carry out this study.

http://dx.doi.org/10.5772/intechopen.77122

Conflict of interest

The authors declare no potential conflicts of interest with respect to the research, authorship, or publication of this manuscript.

Author details

Pedro José Curi-Curi[1]*, Juan Calderón-Colmenero[2], Samuel Ramírez-Marroquín[1] and Jorge Luis Cervantes-Salazar[1]

*Address all correspondence to: pcuricuri001@gmail.com

1 Department of Congenital Heart Disease and Pediatric Cardiac Surgery, "Ignacio Chávez" National Cardiology Institute, Mexico City, Mexico

2 Department of Pediatric Cardiology, "Ignacio Chávez" National Cardiology Institute, Mexico City, Mexico

References

[1] Brix-Christensen V. The systemic inflammatory response after cardiac surgery with cardiopulmonary bypass in children. Acta Anaesthesiologica Scandinavica. 2001;**45**:671-679

[2] Seghaye MC. The clinical implications of the systemic inflammatory reaction related to cardiac operations in children. Cardiology in the Young. 2003;**13**:228-239

[3] Kozik D, Tweddell J. Characterizing the inflammatory response to cardiopulmonary bypass in children. The Annals of Thoracic Surgery. 2006;**81**:S2347-S2354

[4] Kirklin JK, Westaby S, Blackstone EH, Kirklin JW, Chenowelh DE, Pacifico AD. Complement and the damaging effects of cardiopulmonary bypass. The Journal of Thoracic and Cardiovascular Surgery. 1983;**86**:845-847

[5] Seghaye M, Duchateau J, Grabitz RG, Nitsch G, Marcus C, Messmer BJ, von Bernuth G. Complement, leukocytes and leukocyte elastase in full-term neonates undergoing cardiac operation. Journal of Thoracic and Cardiovascular Surgery. 1994;**108**:29-36

[6] Seghaye M, Grabitz RG, Duchateau J, Bussea S, Däbritz S, Koch D, et al. Inflammatory reaction and capillary leak syndrome related to cardiopulmonary bypass in neonates undergoing cardiac operations. The Journal of Thoracic and Cardiovascular Surgery. 1996;**112**:687-697

[7] Ashraf SS, Tian Y, Zacharrias S, Cowan D, Martin P, Watterson K. Effects of cardiopulmonary bypass on neonatal and paediatric inflammatory profiles. European Journal of Cardio-Thoracic Surgery. 1997;**12**:862-868

[8] McBride WT, McBride SJ. The balance of pro- and anti-inflammatory cytokines in cardiac surgery. Current Opinion in Anesthesiology. 1998;**11**:15-22

[9] McBride WT, Armstrong MA, Gilliland H, McMurray TJ. The balance of pro- and anti-inflammatory cytokines in plasma and bronchoalveolar lavage (BAL) at paediatric cardiac surgery. Cytokine. 1996;**8**:724-729

[10] Chevv M, Brandslund I, Brix-Christensen V, et al. Tissue injury and the inflammatory response to pediatric cardiac surgery with cardiopulmonary bypass. Anesthesiology. 2001;**94**:745-753

[11] Finn A, Moat N, Rebuck N, Klein N, Slrobel S, Elliott M. Changes in neutrophil CDllb/CD18 and L-selectin expression and release of interleukin 8 and elastase in paediatric cardiopulmonay bypass. Agents and Actions. 1993;**38**:C44-C46

[12] Brix-Christensen V, Petersen TK, Ravn HB, Hjortdal VE, Andersen NR, Tonnesen E. Cardiopulmonary bypass elicits a pro- and anti-inflammatory response and impaired chemotaxis in neonatal pigs. Acta Anaesthesiologica Scandinavica. 2001;**45**:407-413

[13] Hennein HA, Kiseltepe U, Barst S, Bocchieri KA, Remick DG, et al. Venovenous modified ultrafiltration after cardiopulmonary bypass in children: A prospective randomized study. The Journal of Thoracic and Cardiovascular Surgery. 1999;**117**:496-505

[14] Kern FH, Morana NJ, Sears JJ, Hickey PR. Coagulation defects in neonates during cardiopulmonary bypass. The Annals of Thoracic Surgery. 1992;**54**:541-546

[15] Boga M, Islamoglu F, Badak I, Cikirikcioglu M, Bakalim T, Yagdi T. The effects of modified hemofiltration on inflammatory mediators and cardiac performance in coronary artery bypass grafting. Perfusion. 2000;**15**:143-150

[16] Tassani P, Richter JA, Eising GP, Barabkay A, Braun SL, Haehnel CH, et al. Influence of combined zero-balanced and modified ultrafiltration on the systemic inflammatory response during coronary artery bypass grafting. Journal of Cardiothoracicand Vascular Anesthesia. 1999;**13**:285-291

[17] Pearl JM, Manning PB, McNamara JL, Saucier MM, Thomas DW. Effect of modified ultrafiltration on plasma thromboxane B2, leukotriene B4, endothelin-1 in infants undergoing cardiopulmonary bypass. The Annals of Thoracic Surgery. 1999;**68**:1369-1375

[18] Grunenfelder J, Sund G, Schoeberlein A, Maly FE, Guntli S, Fischer K, et al. Modified ultrafiltration lowers adhesion molecule and cytokine levels after cardiopulmonary bypass without clinical relevance in adults. European Journal of Cardio-Thoracic Surgery. 2000;**17**:77-83

[19] Chew MS. Does modified ultrafiltration reduce the systemic inflammatory response to cardiac surgery with cardiopulmonary bypass? Perfusion. 2004;**19**:S57-S60

[20] Hauser GJ, Ben-Ari J, Colvin MP, Dalton HJ, Hertzog JH, Bearb M, et al. Interleukin-6 levels in serum and lung lavage fluid of children undergoing open heart surgery correlate with postoperative morbidity. Intensive Care Medicine. 1998;**24**:481-486

[21] Gilliland HE, Armstrong MA, McMurray TJ. The inflammatory response to pediatric cardiac surgery: Correlation of granulocyte adhesion molecule expression with postoperative oxygenation. Anesthesia and Analgesia. 1999;**89**:1188-1191

[22] Andreasson S, Góthberg S, Berggren H, Bengtsson A, Eriksson E, Risberg B. Hemofiltration modifies complement activation after extracorporeal circulation in infants. The Annals of Thoracic Surgery. 1993;**56**:1515-1517

[23] Wang W, Chiu I, Chao-Min W, Pei-Lin L, Huand HM, Chung IC, et al. Modified ultrafiltration in pediatric cardiopulmonary bypass. Perfusion. 1998;**13**:304-310

[24] Ming-Jiuh W, Chiu I-S, Chao-Ming W, Pei-Lin L, Chung-I C, Chi-Hsiang H, Shu-Hsun C. Efficacy of ultrafiltration in removing inflammatory mediators during pediatric cardiac operations. The Annals of Thoracic Surgery. 1996;**61**:651-656

[25] Naik S, Knight A, Elliott MJ. A prospective randomized study of a modified technique of ultrafiltration during pediatric open-heart surgery. Circulation. 1991;**84**(suppl III):422-431

[26] Bando K, Turrentine MW, Vijay P, Sharp TG, Lalone BJ, et al. Effect of modified ultrafiltration in high-risk patients undergoing operations for congenital heart disease. The Annals of Thoracic Surgery. 1998;**66**:821-828

[27] Draasima AM, Hazekamp MG, Frank M, Anes N, Schoof PH, Huysmans HA. Modified ultrafiltration after cardiopulmonary bypass in pediatric cardiac surgery. The Annals of Thoracic Surgery. 1997;**64**:521-525

[28] Daggett CW, Lodge AJ, Scarborough JE, Chai PJ, Jaggers J, Ungerleider RM. Modified ultrafiltration versus conventional ultrafiltration: A randomized prospective study in neonatal piglets. The Journal of Thoracic and Cardiovascular Surgery. 1998;**H5**:336-342

[29] Davies MJ, Nguyen K, Gaynor JW, Elliott MJ. Modified ultrafiltration improves left ventricular systolic function in infants after cardiopulmonary bypass. The Journal of Thoracic and Cardiovascular Surgery. 1998;**5**:361-370

[30] Journois D, Israel-Biet D, Pouard P, Rolland B, Silvester W, Vouhe P, Safran D, et al. High-volume, zero-balanced hemofiltration to reduce delayed inflammatory response to cardiopulmonary bypass in children. Anesthesiology. 1996;**85**:965-976

[31] Chew MS, Brix-Christensen V, Ravn H, Brandslund I, Ditlevsen E, Pedersen J, et al. Effect of modified ultrafiltration on the inflammatory response in paediatric open-heart surgery: A prospective, randomized study. Perfusion. 2002;**17**:327-333

[32] Ramamoorthy C, Lynn AM. The use of modified ultrafiltration during pediatric cardiovascular surgery is not a benefit. Journal of Cardiothoracic and Vascular Anesthesia. 1998; **12**(4):483-485

[33] García-Montes JA, Calderón-Colmenero J, Juanico A. Cuidados Intensivos en el niño cardiópata en Attie F. In: Calderón-Colmenero J, Zabal C, Buendía A, editors. Cardiología Pediátrica. México DF: Editorial Médica Panamericana; 2013. p. 203

[34] Curi-Curi PJ, del Villar MRS, Gómez-García L, Vergara BG, Calderón-Colmenero J, Ramírez-Marroquín S, Cervantes-Salazar JL. Impacto intraoperatorio de la ultrafiltración modificada en pacientes pediátricos sometidos a cirugía cardíaca con circulación extracorpórea. Cirugía Cardiovascular. 2016;**23**(4):179-186

Chapter 13

Flow Optimization, Management, and Prevention of LV Distention during VA-ECMO

Cristiano Amarelli, Francesco Musumeci,
Antonio Loforte, Andrea Montalto,
Sveva Di Franco and Jaime Hernandez-Montfort

Additional information is available at the end of the chapter

http://dx.doi.org/10.5772/intechopen.80265

Abstract

Cardiogenic shock (CS) still carries an unacceptably high mortality (30–60%), despite several therapeutic approaches; the SHOCK II trial questioned the benefit of intra-aortic balloon pump (IABP), while IMPRESS and CULPRIT-SHOCK trials confirmed heterogeneity in disease spectrum and patient selection for acute myocardial infarction-related CS requiring acute mechanical circulatory support (AMCS). The heterogeneity of devices employed as AMCS, including temporary micro-axial flow pumps (Impella), percutaneous bypass (TandemHeart), and extracorporeal life support (VA-ECMO), contributed to the actual dramatic scenario, where CS is defined clinically rather than hemodynamically. To date, the role of VA-ECMO is emerging as rapid strategy to mitigate mortality rates of severe refractory states, despite the lack of data regarding the best practices of management and flows control. VA-ECMO's flow represents the "dose" of treatment and higher flows are less tolerated percutaneously requiring, to prevent deleterious pulmonary edema and ventricular distention, additional approaches such as pulmonary, left atrial, or left ventricular unloading. Any efforts have to be directed to (1) determine adequate management of patients on VA-ECMO, (2) define the safer duration of VA-ECMO support, and (3) establish algorithms and techniques to predict and obtain stable weaning from ECMO or ensure fast transition to durable VAD and/or heart transplant.

Keywords: ECMO, myocardial recovery, cardiogenic shock, ventricular unloading, VA-ECMO, Impella, ECLS, ECPELLA, ECMO dose retrieval

1. Introduction

Cardiogenic shock (CS) continues to exhibit a high mortality rate (30–60%), despite several therapeutic approaches; recent data derived from the SHOCK II trial [1] questioned the benefit of intra-aortic balloon pump (IABP) in the treatment of the CS. Subsequently, IMPRESS [2] and CULPRIT-SHOCK [3] confirmed heterogeneity in disease spectrum (using a non-hemodynamic clinical definition for CS) and patient selection for AMI-related cardiogenic shock requiring acute mechanical circulatory support (AMCS) with alternative strategies to counterpulsation such as temporary micro-axial flow pumps (Impella), percutaneous left atrium-aortic bypass (TandemHeart) and venoarterial extracorporeal membrane support (VA-ECMO) [4]. In this dramatic clinical scenario, VA-ECMO is emerging as an alternative strategy to mitigate such elevated mortality. Although a beneficial effect on peripheral perfusion/circulation has been demonstrated with VA-ECMO implantation in patients affected by CS, there is a potential for increasing loading conditions into the left ventricle potentially compromising transition to myocardial recovery. Contemporary VA-ECMO systems are now widely used with a broad spectrum of configurations. Due to case mix and implantation timing differences (from report to report and depending on the institutions), outcomes have wide variability and are limited by its retrospective nature and lack of granular profiling prior and after support. The timing of the implantation potentially accounts for further differences in outcomes between different institutions. Central cannulation, when feasible, warrants the best peripheral flows, the best cardiac perfusion, and unloads adequately both ventricles but is still complicated by a high incidence of bleeding and need of multiple re-sternotomy. Moreover, central VA-ECMO is not always bedside available. Despite the growing experience in the use of VA-ECMO, the target flow has still not been identified, and in literature, there is a lack of data regarding best practices with management. Indeed, VA-ECMO flow represents the "dose" of the treatment: the lower dose corresponding to lower flow may be readily achieved through percutaneous cannulation, while the higher the dose or higher flow can be obtained through larger cannulas (**Figure 1**) and may require modifying VA-ECMO configuration during support aiming to prevent the common complications due to overflow. However, a higher flow warrants optimal peripheral organ perfusion, lower venous pressure, and higher mean pressure. The decongestion of the venous side appears a critical factor in recovery end-organ function and is pivotal both for renal and liver function recovery. The building of the circuit should always aim at the lowest venous pressure to restore a normal perfusion pressure despite low continuous flow pressure. On the other hand, high flow not only induces highly turbulent flows, increasing shear stress, and damaging platelets but also increase the quota of shunt and the left ventricular afterload. The latter mechanism may explain the increased risk of pulmonary edema and moreover the reduced hazard of myocardial recovery [5].

Preventing pulmonary edema is one of the principal targets to reduce the biologic impact of VA-ECMO and possibly to maintain the patients extubated and even ambulatory. A large number of possible approaches have been described to aim through a small-incision pulmonary, left atrial, or left ventricular unloading, thus preventing pulmonary edema. The implantation of a double ECLS (extracorporeal life support) circuit (surgical with CentriMag or percutaneous with TandemHeart) thus aiming to reduce all the possible complications due to the need of an oxygenator [6–8] represents one of the possible solutions.

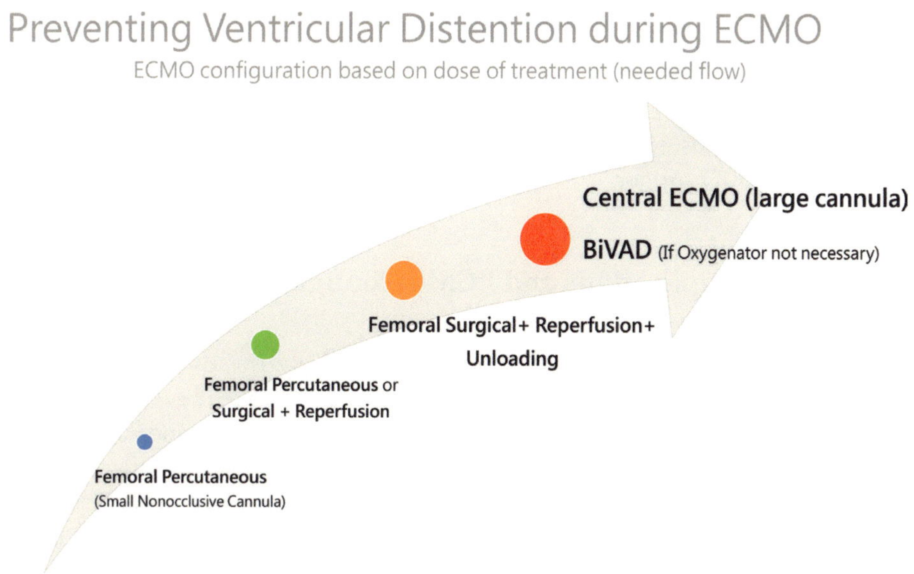

Figure 1. ECMO configuration tailored on needed flow. Representation of the existing relation from type of cannula, site and technique of insertion and flow rates. The figure defines that according to the needed flow the operator may utilize different approaches starting from lower flows provided with a femoral percutaneous small nonocclusive cannula (blue dot) reaching the higher flows with a large cannula in central ECMO or BiVAD.

Today, the first indication of treatment is myocardial recovery as clearly shown both from data coming from leading centers in the VA-ECMO implantation and ELSO registries [9, 10]. This target is more frequently achieved in myocarditis or potentially reversible diseases [11] and stresses the importance of etiological diagnosis at the moment of implantation to define the strategy of implantation. To warrant optimal outcomes, many efforts have to be directed to:

1. Determine adequate management of patients on VA-ECMO.
2. Minimize the time the patient is on VA-ECMO.
3. Establish algorithms and techniques to predict and obtain stable weaning from VA-ECMO.

When pathology is reversible, probably, the quality of myocardial unloading can potentially make an essential difference in the platform for transition (recovery vs. VAD and/or heart transplant). Recent data support the need to reason about a transition to a midterm platform as soon as a stable organ perfusion and function have been warranted, possibly between day 7 [12] and before day 14 [13]. Data emerging on the beneficial effect of early myocardial unloading on the acutely failing hearts with temporary micro-axial flow pumps continue to arise [14–16]; however, there is no clear consensus or longitudinal hemodynamic data to support a specific combination or transition strategy for severe refractory, hemometabolic, and/or biventricular cardiogenic shock, and although it appears that the most commonly described combination is VA-ECMO with LV unloading via an Impella device, the emerging alternative of high-profile biventricular support with combination of Impella 5.0 and RP or percutaneous biatrial VA-ECMO is also possible.

This chapter aims to evaluate best practices and strategies that can be implemented to prevent and reduce ventricular distention and to increase the likelihood of recovery and survival during and after VA-ECMO support.

2. Incidence of complications and ECMO configuration

VA-ECMO currently represents the most effective minimally invasive circulatory support system. VA-ECMO has evolved and can now be placed quickly at the bedside, in the medical unit, or in the cardiac intensive care unit. It provides oxygenation, it is the best option in the setting of associated lung injury, it can be placed peripherally (without thoracotomy), and it is the only percutaneous option for biventricular support. It may provide sufficient support to enable adequate tissue perfusion even in cardiac arrest, and it is a suitable device for acute resuscitation of a patient in shock, even if mortality for cardiogenic shock did not significantly change and is still ranging between 50 and 70% [17].

Moreover, many publications have disclosed a dramatic burden of complications using percutaneous VA-ECMO leading to higher costs and ethical discussions on the right clinical settings for its clinical adoption [9, 18–20].

Looking critically at the landscape of effects and complications of different configurations of mechanical circulatory support and specifically of VA-ECMO emerges the importance to select the right device and the right VA-ECMO's configuration to warrant the best outcome. The crucial factor in selecting the device and the VA-ECMO's configuration is the amount of flow needed to restore organ function. Venous oxygen saturation has been indicated by many authors as a good goal to direct VA-ECMO perfusion [21].

Percutaneous VA-ECMO appears fitted to restore peripheral flows when the patient experiences a moderate reduction of cardiac output. When the patient needs higher flows, the risk of pulmonary edema and left ventricular distention increases [22], and additional cares may be necessary to unload the left ventricle and eventually to restore pulmonary function after pulmonary edema [23–25].

Although a beneficial effect on peripheral perfusion/circulation has been demonstrated with VA-ECMO implantation in patients affected by cardiogenic shock, there is a potential for increasing loading conditions into the left ventricle potentially compromising transition to myocardial recovery. Contemporary VA-ECMO systems are increasingly being used with a wide spectrum of configurations.

3. Destination of VA-ECMO

Contemporary registries and center reports support the ultimate finality of therapy for acute decompensated heart failure being myocardial recovery [26]. When pathology is reversible, the time to recovery on the basis of the etiopathology of the disease plays a pivotal role together with the modality of support aiming to help myocardial healing [27].

Therefore, if during the acute phase of VA-ECMO implantation the "dose" is a critical factor to recovery the end-organ function, the complementary goal is to reduce the biologic impact of support and favor myocardial healing. Many data are emerging in support of a role of myocardial unloading to reach this aim [28]. Data coming out from experimental data on animal and computer simulations seem to support the hypothesis that ventricular unloading is more effective than atrial unloading. Data emerging on the beneficial effect of early myocardial unloading on the acutely failing hearts with temporary micro-axial flow pumps continue to arise; however, there is no clear consensus or data to support a specific combination or transition strategy for severe refractory, hemometabolic, and/or biventricular cardiogenic shock.

VA-ECMO has multiple effects on the left ventricular myocardium:

- The decrease of venous return and the volume work may reduce the wall tension of the heart and subsequently the LVEDV and LVEDP.
- The increase of arterial pressure (MAP) and reduction of venous pressure improve the pressure gradient and then the myocardial perfusion.
- The increase of blood pressure increases afterload and the pressure work of myocardium affecting the Frank-Starling law.

The overall effect of the decrease in volume work and the increase in pressure work depends on the "dose" of VA-ECMO as well as myocardial function and its response to these phenomena. Peripheral ECMO with a high flow may further increase afterload due to the reversal of flow in the most of the aorta [29, 30].

The real question remains if myocardial unloading is always beneficial or potentially detrimental by increasing the complexity of management and when is indeed indicated the transition from ECMO support to ECMO + LV unloading.

Although it appears that the most commonly described combination is VA-ECMO with LV unloading via an Impella device, the emerging alternative of high-profile biventricular support with the combination of Impella 5.0 and RP or percutaneous biatrial ECMO is also possible valuable solutions [31].

Many contradictory data are emerging regarding the effect of VA-ECMO on LV contractile function. LV afterload before ECMO is related to systemic arterial pressure, and the Starling curve generated before initiation of ECMO flow predicts the filling pressure associated with any target SV at that systemic pressure. The addition of ECMO flow or alterations solely in SVR does not alter the relationship between filling pressure and native LV SV, and then the abrupt increase of afterload due to the ECMO flow may be useful to predict ventricular distension during ECMO support [32].

In the presence of severe LV dysfunction, the left ventricle is unable to eject a sufficient volume of blood against the increased afterload caused by the ECMO flow, resulting in impairment of various parameters of LV performance [33–35] and, in extreme situations, the aortic valve can remain closed even during systole.

When VA-ECMO is established due to ongoing cardiogenic shock, it is possible to measure PCWP and LV SV directly. The additional systemic flow conferred by ECMO may be offset by volume reduction of venous return that may cause a reduction in PCWP. When VA-ECMO is established for cardiogenic shock due to right ventricle failure, PCWP is typically low, and the LV is relatively afterload insensitive.

The presence of a pulse pressure depends (without IABP) on the stroke volume of the left ventricle. The absence of arterial pulsatility may prove an appropriate level of support (60–80% of the predicted cardiac output allowing for the remaining 20–40% to pass through the lungs and heart). However, on the other end, it indicates also the inability of the myocardium to overcome the superimposed afterload worsened by a decreased preload and volume work.

When mitral regurgitation is absent, and a significant amount of blood returns in the LV, blood may stagnate within the left ventricle and at the aortic root. The persistent closure of the aortic valve may increase the risk of thrombus formation and subsequent embolic. Besides, the reduction of the stroke volume and of the transmitral flow due to VA-ECMO, the increase of the PCWP, the persistent venous return from thebesian and bronchial veins lead to overdistension of the LV. The distention of the LV measured in terms of LVEDV leads to an LVEDP; impairing coronary perfusion pressure may further worsen the ischemic subendocardial injury to the myocardium. In some instance, left ventricular distension may cause tethering of a previously competent mitral valve causing functional mitral insufficiency due to annular dilation. In this scenario, a pulmonary artery catheter may demonstrate an increase in the telediastolic pulmonary capillary occlusion pressure. The presence of severe mitral regurgitation may worsen left atrial hypertension congesting the pulmonary bed leading to pulmonary edema and even hemorrhage. Functional assessment of the heart in a partially bypassed state can be challenging, but transesophageal echocardiography may aid in confirming aortic valve opening as well as by providing an assessment of the variations of the left ventricular end-diastolic dimension after VA-ECMO institution. The serial evaluation of LVED and of the PCWP should be routinely used during VA-ECMO to give a prompt indication to LV unloading when the simple physiopathologic and/or eventual simulation models do not already suggest the need of an unloading. Recently, the option to first unload and then evaluate the need of VA-ECMO has been prompted. The increase in systemic pressure, in this scenario, is slight, and a modest increase in PCWP would accompany the increase in LV afterload without a significant change in LV SV.

When VA-ECMO is established for cardiogenic shock due to acute LV failure, the magnitude in afterload change depends on the increase of systemic pressure. In this scenario, if PCWP is already high and without a substantial improvement in LV contractility, a dramatic rise in PCWP with LV distension is expected. LV and pulmonary venous distension lead shortly to a massive acute pulmonary edema and blood stasis in the left heart with a serious risk of thrombus formation. Prompt diagnosis and a high suspicion have to be kept in this situation as it is imperative to both unload the central circulation while maintaining a minimal LV SV. The effectiveness of oxygenation and drainage is a vital factor for the diagnosis as if the patient is well drained and perfused; the diagnosis of pulmonary edema may be masked by ECMO. VA-ECMO differs from the standard cardiopulmonary bypass circuit due to the absence of a venous reservoir halting the possibility to control the amount of venous return to the left heart during VA-ECMO; the blood volume bypassing the venous cannula due to incomplete drainage or coursing through the bronchial circulation returns to the left heart; this represents the additional LV output to VA-ECMO flow in the systemic circulation. While this additional flow may be altered by changes in circulating blood volume (e.g., diuresis), the LV will require a preset inflow pressure warranting to deliver a target SV (to prevent blood stasis) depending on the Starling relations. The risk of ventricular distention after initiation of VA-ECMO is related to the preinitiation EF in a setting of high afterload sensitivity as contractile strength is reduced. Even a moderate reduction in pre-ECMO EF (less than 50%) may predict high PCWP after VA-ECMO institution, due to the abrupt increase of systemic pressure and afterload when peripheral cannulation is accomplished.

Placed in the setting of hypotension and cardiogenic shock, the increase in MAP after initiation of VA-ECMO is associated with a significant increase in PCWP and decrease in LV SV, counteracting the emptying of the ventricle and its work.

Careful management of patients on VA-ECMO should include monitoring of intravascular volume status, MAP, and PCWP.

Volume status should be managed in a way to warrant a minimally acceptable LV SV, while the MAP should be kept down acting on VA-ECMO flow rates and by pharmacologic manipulation of SVR. VA-ECMO flows can be reduced in an attempt to reduce afterload. However, this maneuver may not be possible if it compromises oxygen delivery and end-organ perfusion due to the inability of the heart to produce a compensatory increase in native cardiac output. The value of PCWP depends on LV contractility and MAP but not on the method by which MAP is controlled while maintaining a minimal LV SV.

LV overload and distension except for pulmonary edema may induce increased wall stress and myocardial oxygen consumption [36]. During acute decompensation of chronic heart failure leading to cardiogenic shock, the left ventricle is compliant, and the mitral valve is frequently incompetent as a result of chronic annular dilation and mitral valve leaflet tethering. Mitral regurgitation in this setting decompresses the left ventricle to some extent but may result in elevation of left atrial pressure and pulmonary edema [21, 37]. In contrast, acute myocarditis or myocardial infarction is associated with a noncompliant left ventricle and competent mitral valve. LV distension in this setting will result in a significant rise in intraventricular pressure and wall tension, which could be detrimental to the damaged myocardium, and reduced coronary blood flow, causing subendocardial myocardial ischemia [38]. Aortic regurgitation should always be kept into account in ECMO patients due to its potentially detrimental effects [39].

Commonly, myocardial recovery on VA-ECMO support is suggested by an increase in pulse pressure and by improved contractility on echocardiography, but the appearance of pulsatility on the arterial waveform may also reflect a worsening volume overload. Tracking PCWP or repeat echocardiographic assessment may help to ascertain to manage the patient at the best.

The ultimate test of myocardial recovery, however, is accomplished by assessing hemodynamic stability on minimal or no support. Under adequate heparinization, the "dose" of VA-ECMO can be decreased to achieve ~1 L/min of flow or the cannulas can be briefly clamped to ascertain the ability of the native ventricle to handle the full cardiac output. When the myocardium has recovered, during the weaning phases or temporary withdrawal,

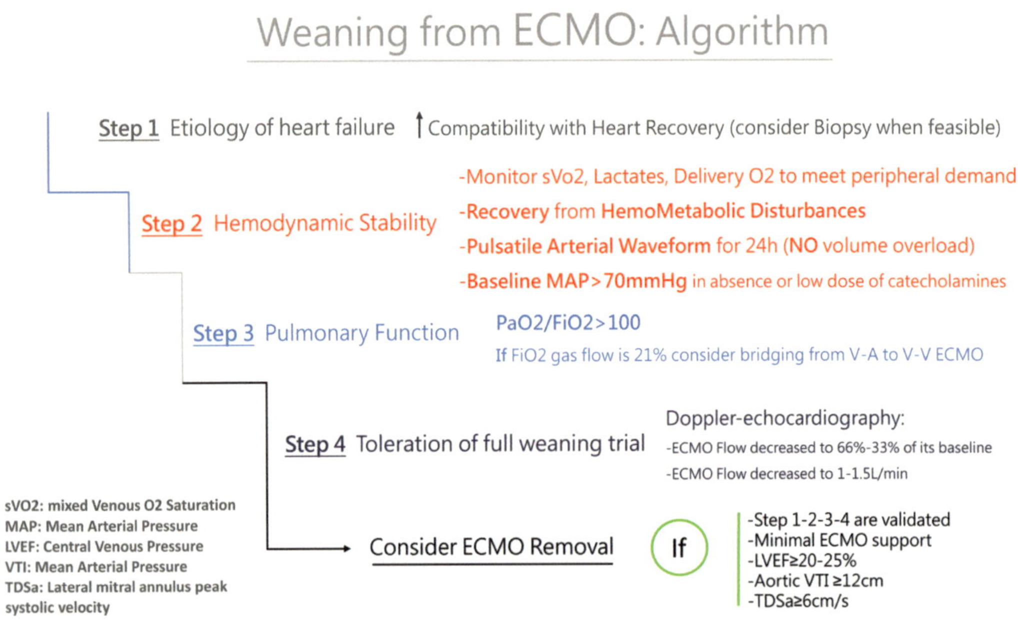

Figure 2. Flow-chart for ECMO management.

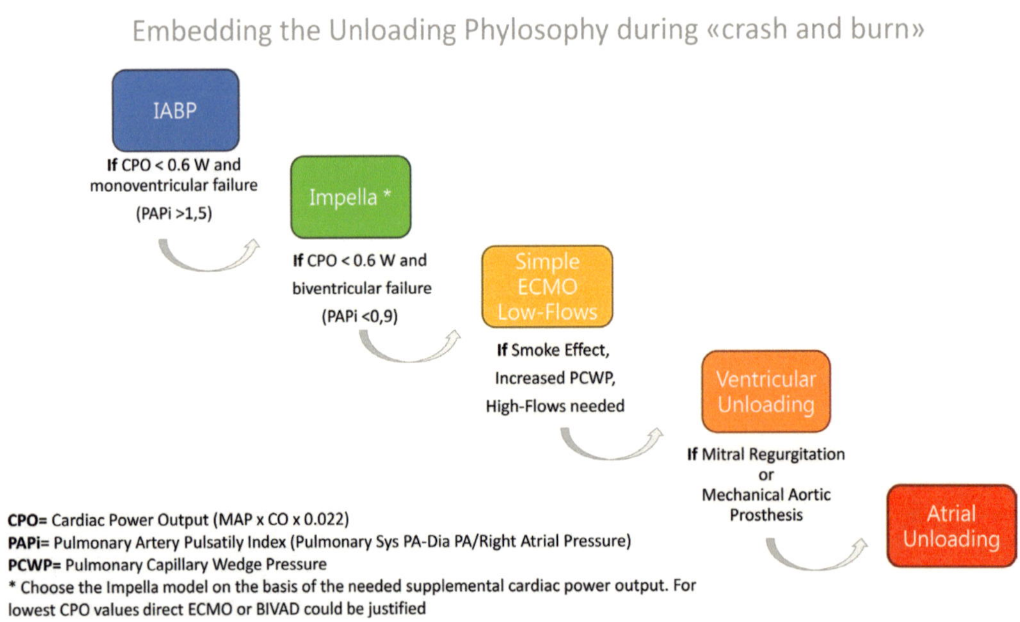

Figure 3. Flow-chart describing the suggested therapeutical strategy according to patient's clinical conditions and needs.

acceptable contractility on echocardiography and stable hemodynamics (MAP, CVP and heart rate) has to be checked. We provide a schematic view of the Flow-chart for ECMO management form step 1 to step 4 and complete weaning (**Figure 2**). Hypotension, a rising

http://dx.doi.org/10.5772/intechopen.80265

CVP, atrial fibrillation, and a poorly contractile myocardium on echocardiography suggest weak recovery and a high risk of need of support [40, 41]. Recently, the group of Esposito and Kapur [42] has suggested a facilitating effect in withdrawal when the patients have an Impella in place to sustain left ventricular function. This knowledge, merged with the knowledge of the need of a short period of ECMO support and to the capability of Impella to interrupt the vicious cycle leading the patient to biventricular failure, may suggest the adoption of Impella when cardiac power output falls under 0.6 and IABP is judged not enough to maintain adequate end-organ perfusion [43], in this case ECMO need has to be evaluated. In **Figure 3**, it has been represented a scheme of the associations between patients' clinical conditions and the suggested therapeutical strategy to face patients' hemodynamic needs.

4. IABP during ECMO

Intra-aortic balloon pump (IABP) has long been clinically applied to augment pulsatility, decrease afterload, and improve blood flow in native coronary arteries and bypass grafts [44, 45].

The inflations and deflations of the 30–50 ml balloon delivered by the IABP device are synchronized with cardiac cycle: the deflation just before systolic ejection aims to decrease afterload and improve LV ejection, while the inflation during diastole warrants increased diastolic perfusion aiming at improve coronary, cerebral, and visceral blood flow.

Despite the controversial data from the Intra-Aortic Balloon Pump in cardiogenic SHOCK (IABP-SHOCK) II trial [1], IABP currently remains one of the most commonly used mechanical circulatory support devices in the treatment of acute heart failure. When administered promptly, it can play a critical role in the rescue of patients with acute myocardial damage, reversing the ongoing vicious cycle leading to death. It has been shown in animal models that IABP may improve several parameters of LV performance during VA-ECMO support [46]. Currently, several centers use IABP during VA-ECMO therapy to reduce LV afterload and warrant pulsatility in the end-organ capillary bed [47]. In a group of 219 patients treated with VA-ECMO after cardiac surgery, Doll et al. [18] found that the use of IABP during ECMO support was associated with a significantly higher survival rate. Ma et al. [48] reported 54 adult patients with acute heart failure who received combined ECMO and IABP support, all of whom showed improvements in terms of overall circulation. Thirty-four of the patients were successfully weaned from mechanical circulatory support, and 21 (39%) survived to hospital discharge. Petroni et al. [49] showed that adding an IABP to peripheral VA-ECMO was associated with improved LV function, and discontinuation of intra-aortic balloon pumping was associated with higher pulmonary artery wedge pressure, increased LV end-, and end-diastolic diameters, while decreasing pulse pressure (15 ± 13 versus 29 ± 22 mmHg; P = 0.02) [49]. Park et al. [50] did not find any mortality or morbidity benefit with IABP in the group of 96 VA-ECMO-treated patients with cardiogenic shock due to acute myocardial infarction. Recent data coming out from the Shock trial suggest that cardiac power output (CPO = cardiac output × MAP × 0.022) may be the best predictor of the effectiveness of IABP during impending cardiogenic shock [51]. Impella or VA-ECMO is needed when CPO is very low or upgrading of the MCS is necessary. Eventually the upgrade to ECMO or ECPELLA

(VA-ECMO + IMPELLA) may portend both optimal perfusion and ventricular unloading aiming to myocardial recovery. Etiologic definition and eventual correction of the cause should be mandatory to increase the chance of recovery.

A marked increase in systemic blood pressure caused by VA-ECMO and retrograde aortic ECMO flow may increase cardiac afterload, together with severe systolic dysfunction, resulting in LV overload with a subsequent increase in left atrial pressure, severe pulmonary edema, myocardial ischemia, elevated pulmonary pressures, blood stasis, and potential thrombus formation, jeopardizing ventricular recovery.

Echocardiographic monitoring should be strictly recommended to detect a fluid overload early, and a Swan-Ganz catheter should be inserted to measure the pulmonary capillary wedge pressure to detect high left ventricular filling pressures as an indicator for left ventricular distension. Ventilation with low tidal volumes and positive end-expiratory pressure (PEEP) has been suggested to keep the lung open. A higher PEEP is advisable in patients with ongoing pulmonary edema. Early extubation is feasible and desired when the patient has a low risk of pulmonary edema because optimal unloading.

To date, there are several possibilities to decrease the likelihood of left ventricular distension on ECMO, but the cohort of patients who benefit from left ventricular venting is unclear.

Decreasing afterload leads to a decrease in workload and O_2 consumption. In case of an extremely poor left ventricular function, it is advisable to administer inotropes with a sufficient mean arterial pressure of 50–60 mmHg. Physiologic lactate levels, normal pH levels, and regular central venous saturations as a guide and flow rates of 2.5–4 L/min are probably sufficient in most cases. Even if sometimes lower pump flow rates also reduce the perfusion-related afterload [21].

Intra-aortic balloon pumping (IABP) concomitant to retrograde aortal perfusion is seen controversial as the inflated balloon in the descending aorta might hinder proper perfusion. IABP counterpulsation is a device that inflates and deflates a 30–50 cm balloon in the descending aorta. The balloon inflations and deflations are synchronized with cardiac cycle, and, therefore, deflation just before systolic ejection may decrease afterload and improve LV ejection. Moreover, increased diastolic pressure on IABP could also improve coronary blood flow [52, 53].

Despite the general expectations that IABP is useful during VA-ECMO for a supposed "perfusion benefit" which indeed is overcome by ECMO blood flow, our belief is that the rationale of the combined use of VA-ECMO and IABP is to provide a pressure unloading to the left ventricle especially when a certain amount of residual SV is provided by the native circulation.

Although in a very unstable patient ECMO can stabilize end organs and restore their function, the lack of left ventricular unloading and reduced ventricular work threaten the myocardium worsening the already impaired myocardial performance superimposing an extremely high afterload further compromising wall tension and myocardial oxygen demand. Multiple studies have shown that coronary perfusion worsens, especially if the patient is cannulated peripherally. Because relative cerebral or coronary hypoxia occurs in many situations due to a "watershed" effect, it is imperative to check blood saturations at multiple sites to determine if perfusion is adequate everywhere to avoid to misdiagnose the "Harlequin syndrome" due to inadequate mixing of the two parallel circulations (ECMO and native heart) [23, 54, 55].

As a matter of fact, IABP should be already in place at the time of VA-ECMO implantation, as stated by ELSO Guidelines 2017 [www.elso.org]. For those patients who do not have one, it should be placed via the contralateral femoral artery, associating earlier the hemodynamic effects of IABP to those of VA-ECMO; from a mechanistic point of view IABP could neutralize some of the unwanted effects of VA-ECMO [56].

The role of IABP in patients suffering from cardiogenic shock should be highlighted as (I) it is rapidly deployable at any hospital and therefore reduces the duration of "uncontrolled shock"; (II) it allows, thereafter, safe transport to MCS units; (III) it does allow foe exploiting the same vascular access for Impella implant; and (IV) it has a major role in weaning from VA-ECMO and therefore reduces the burden of the complications related to ECLS.

Despite the controversial data from the intra-aortic balloon pump in cardiogenic SHOCK (IABP-SHOCK) II trial, which could not demonstrate a survival benefit for the IABP application, IABP currently remains one of the most commonly used mechanical circulatory support devices in the treatment of acute heart failure. The bad news is that for none of the percutaneous devices, used in LV venting, a survival benefit has yet been documented in adequately sized randomized clinical trials (RCTs). A meta-analysis, by Cheng et al., including a total of 100 patients in three small RCTs with the TandemHeart and the Impella PL2.5 pump did not see a survival benefit in comparison to the IABP, despite better hemodynamic effects [57].

When administered in a timely manner, IABP can play a critical role in the rescue of patients with acute myocardial damage. It has been shown in animal models that insertion of IABP during VA-ECMO support may improve several parameters of LV performance and can reduce mean arterial pressure as well as oxygen saturation in the coronary sinus [24].

The combination of IABP and VA-ECMO can be found in the nationwide Japanese Diagnosis Procedure Combination national inpatient database; IABP combined with VA-ECMO was associated with reduced mortality and successful weaning from VA-ECMO. They also concluded, of course, that randomized controlled studies are required to confirm the mortality-reducing effect of the combination of IABP and VA-ECMO [57].

Despite the lack of clarity, in a systematic literature search, the use of concomitant IABP with ECMO is widespread. IABP was present in approximately 55% of all ECMO cases reviewed, stretching across all etiologies of cardiac failure beyond acute myocardial infarction (AMI).

The rationale for concomitant IABP use is primarily for LV venting [58]. The incremental benefit of IABP support for afterload reduction and increasing organ perfusion in the presence of ECMO support is relatively minimal. Regarding improved diastolic pressures and coronary flow, despite the previously held belief of an estimated 11% survival benefit from pooled analyses of retrospective studies of IABP use in AMI, it is now known from the prospective and randomized IABP-SHOCK II study that the use of IABP in this cohort had no survival benefit [59].

Early IABP, or, when CPO is very low and Impella offering the adequate flow, would significantly impact the management of cardiogenic shock as it would avoid the administration of "toxic doses" of inotropes, allowing for smoother transition to VA-ECMO and routine unloading of the LV [44–60].

Even though, the combined use of IABP and VA-ECMO or Impella and VA-ECMO is well described to improve the hemodynamic facilitating and supporting conditions for recovery or ventricular assist device implantation [61, 62].

Recently, a simulation published on the ASAIO Journal [63] has supported the relevance of optimal medical management, fluid removal while minimizing VA-ECMO flow, reducing blood pressure, and eventually adding inotropes to reduce PCWP and prevent pulmonary edema [64]. Recent clinical data support this notion for different clinical settings and do not advocate a routine combination of VA-ECMO and IABP. Clinical studies have shown a slight reduction in PCWP, LV dimensions, and pulmonary edema in-line with the computer simulation [65].

Patients showing PCWP above 25 mmHg or a virtually non-ejecting LV will require interventional or surgical adjunct measures, which theoretically reduce PCWP by more than 5 mmHg. It has to be kept in mind that sometimes when you think of adding an unloading is too late for the patient, a proactive management reasoning on the patient characteristics and hemodynamics is pivotal.

In a recent computer simulation, this combined approach showed only limited LV unloading, although pulsatility and increased stroke volume were noted. The CPO before VA-ECMO implantation and the native heart stroke volume after VA-ECMO implantation could be relevant determinants of the effectiveness of IABP also during VA-ECMO perfusion (**Figure 3**), while a low PAPi may push toward biventricular support with Impella or TandemHeart.

5. Differences between atrial and ventricular unloading

When echocardiographic monitoring discloses surrogates of low contractility, LV distention or high filling pressure (PCWP) of the left ventricle, inotropic support should be considered or up titrated to increase contractility of the myocardium, and volume load should be assessed and eventually treated. Other conditions to be considered as drivers for unloading need have been represented in (**Figure 4**).

There are different drivers for atrial or ventricular unloading (**Figure 5**).

The kind of left side's chamber decompression is strictly related to the mechanism of pulmonary congestion and left ventricular distension. The variables that need to be kept in mind are:

- Adequacy of venous drainage: if the venous drainage may be considered poor, placement of pulmonary artery or left atrial drainage (comprised septostomy) may be sufficient.
- Mitral regurgitation: atrial drainage may be sufficient to unload the ventricle if a significant mitral regurgitation impedes the distension of the left ventricle.

http://dx.doi.org/10.5772/intechopen.80265

- Reversibility of left ventricle damage: ventricular unloading is pivotal to increase the chance of recovery.
- Aortic regurgitation: addressing aortic valve may be needed to avoid blood recirculation and stagnation.

Figure 6 shows the decisional process of management of conditions that may require unloading if not properly treated, the only condition where unloading seems to be mandatory is smoking effect or slow flow through the MV. **Figure 7** shows the possible surgical invasive, minimally invasive and percutaneous approaches aiming at ventricle unloading. When atrial unloading may be sufficient, a percutaneous left atrial septostomy may be accomplished, which allows blood from the LA to drain down its pressure gradient into the right atrium (RA) to then be drained via the venous cannula. This procedure is quite common in many hemodynamic lab especially used to treat pediatric patients. A cannula may also be placed into the LA through a transseptal puncture to facilitate drainage [66]. In addition, the left atrium or left ventricle can be directly cannulated allowing blood to be vented into the venous arm of the ECMO circuit. The transition to a BiVAD (TandemHeart or Centrimag or Rotaflow) could be considered if the oxygenator is no longer needed [67]. Finally, the use of a left ventricular assist device such as the Impella (Abiomed, Danvers, MA) or BiPella (left and right Impella RP) [68] to provide left ventricular decompression as well as forward flow has been described and is gaining success due to its ease also bedside.

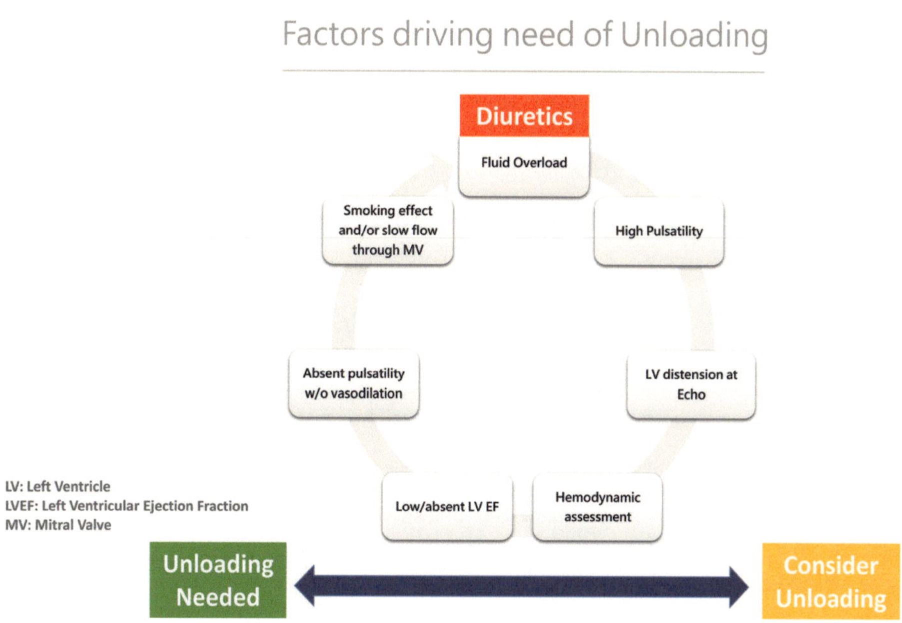

Figure 4. Factors driving unloading need in crash and burn patients. It has to be considered the possibility of unloading LV if signs of fluid overload (high pulsatility and LV distension at Echo and hemodynamic data) are not effectively treated with diuretics. Unloading is needed when there is low or absent LVEF, absent pulsatility without vasodilatation, smoking effect or slow flow through the MV.

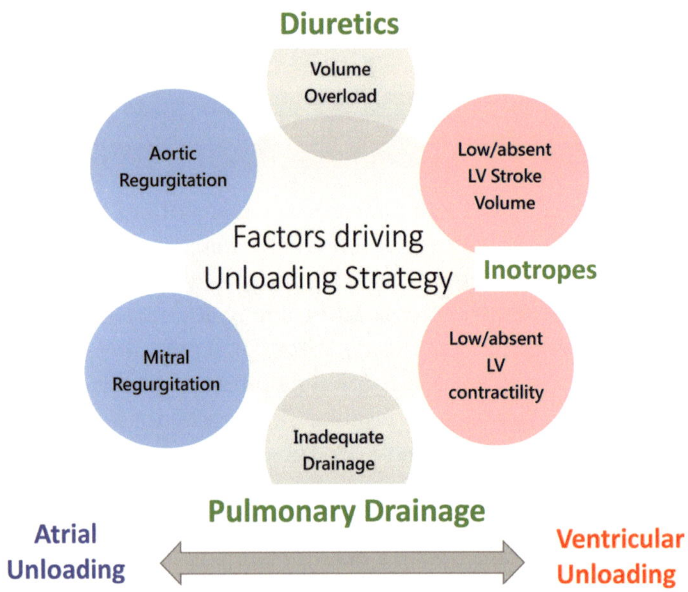

Figure 5. Atrial or ventricular unloading, decision making graph. In the graph, the pathological conditions in the blue dots are drivers of ventricular unloading while that ones in the red dots are drivers for atrial decompression. In green the first step therapy according to etiology.

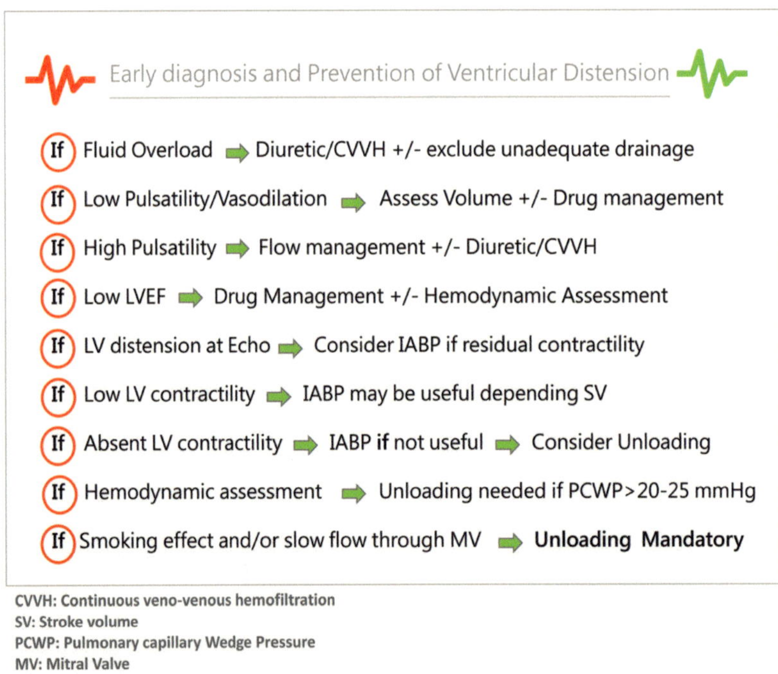

Figure 6. Management of conditions that may require unloading if not properly treated.

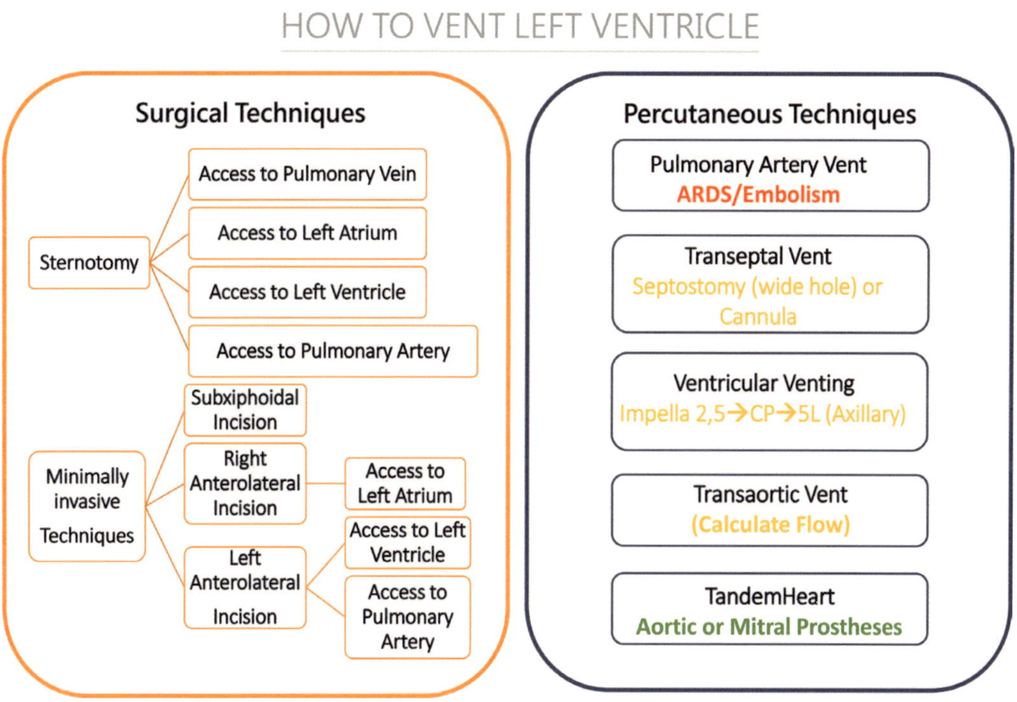

Figure 7. Surgical invasive, minimally invasive and percutaneous approaches to ventricle unloading.

Left-to-right shunt can achieve effective decompression of the left ventricle in the setting of VA-ECMO at the presence of atrial communication (atrial septal defect or patent foramen ovale); atrial shunt can be, however, created also artificially with a percutaneous blade or balloon septostomy [69]. The procedure may be fruitful to induce pulmonary decongestion reducing atrial pressure and pulmonary edema but led to a suboptimal LV decompression.

An alternative way to perform atrial unloading, under guidance by bedside transoesophageal echocardiography, is by transseptal puncture and placement of a drain (8 Fr to 15 Fr). The percutaneous atrial transseptal cannula can then be placed and connected to the inflow part of the ECMO circuit, thus, decompressing the pulmonary circulation [70].

The left ventricle can be vented directly by placing a transaortic vent through the axillary artery or by echocardiography-guided insertion of a pigtail catheter into the left ventricle through the aortic valve and connected to the inflow part of the ECMO circuit [71]. Fumagalli et al. [72] achieved the decompression with a catheter placed percutaneously through the aortic valve into the left ventricle. The blood drained from the left ventricle was pumped into the femoral artery through the VA-ECMO circuit. The normalization of left heart filling pressures led to the resolution of pulmonary edema, and the patient underwent successful heart transplantation. Barbone et al. [73] claimed LV unloading with a 7 Fr pigtail catheter inserted into the left ventricle via the femoral artery contralateral to the arterial outflow cannula. Using this approach in three different patients, the authors described resolution of LV distension and prevention of lung congestion without major complications. However, a so long and tight

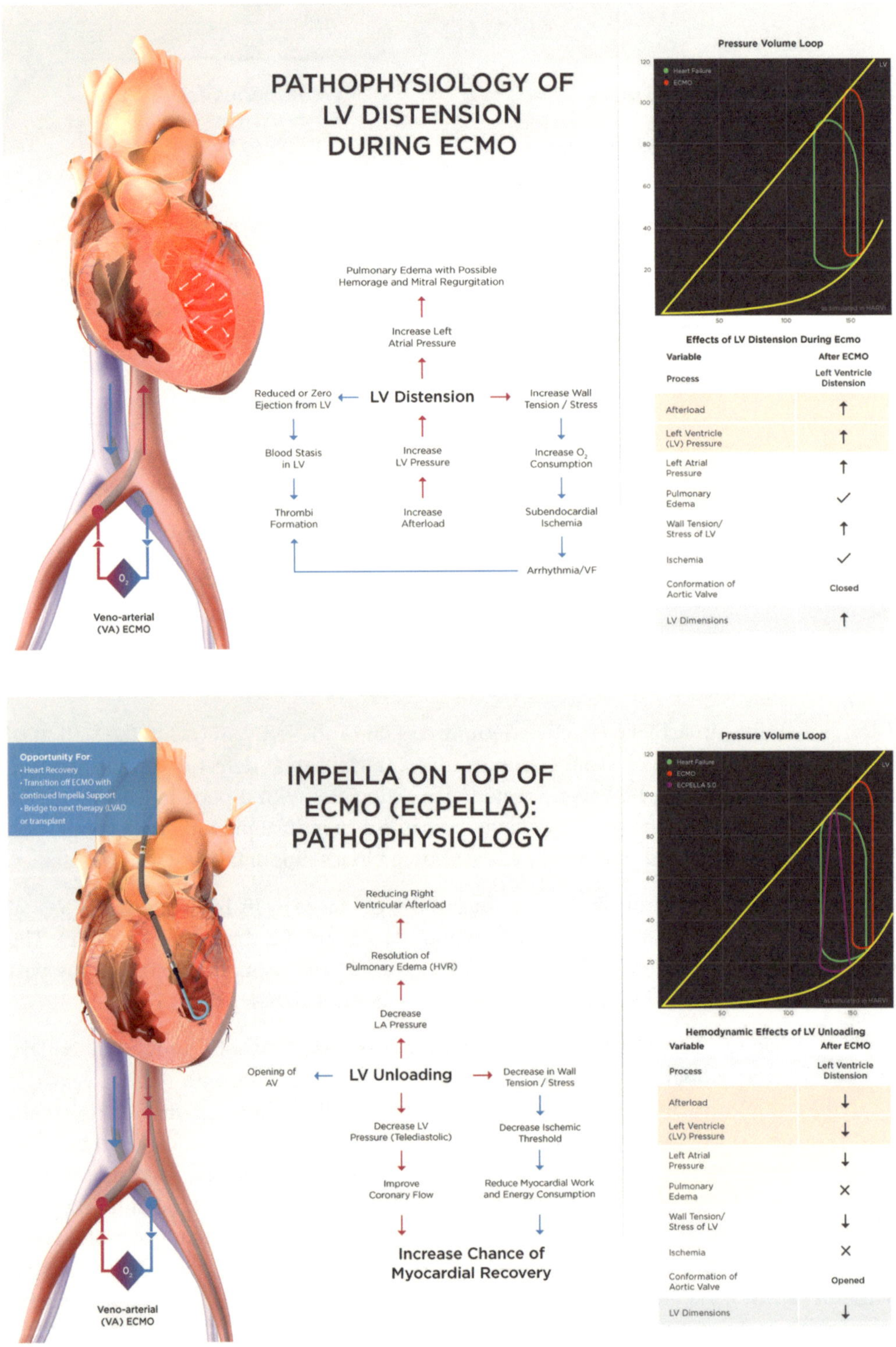

Figure 8. Techniques to unload the heart during ECMO. (1) Pathophysiology of LV distension during ECMO and (2) Impella on top of ECMO (ECPELLA): pathophysiology.

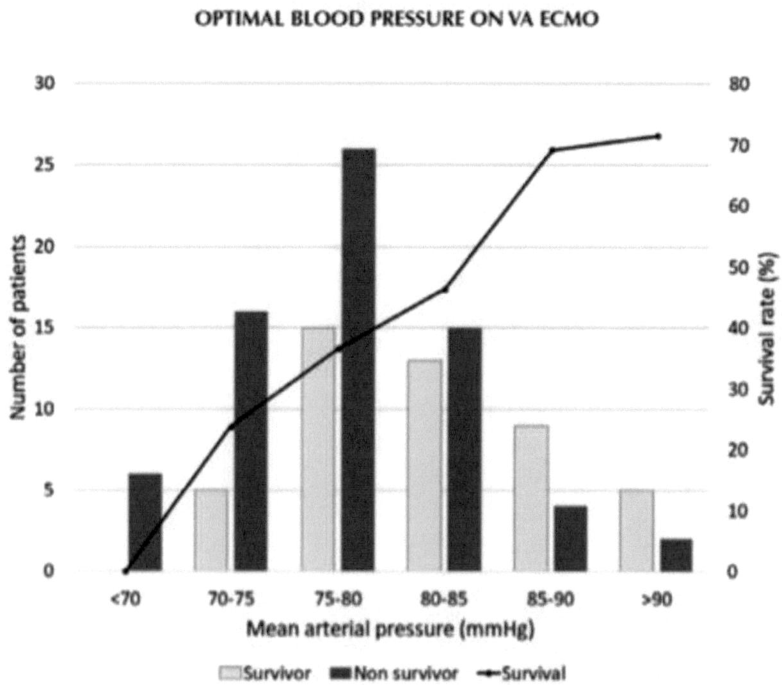

Figure 9. Optimal Arterial Pressure on VA-ECMO (Copyright from ASAIO).

line may be argued ineffective to warrant a large amount of drainage as it is generally needed. Indeed, a recent paper indicates an algorithm to select the right dimension of the pig aiming to reach the right unloading flow [74].

An alternative approach to LV decompression is the percutaneous insertion of a venous cannula into the pulmonary artery and connection of this cannula to the inflow part of the ECMO circuit [75]. A small (15 Fr) venous cannula may be placed percutaneously to the pulmonary artery and connected to the ECMO circuit to decompress the left heart and to facilitate LV function. Surgical minimal invasive access to directly drain the pulmonary artery has been also suggested.

Impella (Abiomed Inc., USA) is a catheter-based transaortic axial flow pump that can be introduced through a percutaneous femoral approach. The device is placed across the aortic valve and pumps up (2.5–5 L/min) of blood on the basis of the model (2.5, CP or 5 L) from the left ventricle to the ascending aorta. The 2.5 and the CP are placed in the groin percutaneously while the 5.0 is generally placed surgically in the right axillary artery to warrant to the patient the possibility to be extubated and ambulatory.

Koeckert et al. [75] reported the use of Impella LP 2.5 for left ventricle decompression in a 70-year-old man with acutely decompensated heart failure who was placed on VA-ECMO for cardiogenic shock with severe pulmonary edema and respiratory failure. Both devices were successfully weaned on day 5 after myocardial recovery. Narain et al. [76] described a case involving 31-year-old man with fulminant myocarditis treated with the Impella device and

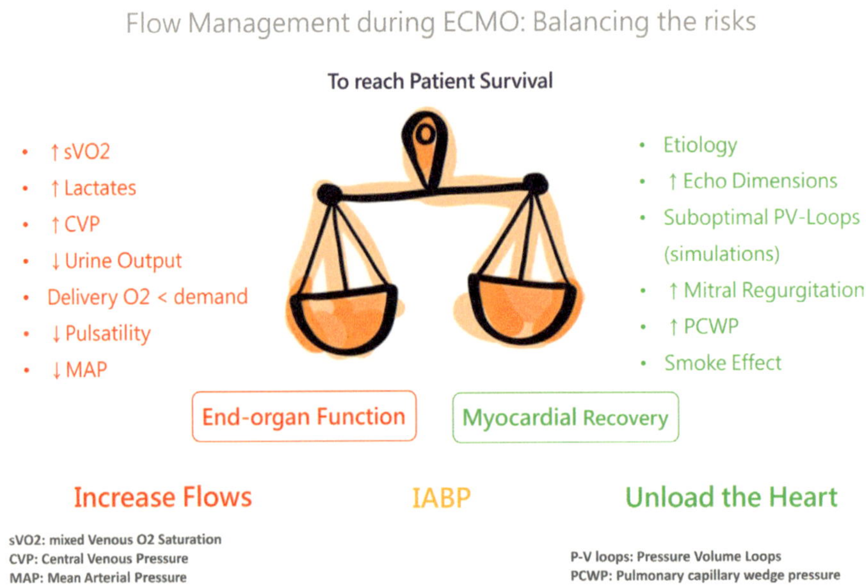

Figure 10. Patient survival from end-organ function to myocardial recovery.

VA-ECMO. On full mechanical circulatory support, the hemodynamic status improved, and both systems were explanted after 48 h. Many centers are now moving toward the adoption of Impella as bailout for weaning and to unload the ventricle during VA-ECMO even if many warnings have been expressed regarding the risks to add more complexity to the management of an already complex patient [77, 78]. **Figure 8** shows the pathophisiology of Left Ventricle distention due to ECMO (**Figure 8-1**) and the effects of adding Impella during ECMO (**Figure 8-2**).

Figure 9 shows all the possible surgical and percutaneous solutions to unload the left circulation, preventing pulmonary edema and, possibly, facilitating the myocardial recovery when the underlying disease is potentially reversible. According to what said before, to reach patient survival, from end-organ function to myocardial recovery, we should balance arterial pressure, flow rate and unloading passing through IABP if necessary. The delicate balance of this therapeutical strategy is described in **Figure 10**.

6. Arterial pressure management during ECMO

While maintenance of flows is crucial to the care of the patient on VA-ECMO, attention must also be paid to the mean arterial pressure, as the end organs require both a cardiac output and a perfusion pressure for optimal function and a low venous pressure. A goal MAP >65 mmHg may be used as a starting point but can be adjusted either lower or higher given individual circumstances keeping in mind that the differential pressure between MAP and LAP is the driving force of organ perfusion and function. On the other side, MAP should never exceed 90 mmHg to limit afterload and to promote forward flow, especially when peripheral cannulation limits the adequacy of drainage and leaves a remarkable amount of blood stagnating in the lung bed. A recent paper on the ASAIO Journal showed an inverse relationship between mortality and MAP in VA-ECMO but not in VV-ECMO (**Figure 10**) [79]. In the hypotensive patient, MAP may be increased by manipulating either CO or SVR. The total cardiac output of the body is composed of native cardiac output and VA-ECMO flows. Thus, hypotension may potentially be corrected by increasing VA-ECMO flows and its contribution to total CO. Assuming a centrifugal pump, this may be achieved by administering volume or by increasing the RPMs of the pump. If the problem is related to SVR, such as with septic shock, a vasoconstrictor may be needed to increase MAP, although this must be weighed against the effect of increased afterload and the increase in pressure work of the left ventricle.

Many different policies exist on the management of arterial pressure during VA-ECMO: one concern is about the equivalence of MAP in patients with or without pulsatility. Physiologic autoregulation is pivotal for end-organ perfusion and particularly for the brain and kidney. Many studies dealt with ideal MAP value in the ICU patient, the most identify a cutoff of 65 mmHg, as a value usually sufficient also if the study [80] suggested a MAP of 75–85 as protective for acute kidney injury in patients with a previous history of hypertension. To our knowledge, however, there has been only few studies examining optimal MAP for patients on ECMO and evidences in support of every practice are still weak.

Clearly, the physiology of VA-ECMO patients is considerably different from other critically ill patients. Several studies identified to determine the optimal pressure on cardiopulmonary bypass (CPB) during cardiac surgery [81–83] and the majority supports a MAP higher than 70 mm Hg on CPB. VA-ECMO is quite different from CPB: CPB is usually initiated electively for patients on stable patients, while VA-ECMO intervenes on an unstable circulatory condition. Moreover, the circuit is not open as in the CPB, the heart is not arrested, and there is not a reservoir to avoid pulmonary fluid overload. The heart is in a dynamic parallel circulation with ECMO aiming to reach an equilibrium to eject against incoming blood flow from the ECMO circuit. The amount of workload may often be incompatible with the failing heart performance of most VA-ECMO patients. VA-ECMO could induce increased afterload and further worsen myocardial dysfunction. If a lower MAP could have the rationale to permit the heart to eject against a lower resistance decreasing the myocardial oxygen demand, the clinical impact of hypotension on the patient in cardiogenic shock has to be carefully judged. Furthermore, it may not be suitable to compare the MAP of patients with and without pulsatility because patients without pulsatility may require a higher MAP for end-organ perfusion. It may not be suitable to compare the MAP of patients with and without pulsatility because patients without pulsatility may require a higher MAP for end-organ perfusion.

Pulsatility is a dynamic property due to the interaction between the two concurrent parallel circulations; indeed a loss of pulsatility may signal worsening myocardial function, while the appearance of pulsatility or an improvement in pulse pressure may signal recovery. However, the loss of pulsatility may also suggest that VA-ECMO flows are too high, so reducing the amount of blood managed from the impaired native circulation. The higher the ECMO flows, the more blood that drains into the circuit causing a more significant decrease in LV preload, stroke volume, and pulse pressure. Total bypass, where the ECMO circuit takes over 100% of the cardiac output, creates a flat, non-pulsatile arterial tracing and signifies the lack of ejection of blood from the left ventricle. A recent study from Sakir Akin and the Erasmus group has shown how the peripheral recovery of pulsatility is a predictor of recovery that should push to weaning of ECMO [84].

Reduced pulsatility may also reflect a decrease in intravascular volume or a mechanical cause of decreased venous return (i.e., atrial tamponade) that may cause a decrease in LV preload leading decreased stroke volume and pulse pressure.

VA-ECMO reduces the volume work of the right ventricle through the decreased RV preload, while pulmonary edema may cause hypoxic pulmonary vasoconstriction worsening pulmonary hypertension and increasing RV pressure work. If this setting, the right ventricle may be unable to pump to the left side of the heart, flattening arterial pressure waveform and decreasing the stroke volume. Nitric oxide with inodilators such as milrinone and dobutamine (which will also provide inotropic assistance) are needed. If systemic pressures allow, nitroglycerin or nitroprusside may also be utilized.

7. Conclusions

Today, the first indication of treatment is weaning from ECMO and myocardial recovery. This target is more frequently achieved in myocarditis or potentially reversible diseases and stresses the importance of etiological diagnosis at the moment of implantation to define the strategy of implantation. In **Figure 11** there is a flow chart that clarifies how VA-ECMO should be managed, according to the etiology, to reach the weaning from ECMO goal and myocardial recovery, analysing the phases of the hemodynamic support and detecting unloading need at the right time.

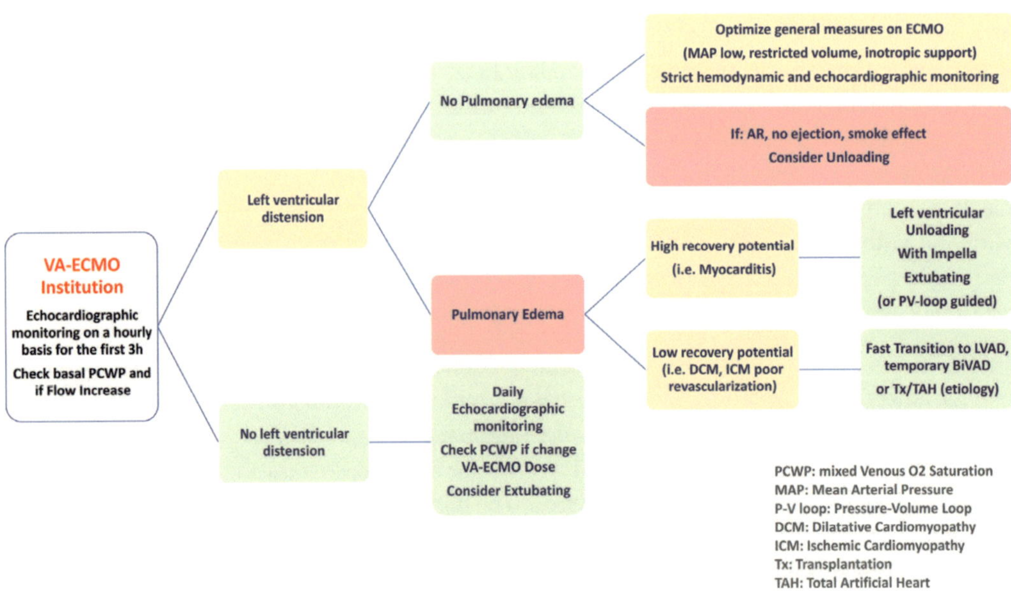

Figure 11. Flow chart on VA-ECMO management according to etiology.

http://dx.doi.org/10.5772/intechopen.80265

VA-ECMO has to be deemed as temporary short-term support, and the risks related to the permanence of an oxygenator must focus on a rapid transition to further MCS systems. The assessment of left atrial pressure (direct or indirect) should be a mandatory tool in patients with VA-ECMO to increase the chance of recovery or transition to next support or treatment. When left atrial pressure is deemed increased in surgical unloading, or percutaneous unloading has to be considered preferring whenever possible ventricular unloading especially when mitral regurgitation is absent.

Randomized trials and registries will have to answer some of the open questions the clinician has to solve daily, dealing with the patient on VA-ECMO:

- Which goal directs the "dose" of VA-ECMO?
- Does one VA-ECMO configuration fit all?
- When unload before and when after VA-ECMO institution?
- Which clinical and hemodynamic profiles favor upfront VA-ECMO with LV venting?
- To vent or not to vent?
- When is vent mandatory?
- How vent without harm the patient?
- Should we transition to durable LVAD or BiVAD as soon as the end organs recovers?
- What are the granular aspects of management that should be included in trial design for VA-ECMO and LV venting?

Acknowledgements

Cristiano Amarelli acknowledges the Abiomed for the figures freely provided on the association between ECMO and Impella.

This section of your manuscript may also include funding information.

Conflict of interest

No conflict of interest to declare.

Notes/thanks/other declarations

Thanks to IntechOpen for trusting and awaiting for the work to be finished.

Author details

Cristiano Amarelli[1]*, Francesco Musumeci[2], Antonio Loforte[3], Andrea Montalto[2], Sveva Di Franco[4] and Jaime Hernandez-Montfort[5]

*Address all correspondence to: camarell@tiscali.it

1 Department of Cardiac Surgery and Transplants, Monaldi Azienda dei Colli, Napoli, Italy

2 Department of Heart and Vessels, Cardiac Surgery Unit and Heart Transplantation Center, S. Camillo-Forlanini Hospital, Rome, Italy

3 Department of Cardiovascular Surgery and Transplantation, S. Orsola-Malpighi Hospital, Bologna University, Bologna, Italy

4 Department of Anaesthesiology and Critical Care Medicine, L. Vanvitelli University, Naples, Italy

5 Department of Cardiology, University of Texas Medical Branch, Galveston, USA

References

[1] Thiele H, Zeymer U, Neumann F-J, Ferenc M, Olbrich H-G, Hausleiter J, et al. Intraaortic balloon support for myocardial infarction with cardiogenic shock. New England Journal of Medicine. 2012;**367**(14):1287-1296. DOI: 10.1056/NEJMoa1208410

[2] Ouweneel DM, Eriksen E, Sjauw KD, van Dongen IM, Hirsch A, Packer EJS, et al. Impella CP versus intra-aortic balloon pump in acute myocardial infarction complicated by cardiogenic shock: The IMPRESS trial. Journal of the American College of Cardiology. 2017;**69**(3):278-287. DOI: 10.1016/j.jacc.2016.10.022. [Epub 2016 Oct 31]

[3] Thiele H, Akin I, Sandri M, Fuernau G, de Waha S, Meyer-Saraei R, et al. PCI strategies in patients with acute myocardial infarction and cardiogenic shock. New England Journal of Medicine. 2017;**377**(25):2419-2432. DOI: 10.1056/NEJMoa1710261

[4] Csepe TA, Kilic A. Advancements in mechanical circulatory support for patients in acute and chronic heart failure. Journal of Thoracic Disease. 2017;**9**(10). Retrieved from: http://jtd.amegroups.com/article/view/16372

[5] Kawashima D, Gojo S, Nishimura T, Itoda Y, Kitahori K, Motomura N, et al. Left ventricular mechanical support with impella provides more ventricular unloading in heart failure than extracorporeal membrane oxygenation. ASAIO Journal. 2011;**57**(3):169-176. DOI: 10.1097/MAT.0b013e31820e121c. Retrieved from: https://journals.lww.com/asaiojournal/Fulltext/2011/05000/Left_Ventricular_Mechanical_Support_with_Impella.5.aspx

[6] Amarelli C, Mastroianni C, Brechot N. Prompt diagnosis of a new clinical entity: Membrane oxygenator infection during ECMO. ASAIO Journal. 2013;**59**(4):367. DOI: 10.1097/MAT.0b013e31829c5d21

[7] Beely BM, Campbell JE, Meyer A, Langer T, Negaard K, Chung KK, et al. Electron microscopy as a tool for assessment of anticoagulation strategies during extracorporeal life support: The proof is on the membrane. ASAIO Journal. 2016;**62**(5):525-532. DOI: 10.1097/MAT.0000000000000394. Retrieved from: https://journals.lww.com/asaiojournal/Fulltext/2016/09000/Electron_Microscopy_as_a_Tool_for_Assessment_of.5.aspx

[8] Wilm J, Philipp A, Müller T, Bredthauer A, Gleich O, Schmid C, et al. Leukocyte adhesion as an indicator of oxygenator thrombosis during extracorporeal membrane oxygenation therapy? ASAIO Journal. 2018;**64**(1):24-30. DOI: 10.1097/MAT.0000000000000586. Retrieved from https://journals.lww.com/asaiojournal/Fulltext/2018/01000/Leukocyte_Adhesion_as_an_Indicator_of_Oxygenator.4.aspx

[9] Karagiannidis C, Brodie D, Strassmann S, et al. Extracorporeal membrane oxygenation: Evolving epidemiology and mortality. Intensive Care Medicine. 2016;**42**:889-896

[10] Smith M, Vukomanovic A, Brodie D, Thiagarajan R, Rycus P, Buscher H. Duration of veno-arterial extracorporeal life support (VA ECMO) and outcome: An analysis of the extracorporeal life support organization (ELSO) registry. Critical Care. 2017;**21**(1):45. DOI: 10.1186/s13054-017-1633-1

[11] Nakamura T, Ishida K, Taniguchi Y, Nakagawa T, Seguchi M, Wada H. Prognosis of patients with fulminant myocarditis managed by peripheral venoarterial extracorporeal membranous oxygenation support: A retrospective single-center study. Journal of Intensive Care. 2015;**3**(1). DOI: 10.1186/s40560-014-0069-9

[12] Rousse N, Juthier F, Pinçon C, Hysi I, Banfi C, Robin E, et al. ECMO as a bridge to decision: Recovery, VAD, or heart transplantation? International Journal of Cardiology. 2015;**187**(1):620-627. DOI: 10.1016/j.ijcard.2015.03.283

[13] Durinka JB, Bogar LJ, Hirose H, Brehm C, Koerner MM, Pae WE, et al. End organ recovery is key to success for extracorporeal membrane oxygenation as a bridge to implantable left ventricular assist device. ASAIO Journal (American Society for Artificial Internal Organs: 1992). 2014;**60**(2):189-192. DOI: 10.1097/MAT.0000000000000043

[14] Cheng A, Swartz MF, Massey HT. Impella to unload the left ventricle during peripheral extracorporeal membrane oxygenation. ASAIO Journal. 2013;**59**(5):533-536. DOI: 10.1097/MAT.0b013e31829f0e52

[15] Pappalardo F, Schulte C, Pieri M, Schrage B, Contri R, Soeffker G, et al. Concomitant implantation of Impella® on top of veno-arterial extracorporeal membrane oxygenation may improve survival of patients with cardiogenic shock. European Journal of Heart Failure. 2017;**19**(3):404-412. DOI: 10.1002/ejhf.668

[16] Patel SM, Lipinski J, Al-Kindi SG, Patel T, Saric P, Li J, et al. Simultaneous venoarterial extracorporeal membrane oxygenation and percutaneous left ventricular decompression therapy with impella is associated with improved outcomes in refractory cardiogenic shock. ASAIO Journal. 2018:1. DOI: 10.1097/MAT.0000000000000767. [Epub ahead of print]

[17] Goldberg RJ, Spencer FA, Gore JM, Lessard D, Yarzebski J. Thirty-year trends (1975 to 2005) in the magnitude of, management of, and hospital death rates associated with cardiogenic shock in patients with acute myocardial infarction a population-based perspective. Circulation. 2009;**119**(9):1211-1219. DOI: 10.1161/CIRCULATIONAHA.108.814947

[18] Doll N, Kiaii B, Borger M, et al. Five-year results of 219 consecutive patients treated with extracorporeal membrane oxygenation for refractory postoperative cardiogenic shock. The Annals of Thoracic Surgery. 2004;**77**:151-157

[19] Sauer CM, Yuh DD, Bonde P. Extracorporeal membrane oxygenation use has increased by 433% in adults in the United States from 2006 to 2011. ASAIO Journal. 2015;**61**(1):31-36. DOI: 10.1097/MAT.0000000000000160

[20] Han JJ, Swain JBD. The perfect ECMO candidate. Journal of the American College of Cardiology. 2018;**71**(10):1178-1182. DOI: 10.1016/j.jacc.2018.02.001

[21] Chung M, Shiloh AL, Carlese A. Monitoring of the adult patient on venoarterial extracorporeal membrane oxygenation. The Scientific World Journal. 2014;**2014**:393258. DOI: 10.1155/2014/393258

[22] Truby LK, Takeda K, Mauro C, Yuzefpolskaya M, Garan AR, Kirtane AJ, et al. Incidence and implications of left ventricular distention during venoarterial extracorporeal membrane oxygenation support. ASAIO Journal. 2017;**63**(3):257-265. DOI: 10.1097/MAT.0000000000000553

[23] Rupprecht L, Flörchinger B, Schopka S, et al. Cardiac decompression on extracorporeal life support: A review and discussion of the literature. ASAIO Journal. 2013;**59**(6):547-553. DOI: 10.1097/MAT.0b013e3182a4b2f6

[24] Strunina S, Ostadal P. Left ventricle unloading during veno-arterial extracorporeal membrane oxygenation. Current Research: Cardiology. 2016;**3**(1):5-8

[25] Bernhardt AM, Hillebrand M, Yildirim Y, Hakmi S, Wagner FM, Blankenberg S, et al. Percutaneous left atrial unloading to prevent pulmonary oedema and to facilitate ventricular recovery under extracorporeal membrane oxygenation therapy. Interactive Cardiovascular and Thoracic Surgery. 2018;**26**(1):4-7. DOI: 10.1093/icvts/ivx266

[26] Flecher E, Anselmi A, Corbineau H, Langanay T, Verhoye J-P, Felix C, et al. Current aspects of extracorporeal membrane oxygenation in a tertiary referral Centre: Determinants of survival at follow-up. European Journal of Cardio-Thoracic Surgery. 2014;**46**(4):665-671. DOI: 10.1093/ejcts/ezu029

[27] Meani P, Pappalardo F. The step forward for VA ECMO: Left ventricular unloading! Journal of Thoracic Disease. 2017;**9**(11):4149-4151. http://doi.org/10.21037/jtd.2017.10.14

[28] Hireche-Chikaoui H, Grübler MR, Bloch A, Windecker S, Bloechlinger S, Hunziker L. Nonejecting hearts on femoral veno-arterial extracorporeal membrane oxygenation. Critical Care Medicine. 2018;**1**:e459-e464. DOI: 10.1097/CCM.0000000000002966

[29] Hékimian G, Jovanovic T, Bréchot N, Lebreton G, Leprince P, Trouillet J, et al. When the heart gets the flu. Journal of Critical Care. 2018;**47**:61-64

[30] Stevens MC, Callaghan FM, Forrest P, Bannon PG, Grieve SM. Flow mixing during peripheral veno-arterial extra corporeal membrane oxygenation—A simulation study. Journal of Biomechanics. 2017;**55**:64-70. DOI: 10.1016/j.jbiomech.2017.02.009

[31] Meani P, Gelsomino S, Natour E, Johnson DM, Rocca HPBL, Pappalardo F, et al. Modalities and effects of left ventricle unloading on extracorporeal life support: A review of the current literature. European Journal of Heart Failure. 2017;**19**:84-91. DOI: 10.1002/ejhf.850

[32] Dickstein ML. The starling relationship and veno-arterial ECMO. ASAIO Journal. 2018;**64**(4):497-501. DOI: 10.1097/MAT.0000000000000660

[33] Ostadal P, Mlcek M, Kruger A, et al. Increasing venoarterial extracorporeal membrane oxygenation flow negatively affects left ventricular performance in a porcine model of cardiogenic shock. Journal of Translational Medicine. 2015;**13**:266

[34] Aissaoui N, Guerot E, Combes A, et al. Two-dimensional strain rate and Doppler tissue myocardial velocities: Analysis by echocardiography of hemodynamic and functional changes of the failed left ventricle during different degrees of extracorporeal life support. Journal of the American Society of Echocardiography. 2012;**25**:632-640

[35] Soleimani B, Pae WE. Management of left ventricular distension during peripheral extracorporeal membrane oxygenation for cardiogenic shock. Perfusion. 2012;**27**:326-331

[36] Fuhrman BP, Hernan LJ, Rotta AT, Heard CMB, Rosenkranz ER. Pathophysiology of cardiac extracorporeal membrane oxygenation. Artificial Organs. 1999;**23**:966-969

[37] Burkhoff D, Sayer G, Doshi D, Uriel N. Hemodynamics of mechanical circulatory support. Journal of the American College of Cardiology. 2015;**66**(23):2663-2674. DOI: 10.1016/j.jacc.2015.10.017

[38] Doufle G, Ferguson ND. Monitoring during extracorporeal membrane oxygenation. Current Opinion in Critical Care. 2016;**22**(3):230-8. DOI: 10.1097/MCC.0000000000000309

[39] Sidebotham D, Allen S, McGeorge A, Beca J. Catastrophic left heart distension following initiation of venoarterial extracorporeal membrane oxygenation in a patient with mild aortic regurgitation. Anaesthesia and Intensive Care. 2012;**40**:568-569

[40] Douflé G, Roscoe A, Billia F, Fan E. Echocardiography for adult patients supported with extracorporeal membrane oxygenation. Critical Care. 2015;**19**:326. DOI: 10.1186/s13054-015-1042-2

[41] Donker DW, Meuwese CL, Braithwaite SA, Broomé M, van der Heijden JJ, Hermens JA, et al. Echocardiography in extracorporeal life support: A key player in procedural guidance, tailoring and monitoring. Perfusion (United Kingdom). 2018;**33**(1_suppl):31-41. DOI: 10.1177/0267659118766438

[42] Esposito ML, Kapur NK. Acute mechanical circulatory support for cardiogenic shock: The "door to support" time. F1000Research. 2017;**6**:737. DOI: 10.12688/f1000research.11150.1

[43] Truesdell AG, Tehrani B, Singh R, Desai S, Saulino P, Barnett S, et al. "Combat" approach to cardiogenic shock. Interventional Cardiology Review. 2018;**13**(2):81-86. http://doi.org/10.15420/icr.2017:35:3

[44] Williams DO, Korr KS, Gewirtz H, Most AS. The effect of intraaortic balloon counterpulsation on regional myocardial blood flow and oxygen consumption in the presence of coronary artery stenosis in patients with unstable angina. Circulation. 1982;**66**(3):593-597. DOI: 10.1161/01.CIR.66.3.593

[45] Marra C, De Santo LS, Amarelli C, Della Corte A, Onorati F, Torella M, et al. Coronary artery bypass grafting in patients with severe left ventricular dysfunction: A prospective randomized study on the timing of perioperative intraaortic balloon pump support. International Journal of Artificial Organs. 2002;**25**(2):141-146

[46] Zobel G, Dacar D, Kuttnig M, Rodl S, Rigler B. Mechanical support of the left ventricle in ischemia induced left ventricular failure: An experimental study. The International Journal of Artificial Organs. 1992;**15**(2):114-119

[47] Werdan K, Gielen S, Ebelt H, Hochman JS. Mechanical circulatory support in cardiogenic shock. European Heart Journal. 2014;**35**(3):156-167. DOI: 10.1093/eurheartj/eht248. [Epub 2013 Sep 7]

[48] Ma P, Zhang Z, Song T, Yang Y, Meng G, Zhao J, et al. Combining ECMO with IABP for the treatment of critically ill adult heart failure patients. Heart Lung and Circulation. 2014;**23**(4):363-368. DOI: 10.1016/j.hlc.2013.10.081

[49] Petroni T, Harrois A, Amour J, et al. Intra-aortic balloon pump effects on macrocirculation and microcirculation in cardiogenic shock patients supported by venoarterial extracorporeal membrane oxygenation. Critical Care Medicine. 2014;**42**:2075-2082

[50] Park TK, Yang JH, Choi SH, et al. Clinical impact of intra-aortic balloon pump during extracorporeal life support in patients with acute myocardial infarction complicated by cardiogenic shock. BMC Anesthesiology. 2014;**14**:27

[51] Fincke R, Hochman JS, Lowe AM, Menon V, Slater JN, Webb JG, et al. Cardiac power is the strongest hemodynamic correlate of mortality in cardiogenic shock: A report from the SHOCK trial registry. Journal of the American College of Cardiology. 2004;**44**(2):340-348. DOI: 10.1016/j.jacc.2004.03.060

[52] De Silva K, Lumley M, Kailey B, Alastruey J, Guilcher A, Asrress KN, et al. Coronary and microvascular physiology during intra-aortic balloon counterpulsation. JACC: Cardiovascular Interventions. 2014;**7**(6):631-640. DOI: 10.1016/j.jcin.2013.11.023

[53] Scandroglio AM, Pieri M, Pappalardo F, Landoni G. Intra-aortic balloon pump during venoarterial extracorporeal membrane oxygenation: Still a matter of debate? Contemporary multi-device approach to cardiogenic shock. Journal of Thoracic Disease. 2017;**9**(5):E522-E524

[54] Shishehbor MH, Moazami N, Tong MZY, Unai S, Tang WHW, Soltesz EG. Cardiogenic shock: From ECMO to Impella and beyond. Cleveland Clinic Journal of Medicine. 2017;**84**(4):287-295. DOI: 10.3949/ccjm.84gr.17002

[55] Hoeper MM, Tudorache I, Kühn C, Marsch G, Hartung D, Wiesner O, et al. Extracorporeal membrane oxygenation watershed. Circulation. 2014;**130**(10):864-865. DOI: 10.1161/CIRCULATIONAHA.114.011677

[56] Lin LY, Liao CW, Wang CH, Chi NH, Yu HY, Chou NK, et al. Effects of additional intra-aortic balloon counter-pulsation therapy to cardiogenic shock patients supported by extra-corporeal membranous oxygenation. Scientific Reports. 2016;**6**:23838 DOI: 10.1038/srep23838

[57] Cheng JM, den Uil CA, Hoeks SE, et al. Percutaneous left ventricular assist devices vs. intra-aortic balloon pump counterpulsation for treatment of cardiogenic shock: A meta-analysis of controlled trials. European Heart Journal. 2009;**30**:2102-2108

[58] Nuding S, Werdan K. IABP plus ECMO—Is one and one more than two? Journal of Thoracic Disease. 2017;**9**(4):961-964

[59] Sauren LDC, Accord RE, Hamzeh K, De Jong M, Van Der Nagel T, Van Der Veen FH, et al. Combined Impella and intra-aortic balloon pump support to improve both ventricular unloading and coronary blood flow for myocardial recovery: An experimental study. Artificial Organs. 2007;**31**(11):839-842. DOI: 10.1111/j.1525-1594.2007.00477.x

[60] O'Connor CM, Rogers JG. Evidence for overturning the guidelines in cardiogenic shock. New England Journal of Medicine. 2012;**367**(14):1349-1350. DOI: 10.1056/NEJMe1209601

[61] Gaudard P, Mourad M, Eliet J, Zeroual N, Culas G, Rouvière P, et al. Management and outcome of patients supported with Impella 5.0 for refractory cardiogenic shock. Critical Care. 2015;**19**(1). DOI: 10.1186/s13054-015-1073-8

[62] Pieri M, Contri R, Winterton D, Montorfano M, Colombo A, Zangrillo A, et al. The contemporary role of Impella in a comprehensive mechanical circulatory support program: A single institutional experience. BMC Cardiovascular Disorders. 2015;**15**(1):126. DOI: 10.1186/s12872-015-0119-9

[63] Donker DW, Brodie D, Henriques JPS, Broomé M. Left ventricular unloading during veno-arterial ECMO. ASAIO Journal. 2018. DOI: 10.1097/MAT.0000000000000755. [Epub ahead of print]

[64] Bréchot N, Demondion P, Santi F, Lebreton G, Pham T, Dalakidis A, et al. Intra-aortic balloon pump protects against hydrostatic pulmonary oedema during peripheral venoarterial-extracorporeal membrane oxygenation. European Heart Journal: Acute Cardiovascular Care. 2018;**7**(1):62-69. DOI: 10.1177/2048872617711169. [Epub 2017 Jun 2]

[65] Cheng R, Hachamovitch R, Makkar R, Ramzy D, Moriguchi JD, Arabia FA, et al. Lack of survival benefit found with use of intraaortic balloon pump in extracorporeal membrane oxygenation: A pooled experience of 1517 patients. Journal of Invasive Cardiology. 2015;**27**(10):453-458

[66] Baruteau A-E, Barnetche T, Morin L, Jalal Z, Boscamp NS, Le Bret E, et al. Percutaneous balloon atrial septostomy on top of venoarterial extracorporeal membrane oxygenation results in safe and effective left heart decompression. European Heart Journal: Acute Cardiovascular Care. 2018;**7**(1):70-79. DOI: 10.1177/2048872616675485. [Epub 2016 Oct 14]

[67] Saffarzadeh A, Bonde P. Options for temporary mechanical circulatory support. Journal of Thoracic Disease. 2015;**7**(12):2102-2111. DOI: 10.3978/j.issn.2072-1439.2015.09.14

[68] Kuchibhotla S, Esposito ML, Breton C, Pedicini R, Mullin A, O'Kelly R, et al. Acute biventricular mechanical circulatory support for cardiogenic shock. Journal of the American Heart Association. 2017;**6**(10). pii:e006670. DOI: 10.1161/JAHA.117.006670

[69] Seib PM, Faulkner SC, Erickson CC, Van Devanter SH, Harrell JE, Fasules JW, et al. Blade and balloon atrial septostomy for left heart decompression in patients with severe ventricular dysfunction on extracorporeal membrane oxygenation. Catheterization and Cardiovascular Interventions. 1999;**46**(2):179-186. DOI: 10.1002/(SICI)1522-726X(199902)46:2<179::AID-CCD13>3.0.CO;2-W

[70] Aiyagari RM, Rocchini AP, Remenapp RT, Graziano JN. Decompression of the left atrium during extracorporeal membrane oxygenation using a transseptal cannula incorporated into the circuit. Critical Care Medicine. 2006;**34**(10):2603-2606. DOI: 10.1097/01.CCM.0000239113.02836.F1

[71] Avalli L, Maggioni E, Sangalli F, Favini G, Formica F, Fumagalli R. Percutaneous left-heart decompression during extracorporeal membrane oxygenation: An alternative to surgical and transeptal venting in adult patients. ASAIO Journal. 2011;**57**(1):38-40. DOI: 10.1097/MAT.0b013e3181fe5d0b

[72] Fumagalli R, Bombino M, Borelli M, Rossi F, Colombo V, Osculati G, et al. Percutaneous bridge to heart transplantation by venoarterial ECMO and transaortic left ventricular venting. International Journal of Artificial Organs. 2004;**27**(5):410-413. DOI: 10.1177/039139880402700510

[73] Barbone A, Malvindi PG, Ferrara P, Tarelli G. Left ventricle unloading by percutaneous pigtail during extracorporeal membrane oxygenation. Interactive Cardiovascular and Thoracic Surgery. 2011;**13**(3):293-295. DOI: 10.1510/icvts.2011.269795

[74] Kim WH, Hong TH, Byun JH, Kim JW, Kim SH, Moon SH, et al. Flow rate through pigtail catheter used for left heart decompression in an artificial model of extracorporeal membrane oxygenation circuit. ASAIO Journal. 2017;**63**(3):346-350. DOI: 10.1097/MAT.0000000000000472

[75] Koeckert MS, Jorde UP, Naka Y, Moses JW, Takayama H. Impella LP 2.5 for left ventricular unloading during venoarterial extracorporeal membrane oxygenation support. Journal of Cardiac Surgery. 2011;**26**:666-668

[76] Narain S, Paparcuri G, Fuhrman TM, Silverman RB, Peruzzi WT. Novel combination of Impella and extra corporeal membrane oxygenation as a bridge to full recovery in fulminant myocarditis. Case Reports in Critical Care. 2012;**2012**:1-3. DOI: 10.1155/2012/459296

[77] Camboni D, Schmid C. To vent or not on veno-arterial extracorporeal membrane oxygenation, does it improve myocardial recovery and outcome? Journal of Thoracic Disease. 2017;**9**(12):4915-4918. https://doi.org/10.21037/jtd.2017.11.98

[78] Akanni OJ, Takeda K, Truby LK, Kurlansky PA, Chiuzan C, Han J, et al. EC-VAD: Combined use of extracorporeal membrane oxygenation and percutaneous microaxial pump left ventricular assist device. ASAIO Journal. 2018. DOI: 10.1097/MAT.0000000000000804 [Epub ahead of print]. Retrieved from: https://journals.lww.com/asaiojournal/Fulltext/onlinefirst/EC_VAD_Combined_Use_of_Extracorporeal_Membrane.98870.aspx

[79] Tanaka D, Shimada S, Mullin M, Kreitler K, Cavarocchi N, Hirose H. What is the optimal blood pressure on Veno-arterial extracorporeal membrane oxygenation? Impact of mean arterial pressure on survival. ASAIO Journal. 2018. DOI: 10.1097/MAT.0000000000000824. [Epub ahead of print]. Retrieved from: https://journals.lww.com/asaiojournal/Fulltext/onlinefirst/What_Is_the_Optimal_Blood_Pressure_on.98853.aspx

[80] Leone M, Asfar P, Radermacher P, Vincent JL, Martin C. Optimizing mean arterial pressure in septic shock: A critical reappraisal of the literature. Critical Care. 2015;**19**:101. DOI: 10.1186/s13054-015-0794-z

[81] Gold JP, Charlson ME, Williams-Russo P, Szatrowski TP, Peterson JC, Pirraglia PA, et al. Improvement of outcomes after coronary artery bypass: A randomized trial comparing intraoperative high versus low mean arterial pressure. The Journal of Thoracic and Cardiovascular Surgery. 1995;**110**(5):1302-1314. DOI: 10.1016/S0022-5223(95)70053-6

[82] Murphy GS, Hessel EA, Groom RC. Optimal perfusion during cardiopulmonary bypass: An evidence-based approach. Anesthesia and Analgesia. 2009;**108**(5):1394-1417. DOI: 10.1213/ane.0b013e3181875e2e

[83] Levin MA, Lin HM, Castillo JG, Adams DH, Reich DL, Fischer GW. Early on-cardiopulmonary bypass hypotension and other factors associated with vasoplegic syndrome. Circulation. 2009;**120**(17):1664-1671. DOI: 10.1161/CIRCULATIONAHA.108.814533

[84] Akin S, dos Reis Miranda D, Caliskan K, Soliman OI, Guven G, Struijs A, et al. Functional evaluation of sublingual microcirculation indicates successful weaning from VA-ECMO in cardiogenic shock. Critical Care. 2017;**21**(1):265. DOI: 10.1186/s13054-017-1855-2

Chapter 14

Extracorporeal Membrane Oxygenation (ECMO) for Long-Term Support: Recent Advances

R. Gregory Conway, Douglas Tran,
Bartley P. Griffith and Zhongjun J. Wu

Additional information is available at the end of the chapter

http://dx.doi.org/10.5772/intechopen.76506

Abstract

Considerable progress has been made in component technology, circuitry, and clinical practice related to extracorporeal membrane oxygenation (ECMO). These advances allow prolonged support with fewer complications when compared to the past eras. Long-term support cases were frequently reported with indications including respiratory failure, cardiac failure, bridge to transplantation, extracorporeal cardiopulmonary resuscitation (ECPR), and even ambulatory extracorporeal membrane oxygenation (ECMO) support. The common complications associated with ECMO, including thrombosis, hemorrhage, nosocomial infection, neurological injury, vessel injury, multiple organ failure and mechanical failure, and the disease process of patients remain limiting factors. In spite of the complications, ECMO remains the only possible option in treatments for patients requiring long-term respiratory or cardiopulmonary support. In this chapter, the recent advances in long-term ECMO support are reviewed. Clinical etiology of patients placed on long-term ECMO support, the various circuit configurations, clinical and technical issues, management aspects, and clinical outcomes are discussed.

Keywords: extracorporeal membrane oxygenation (ECMO), long-term ECMO, critical care medicine, respiratory failure, cardiopulmonary failure, cardiac failure, blood oxygenator, blood pump

1. Introduction

In its earliest application, extracorporeal membrane oxygenation (ECMO) was used as a rescue therapy in support of patients with acute circulatory or respiratory failure. The first reported use of ECMO was to support a 24-year-old trauma patient suffering from acute respiratory failure, where venoarterial ECMO provided 75 h of life-sustaining support in 1972 [1]. Despite initial barriers to widespread adoption, by the 1990s, a growing body of literature demonstrated a clinical benefit to ECMO in certain patients. Advances in ECMO technology, critical care, rehabilitation, and comorbidity management have resulted in increased adoption of ECMO, with ever-increasing duration of ECMO runs. In 2003, there were 1606 patients supported with ECMO [2], with this number increasing to 2895 by 2011 [3] and more than 6600 cases in 2015 [4]. Although the mean duration of ECMO support is approximately 1 week, reports of over 7 months exist in the literature. Long-term ECMO, defined as 3 weeks or longer of ECMO support, has become increasingly prevalent, with many centers reporting success in long-term support.

In general, the initial indications for long-term ECMO support are the same as short-term ECMO support, and it is the patient's recovery which dictates the duration of use. **Table 1** lists respiratory indications for ECMO support, with diagnosis, average run duration, and percent survival stratified by age group. Despite the ability of ECMO to treat both respiratory and circulatory conditions, it is the patients with severe respiratory failure who are most commonly supported on long-term ECMO. In contrast, patients with cardiogenic shock are typically transitioned to ventricular assist device (VAD) therapy or heart transplant prior to 3 weeks of ECMO support. The most prevalent respiratory indications for long-term ECMO include bacterial and viral pneumonia, acute respiratory distress syndrome (ARDS), and acute respiratory failure in the adult and pediatric populations. In the neonatal patient

Age group	Diagnosis	Average run duration (h)	% survival
Neonatal	Congenital diaphragmatic hernia	257	51
	Persistent pulmonary hypertension of newborn	155	77
	Sepsis	144	72
	Respiratory distress syndrome of newborn	136	84
	Meconium aspiration syndrome	133	94
Pediatric	Viral pneumonia	317	66
	Bacterial pneumonia	283	60
	Aspiration pneumonia	242	69
	Acute respiratory failure, non-ARDS	226	52
Adult	Viral pneumonia	325	65
	ARDS, non-post-op/trauma	313	54
	Acute respiratory failure, non-ARDS	275	55
	Bacterial pneumonia	261	61
	ARDS, postop/trauma	256	57

Table 1. Average ECMO run duration and % survival by age group and diagnosis, 2016 data [4].

http://dx.doi.org/10.5772/intechopen.76506

population, meconium aspiration syndrome, persistent pulmonary hypertension of the newborn, congenital diaphragmatic hernia, sepsis, and respiratory distress syndromes are more prevalent.

2. Indications and outcomes

The decision to support a patient with ECMO is based on the severity of cardiopulmonary dysfunction, the response to conventional therapy, as well as patient and family preferences for the aggressiveness of treatment. The duration of ECMO use, in contrast, is dependent on patient recovery and the patient's ability to transition to alternative therapies. Indeed, patient and family preferences for the duration of aggressive critical care must be considered, and honest explanations of ECMO outcomes must be provided.

Unfortunately, the data necessary to predict patient outcomes on long-term ECMO support remain limited. Instead, case series and case reports guide much of the decision-making, and key examples are described later.

2.1. Respiratory failure

Respiratory failure remains the condition most commonly supported with long-term ECMO, with ARDS the inciting respiratory insult in many cases. When supporting a patient with severe respiratory failure with ECMO, clinicians must consider strategies for decannulation, which currently include patient recovery and lung transplantation. Despite increased acceptance of ECMO as a long-term therapy, it is currently unable to support patients outside of the intensive care unit (ICU), and does not allow for patients to return to activities of daily living. The ideal scenario for these patients is a full recovery, and there are increasing reports of patients recovering from long-term ECMO support for severe respiratory failure. The longest reported ECMO run with recovery is in a 26-year-old drowning victim, who was supported for 117 days on ECMO [5].

In patients unlikely to recover their native pulmonary function, or in patients with progressive underlying respiratory failure, ECMO may be utilized as a bridge to lung transplantation. The longest reported successful bridge to transplant required ECMO support of 155 days [6]. In these cases, ECMO provides the needed gas-exchange function, allowing for reduced reliance on mechanical ventilation. The principle advantage of this strategy lies in the ability to liberate patients from mechanical ventilation, allowing some patients to talk, eat, and ambulate, which serve to prevent pre-transplant deconditioning. There are two patient populations who receive ECMO as a bridge to lung transplantation: patients with chronic respiratory failure who are listed for transplantation prior to ECMO initiation and those patients without history of respiratory failure, who are only listed for transplantation after ECMO therapy has begun.

In the setting of acute respiratory decompensation, it is unlikely for a patient's transplant candidacy to improve beyond their baseline—instead, the role of ECMO in these patients is to prevent their deconditioning and to avoid transplant-precluding complications. As such, the contemporary management of patients with respiratory failure exceeding the abilities of conventional support measures involves ECMO support followed by urgent lung transplantation, as the prolonged ECMO use continuously exposes patients to the risk of complication.

Acute respiratory decompensation occurs not infrequently in patients who are listed for lung transplantation. For these patients, the use of ECMO provides necessary gas-exchange function in the setting of inadequate native lung function. The use of ECMO in these patients has been widely reported, and the algorithms guiding this management strategy are maturing. One single-center experience reports the use of ECMO as a bridge to lung transplant over a 9-year period, in which the median duration of ECMO use was 12 days (interquartile range—IQR 6.25 to 18.75) [7]. In the series of 72 patients, 56% of patients were successfully bridged to transplant, with 38% surviving for up to 2 years. Notably, the patients were free from mechanical ventilation for a mean time of 10.2 days (SD 18.8 days), and 69% of patients were ambulatory while on ECMO. A similar experience was reported on 31 patients who were bridged to lung transplantation using ECMO over a 5-year period at two institutions [8]. They report ambulation while on ECMO in 18 patients, liberation from the ventilator in 3 patients, and a median duration of ECMO use of 11 days (IQR 3.5–17). Five patients were on ECMO for over 21 days, with one patient requiring 53 days of support. Of note, 7 of the 31 patients were not listed for transplantation prior to ECMO cannulation.

The decision to support patients with acute or acute-on-chronic respiratory failure with ECMO is a challenging one, and no single guideline exists to aid in decision-making. Even so, multiple high-volume pulmonary transplant and ECMO centers have published their experience with ECMO as a bridge to transplant. A typical decision tree is shown in **Figure 1** (adapted from Biscotti et al. [7] and Hoopes et al. [8]). Note that the clinical management decisions are highly center specific, and these treatment algorithms must be adapted to appropriately fit the clinical setting.

Continuous advancement in the technology of ECMO as well as improvements in critical care and rehabilitation have improved the outcomes of all ECMO patients, including those requiring long-term support. A study describing the course of 127 patients placed on ECMO for respiratory failure between 2006 and 2010 found an overall survival to decannulation of 64%. In the stratified analysis, they found that 59, 31, and 52% of patients survived after being placed on ECMO for 10 days or less, 11–20 days, or more than 21 days, respectively. They found no statistically significant difference in survival between the 45 patients who were supported on ECMO for 10 days or less, and the 10 patients who were supported long term ($p = 0.39$) [9]. Similarly, a study of 55 patients placed on ECMO for severe ARDS demonstrated no significant difference in hospital or 30-day mortality, with 27% of patients supported for 3 or more weeks expiring versus 43% of patients supported less than 3 weeks [10]. These data, albeit limited, provide evidence for cautious optimism in the care of patients with severe respiratory failure.

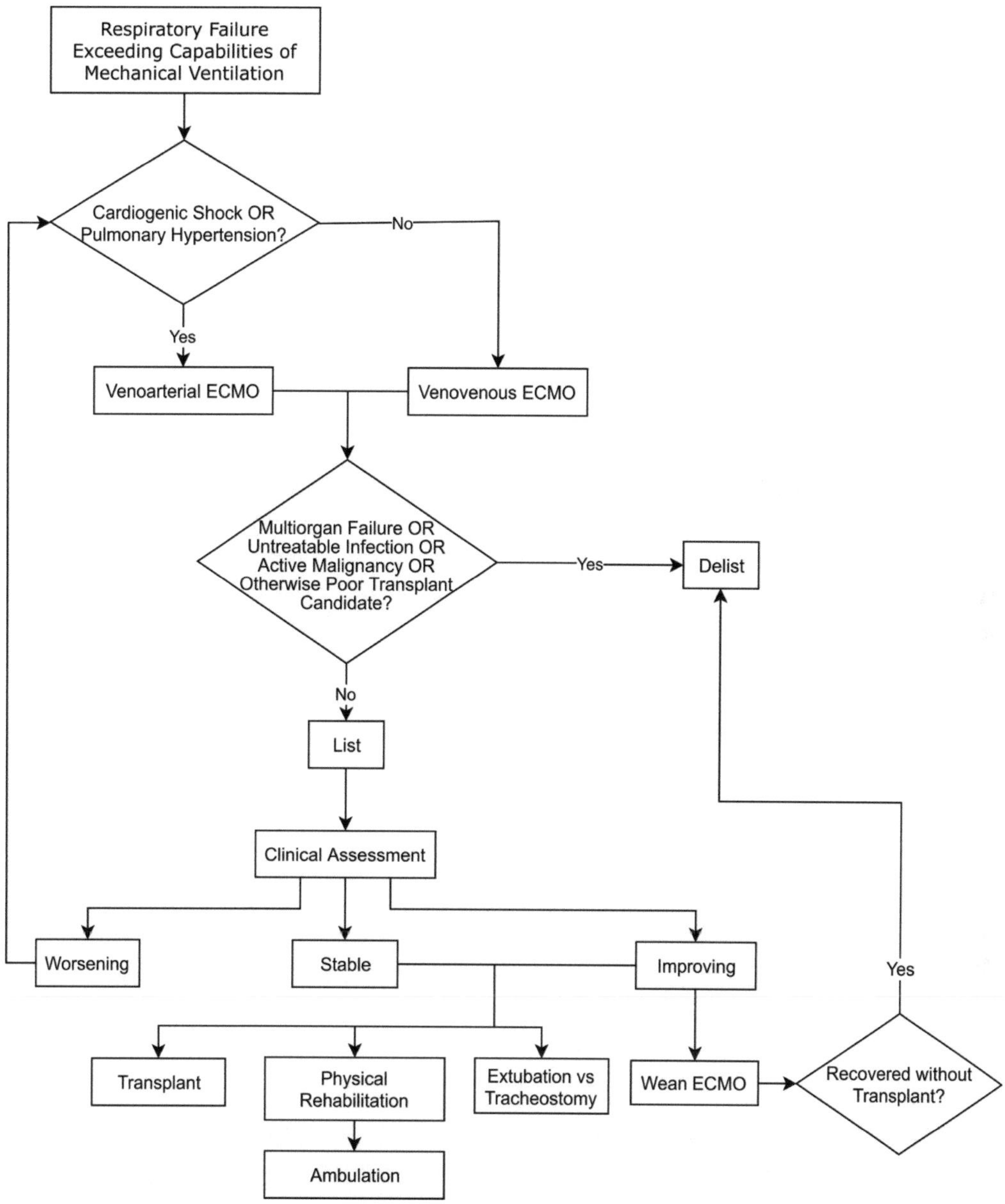

Figure 1. General treatment algorithm for ECMO as a bridge to lung transplant. Note that implementation details are highly dependent on clinical setting.

2.2. Circulatory collapse

The use of long-term ECMO for the treatment of cardiogenic shock is less common than for respiratory failure, as many are transitioned to VAD therapy before their tenure on ECMO would be considered long term (21 days). Reports of patients being supported on venoarterial ECMO for prolonged durations do exist in the literature, however. In one study, a patient unable to wean from cardiopulmonary bypass following re-do sternotomy and aortic valve replacement was supported with venoarterial ECMO for 33 days postoperatively before being successfully weaned and decannulated [11]. Unfortunately, this patient ultimately suffered a cerebrovascular accident and died in a high-dependency unit. In a cohort of 98 patients receiving ECMO for refractory cardiogenic shock, Rousse et al. reported a median duration of ECMO use of 8 days, with the maximum duration of 81 days [12]. This cohort suffered 50% mortality, with 30% of patients recovering to normal cardiac function, 13% of patients receiving a heart transplant, and 7% of patients transitioned to VAD therapy.

The decision to provide long-term ECMO support for these patients is largely dependent on their presumed recovery path, and it is the patients who are poor candidates for VAD support who are typically supported on venoarterial ECMO in the long term. These patients must be aggressively medically optimized, as the goal of the ECMO therapy is in recovery of native cardiac function prior to decannulation. Indeed, some patients will not recover native cardiac function, will never become transplant candidates, and are unsuitable for VAD as a destination therapy. Management of these patients is a significant challenge both medically and ethically, and the family must frequently be updated in the plan of care.

3. ECMO circuit configuration

3.1. Cannulation strategies

Initial cannulation strategies for long-term ECMO are identical to short-term ECMO support, with the goal of achieving adequate blood flow to support gas-exchange requirements, while minimizing recirculation between the cannulae. For patients with isolated respiratory failure, venovenous cannulation is possible. If hemodynamic support is required, or if there is significant pulmonary hypertension, venoarterial ECMO may be necessary. For the expeditious initiation of ECMO, percutaneous cannulation of femoral and jugular vessels is preferred, as it allows for initiation of ECMO at the bedside in a rapid manner.

As the patient's tenure on ECMO becomes prolonged, however, cannulation must not only provide appropriate cardiopulmonary support but must also provide long-term stability and allow for rehabilitation with possible ambulation. In general, long-term femoral cannulation is not preferred due to infectious risk as well as relative limit to mobility associated with access to the femoral vessels.

For isolated respiratory support, early transition to a double-lumen internal jugular cannula (Avalon Elite®), placed under echocardiographic or fluoroscopic guidance, has proven to be beneficial in many centers. Since the double-lumen internal jugular cannula allows for full mobility of the lower extremities, these patients are able to ambulate and undergo physical therapy with the goal of limiting deconditioning. This double-lumen cannula does impose a restriction to flow, however, and careful patient selection is required.

For patients with cardiogenic shock or pulmonary hypertension, the cannulation options are more limited. In principle, the cannulae must provide venous drainage as well as return of oxygenated blood to the arterial system with adequate return pressure to provide end-organ perfusion. In the acute cannulation of patients with cardiopulmonary collapse, the common femoral artery is the preferred vessel for arterial cannulation in adults. Of note, the presence of the arterial cannula in the common femoral artery can compromise distal limb perfusion, and insertion of a distal perfusion catheter is often required. Unfortunately, the groin access required for cannulation of the common femoral artery limits mobility and may be deleterious to rehabilitation.

Although there is no commonly accepted cannulation site for long-term venoarterial access, one reported technique is cannulation of subclavian vessels [13]. This technique is reported to provide adequate flows and improved ambulation options. Technically, this cannulation method requires a small infraclavicular incision, anastomosis of a synthetic arterial graft with the subclavian artery in an end-to-side fashion, and direct insertion of the cannula into the arterial graft. Naturally, decannulation from this arrangement requires a surgical procedure with either explant or close ligation of the arterial graft.

In cases where there is right heart dysfunction or severe pulmonary hypertension, venoarterial ECMO through femoral vein and femoral artery is the traditional means of decompressing the right ventricle. In patients with a congenital atrial septal defect, a less invasive technique can be employed, in which a dual-lumen cannula is placed under fluoroscopic or echocardiographic guidance [14]. This goal of this configuration is to direct the oxygenated blood returned from the ECMO circuit through the atrial septal defect and into the left atrium, thus reducing the blood delivered through the right ventricle. This configuration promotes ambulation, as the dual-lumen venovenous cannula is inserted through the internal jugular vein. Both animal and human studies have shown success with creation of an atrial septostomy in conjunction with venovenous ECMO for the treatment of pulmonary hypertension [15]. If this technique cannot provide adequate right ventricular unloading, central cannulation is required, with two primary configurations.

The first central cannulation technique involves venous drainage from the right atrium and return of oxygenated blood into the pulmonary artery. Technically, this is accomplished through a median sternotomy or thoracotomy, with insertion of the venous drainage cannula into the right atrial appendage, and a synthetic arterial graft is anastomosed to the main pulmonary artery in an end-to-side fashion. The arterial cannula is inserted into this graft. In the patient with pulmonary hypertension, this configuration requires that the ECMO circuit pumps against this high-resistance pulmonary vasculature. This is rarely an issue, however, as even the vasculature of severe pulmonary hypertension has a lower driving pressure than systemic arterial pressure, and modern ECMO circuits have little difficulty driving blood through the systemic circulation. One major advantage of this configuration is that it places the arterial return in the main pulmonary artery, benefiting from the systemic-embolus protection afforded by the pulmonary vasculature. Additionally, cannulae can be tunneled out of the subcutaneous tissues and skin without access to upper or lower limbs, promoting mobility.

Central cannulation between the right atrium and left atrium can also be a strategy to mitigate pulmonary hypertension or right heart dysfunction [16]. In this case, venous blood is drained from the right atrial appendage, passed through the ECMO circuit for gas exchange, and oxygenated blood is returned to the left atrium. Again, cannulae for this technique can be tunneled allowing for mobility. Unfortunately, the invasiveness of the thoracotomy or median sternotomy is required, and there is no "pulmonary filter" to mitigate the consequences of ECMO circuit embolism, with a theoretical increase in the risk of stroke.

In a long-term ECMO patient, physicians may need to transition between cannulation sites, due to changes to patient's support needs, desire to promote mobility, as well as cannulation site complications such as infection, hemorrhage, or inadequate distal perfusion. Continuous reevaluation of the appropriateness of cannulation must be performed, as a highly mobile patient on venovenous ECMO will likely fare better than a bedbound patient supported by a venoarterial configuration. Additionally, long-term ECMO patients may suffer unusual cannulation site and hardware complications. The securing sutures of cannula must be frequently examined, as they may pull from the skin or break during long-term support. Additionally, cannulae are subject to prolonged periods of fatigue, which may lead to early failure. In this author's experience

Drainage	Return	Cannulation	Mobility	Decannulation	Embolization Site	Comments
Femoral vein	Jugular vein	Rapid, bedside	Low	Bedside	Pulmonary	
Jugular vein	Jugular vein	Rapid, bedside	High	Bedside	Pulmonary	
Jugular vein	Jugular vein with atrial septostomy	Lengthy, OR	High	Bedside	Systemic	Requires fluoroscopy or transesophageal echocardiography for positioning
Femoral vein	Femoral artery	Rapid, bedside	Low	Bedside vs. OR	Systemic	Possible limb ischemia, Consider distal perfusion catheter
Subclavian vein	Subclavian or axillary artery	Lengthy, OR	High	OR	Systemic	Possible limb ischemia, vascular complications
Right atrium	Pulmonary artery	Lengthy, OR	High	OR	Pulmonary	Requires chest exploration for bleeding
Right atrium	Left atrium	Lengthy, OR	High	OR	Systemic	Requires chest exploration for bleeding
Right atrium	Aorta	Lengthy, OR	High	OR	Systemic	Requires chest exploration for bleeding

Table 2. Possible cannulation sites.

with long-term cannulation in an ovine model, evidence of impending cannula failure has been detected (and repaired) on multiple occasions (unpublished data) (**Table 2**).

3.2. Circuit maintenance and component exchange

Due to the prolonged duration of component use in patients on long-term ECMO, component failure is a realistic possibility. Catastrophic failures, such as component rupture and hemorrhage, are managed through emergent circuit exchange. As such, a primed backup circuit should be available for emergent exchange at all times.

More gradual failures can occur in both the pump and the oxygenator, requiring exchange of these components. For the pump, failure can occur due to thrombus formation (typically on the impeller or bearing) causing decreased pump performance and increased hemolysis. This can be detected by trending pump rotational speed, blood flows, and plasma-free hemoglobin (PFH). A PFH level of approximately 10 mg/dL is generally acceptable, with a level over 50 mg/dL suggestive of excess hemolysis [18]. Rapid changes in PFH are perhaps more informative than the absolute value, and any rapid increase in PFH should be investigated. Of note, it is critical that blood samples be obtained gently while measuring PFH, as hemolysis can occur during sample acquisition causing an erroneously high reading.

Oxygenator failure can occur as a result of several conditions. The most acute failure is rupture of the fiber bundle, allowing sweep gas to enter the blood path and placing the patient at risk for an air embolism. Slow decline in oxygenator performance can occur due to protein deposition on the membrane, condensation buildup inside the gas passage, or the development of thrombus within the oxygenator. Condensation buildup can be prevented by periodically increasing the sweep gas to a high flow rate (10 LPM) for several seconds to blow the condensate into the exhaust. Care must be taken not to reduce the patient's CO_2 by maintaining this high sweep for a prolonged period. A flashlight can be used to examine the oxygenator (and tubing) for thrombus. Any thrombus visible on the oxygenator outlet side is impetus for oxygenator exchange, as this thrombus is at risk of embolization. Any other thrombus greater than 5 mm or enlarging may also warrant component or circuit exchange [17]. Finally, oxygenator performance may slowly decline as a result of protein deposition on the membrane. There is no reliable test to identify this as the cause of poor oxygenator performance, thus any oxygenator that cannot generate an exhaust oxyhemoglobin saturation of at least 95% is a candidate for exchange [18].

4. Complications

The use of ECMO for long-term support can lead to any number of complications. Although a multitude of complications can occur during long-term ECMO support, the typical complications are related either to cannulation, anticoagulation, concomitant organ failure, or infection. A meta-analysis by Cheng et al. reports complication rates on 1866 adult patients receiving ECMO as rescue therapy for the treatment of cardiogenic shock [18]. The rates of complications from this analysis are as follows: lower extremity ischemia—16.9%, lower extremity fasciotomy or compartment syndrome—10.3%, lower extremity amputation—4.7%, stroke—5.9%, neurologic complication—13.3%, acute kidney injury—55.6%, kidney injury requiring renal replacement therapy—46.0%, major bleeding—40.8%, re-thoracotomy for bleeding or tamponade—41.9%, and significant infection—30.4%. These complications are discussed below.

4.1. Vascular complications

Vascular trauma secondary to cannulation is highly dependent on the selected cannulation strategy. Complications such as perforation of major vessels and arterial dissection are serious issues that can lead to extensive local bleeding, retroperitoneal hematoma formation, and limb ischemia. Perforation of the right atrium is relatively rare, while perforation or dissection of the femoral vessels, subclavian vein, or carotid artery is the more common form of vascular trauma [19, 20].

Compartment syndrome of the cannulated limb can occur in a subset of patients. Secondary complications of compartment syndrome include, but are not limited to, limb ischemia, neurologic deficits, or amputation of the affected limb. The first line of treatment for compartment syndrome is an urgent fasciotomy of the affected limb to release the elevated pressure and restore tissue perfusion [18, 19, 21]. Often, it is the detection of compartment syndrome that is challenging, especially if the patient is intubated and sedated, as they cannot report the altered sensation. As such, it is prudent to document distal perfusion after cannulation with a pulse exam (and Doppler if necessary) and to reexamine at frequent intervals (every few hours by nursing). Laboratory signs such as an elevated lactate, creatine phosphokinase, or myoglobin may be suggestive of compartment syndrome, and further investigation may be necessary. Of note, measurement of compartment pressures often provides little clinical guidance.

Limb ischemia can occur in the absence of compartment syndrome and is a frequent complication of ECMO therapy. The presence of a cannula within an artery (especially with percutaneous femoral artery cannulation) may lead to inadequate distal perfusion. This inadequate perfusion is exacerbated by hemodynamic instability, the need for vasopressors, thromboembolism, compression of the femoral artery and vein, or vascular trauma during cannulation. This risk is mitigated by the usage of a distal perfusion cannula, which is a standard practice at many high-volume ECMO centers [20].

4.2. Hemorrhage

Despite widespread use of antithrombotic surface coatings on ECMO equipment, it remains standard of care that patients on ECMO are on therapeutic anticoagulation. In the majority of patients, unfractionated heparin is used to mitigate the risk of thrombotic events, with the subsequent increased risk of both minor and major bleeding events. The 2014 Extracorporeal Life Support Organization (ELSO) guidelines on anticoagulation therapy provide definitions of both major and minor bleeding events. Major bleeding events are defined as a drop in hemoglobin by at least 2 g/dL within 24 hours, loss of 20 mL/kg of blood within 24 hours, the requirement of at least one 10 mL/kg packed red blood cells (PRBC) transfusion within 24 hours, or the need for reoperation or re-cannulation secondary to bleeding [22]. Blood loss

http://dx.doi.org/10.5772/intechopen.76506

in ECMO patients may present as bleeding at cannulation sites (or at the sites of other vascular access), or may present as a retroperitoneal hematoma, mediastinal hemorrhage (especially in post-operative patients), cardiac tamponade, pulmonary hemorrhage, gastrointestinal (GI) bleeds, intracranial hemorrhage, epistaxis, and hematuria, among others [18].

Minor bleeding is defined by ELSO as a loss of less than 20 mL/kg/day of blood or a requirement of 10 mL/kg or less of PRBC transfusion per day. The most significant concern of minor bleeding events is progression to a major bleeding event, and thus these harbingers must be investigated. Any major bleeding event while on ECMO therapy is known to greatly increase patient mortality [22].

4.3. Thrombosis

Thrombosis is a common occurrence and a concern for patients on prolonged ECMO therapy. Exposure of the patient's blood to foreign substances, non-physiological shear stress, endothelial injury, immobility, alteration of normal blood flows, and critical illness increases the risk of a thrombotic event. In order to mitigate this risk, most modern ECMO circuits are lined with antithrombotic surface coatings that reduce the risk of thrombosis. While cannulated, patients are typically anticoagulated with unfractionated heparin, although there is the risk of developing heparin-induced thrombocytopenia. For these patients, or other patients with a contraindication to unfractionated heparin, direct thrombin inhibitors or factor XIIa inhibitors should be used. Naturally, these options carry a risk of hemorrhagic complication, may be more difficult to titrate, and may pose difficulty in the reversal of anticoagulation if necessary for hemorrhage or procedures [22].

The development of thrombus not only occurs within the patient's native vasculature, but thrombus can develop throughout the ECMO circuit. Oxygenators, connectors, and stopcocks are needed for thrombus formation, due to disrupted local blood flow patterns, non-physiologic shear stresses, and foreign surfaces. Thrombus developed within the ECMO circuit can embolize, and cerebrovascular event such as ischemic stroke and limb ischemia secondary to thromboembolism are of major concern [19].

4.4. Cerebrovascular events

Cerebrovascular events, while on prolonged ECMO therapy can be devastating, leading to increased mortality, permanent neurological deficits, and, in bridge-to-transplant patients, loss of transplant candidacy. Any sudden change to neurologic function in the ECMO patient warrants further workup, including full neurological examination and imaging. If applicable, sedation should be weaned to facilitate accurate neurological examination. Cerebrovascular events can be broadly categorized into hemorrhagic or ischemic stroke. The prolonged exposure to therapeutic anticoagulation places these patients at an increased risk of hemorrhagic stroke [19]. As discussed, hemorrhagic stroke is classified as a major bleeding event, and immediate management is necessary.

Despite therapeutic anticoagulation, patients are also at risk for ischemic stroke, as a result of thromboembolism. As discussed in the section on thrombosis, prolonged ECMO therapy creates disturbances to blood flow, presence of a foreign body, endothelial injury, chronic illness, and non-physiologic shear stress—all of which increase the risk of thromboembolism. For patients on venoarterial ECMO, or in patients with an atrial septal defect or pulmonary arteriovenous malformation, thrombus from the ECMO circuit can travel to the systemic circulation and potentially embolize in the cerebral vasculature.

Cerebral ischemia can also occur without embolus. In patients on venoarterial ECMO with blood return in the femoral artery, it is possible for the great vessels to receive poorly oxygenated blood from the dysfunctional lungs, while the remainder of the body is perfused by well-oxygenated blood from the ECMO circuit. This phenomenon, known as Harlequin syndrome, can lead to chronic cerebral hypoxia [23]. Like other cerebrovascular events, this condition warrants immediate investigation and remedy. There are multiple solutions to this inadequate mixing, ranging from repositioning of the arterial return cannula within the femoral artery, conversion to veno-venoarterial ECMO (which delivers oxygenated blood to the right atrium as well as the arterial circulation), central cannulation of the aorta, or operative cannulation of the subclavian vessels.

4.5. Acute kidney injury

Acute kidney injury (AKI) secondary to ECMO therapy is a relatively common occurrence and is associated with a fourfold increase in mortality when it progresses to chronic kidney disease or end-stage renal failure. The development of AKI is common in critical illness and the underlying disease process necessitating ECMO initiation places the patient at risk for AKI. Additionally, ECMO itself can exacerbate the progression of AKI, due to potential changes to renal perfusion, chronic inflammation resulting in renal injury, changes to endocrine homeostasis, as well as the risk of exposure to nephrotoxic substances during a period of prolonged critical care [24].

4.6. Infection

Patients on long-term ECMO therapy are at significant risk of infectious complications. The combined presence of critical illness, chronic blood-contacting medical devices, and an ICU stay greatly increase the likelihood of infection. Patients on long-term ECMO who develop a systemic infection have an increased mortality rate, possibility for loss of transplant candidacy, and increased complexity of care. Many patients decompensate to a level requiring ECMO as a result of an infectious process, with pneumonia a common presenting condition. Due to the presence of indwelling cannulae, bloodstream infection is a major concern in caring for the ECMO patient. For the long-term ECMO patient, prolonged exposure to nosocomial pathogens is of particular concern, as these pathogens are likely to exhibit multidrug resistance. Cannula site infections may also occur, which require re-cannulation at a distant site, as well as debridement and drainage of the infected cannulation site. Infection at a cannulation site places patients at risk for vascular complications, such as hemorrhage, hematoma, arteriovenous fistula formation, or development of an aneurysm or pseudoaneurysm. Treatment of the infected ECMO patient can be a particular challenge, and consultation with Infectious Disease specialists is often required. The gas exchange requirements of the ECMO circuit result in the development of a large surface area, which results in a large foreign attachment site for bacteria.

Development of biofilms and reduced antimicrobial penetration within the ECMO circuit are factors which contribute to difficult treatment of these patients [18, 19, 25, 26].

5. Rehabilitation

Like all patients with organ failure, patients requiring ECMO therapy for cardiac or respiratory failure are critically ill and are subject to ICU-related complications, deconditioning, and muscle wasting. In the earliest applications of ECMO, patients were highly sedated and immobilized. With technological developments and advancements in ECMO patient management, the once sedated ECMO patient has now been awakened and extubated. In the population of patients with respiratory failure, the awake ECMO technique showed promising results, with improved survival over sedated ECMO patients and mechanically ventilated patients. Currently, patients on ECMO frequently receive physical therapy, with ambulatory physical therapy the goal for many patients.

Physical therapy in the ECMO patient begins with stationary strengthening and mobility exercises, performed supine while in their ICU bed. These typically consist of core strengthening, limb raises, and stretching. The patient is then progressed to exercises while sitting on their bed, with strengthening of their core and limbs, as well as sitting balance as a goal. When tolerating this, the patient can be transitioned to a chair to be out of bed for a period of each day. With assistance, the patient on ECMO can stand and then ambulate [27].

Patients who cannot ambulate due to either preexisting mobility deficits or incompatible cannulation sites can exercise using a stationary bicycle or an upper body hand bike. In general, access of the femoral vessels limits the ability of patients to ambulate while on ECMO, and for the long-term ECMO patient, transition to other cannulation sites may be necessary. Notably, femoral cannulation is not an absolute contraindication to ambulation, and many centers ambulate patients on ECMO despite venous and arterial access to the femoral vessels.

The approach to ambulatory physical therapy begins with patient preparation, with many centers electing to free the femoral vessels from cannulation as a first step. With adequate ECMO oxygenation, patients may then be extubated if possible; if patients are not candidates for extubation, placement of a tracheostomy can facilitate secretion management, weaning from the ventilator, and weaning of sedation. Following these preparatory procedures, the patient is ready to begin active physical therapy, culminating in ambulation. This is a resource-intensive task, requiring physicians, nurses, perfusionists, respiratory therapists, physical therapists, and assistants. Particular attention must be paid to cannula management, as cannula dislodgement has significant adverse consequences [28].

6. Ethical considerations

Since the earliest use of ECMO for short-term life support, the technology has produced ethical dilemmas. The earliest ECMO systems exposed patients to significant risk of morbidity and mortality, and it was not until maturation of the technology and critical care that ECMO could clearly demonstrate benefit to patients. The decision to cannulate a patient and initiate ECMO therapy is viewed as the pinnacle of aggressive modern critical care, and early identification of a decannulation strategy can pose an ethical concern. This is particularly important for patients who are unlikely to recover and will not be a candidate for transplantation. For the patient supported on ECMO for a prolonged duration, the principle ethical concern arises when determining that continuation of ECMO therapy is futile, and this section explores the concept. Indeed, the ethical dilemmas surrounding ECMO may have contributed to the use of ECMO for long-term treatment, as disagreements between the patient's family and treatment teams can result in prolonged duration of ECMO therapy.

A reported case of a 44-year-old patient who received 37 days of venovenous ECMO for severe *Klebsiella pneumonia* offers an insight into the ethical conundrum facing patients, their family, and the medical team. The case reports that the patient was not a candidate for lung transplant and was treated with long-term venovenous ECMO due to severe respiratory failure. With radiographic signs of irreversible lung damage, the treatment team recommended discontinuation of ECMO. The patient's family would not accept this outcome, however, and despite support from the hospital ethics board to withdraw care, threats of medicolegal action challenged the transition to comfort care. Ultimately, the patient died on day 88 of ECMO after deteriorating with septic shock. This case highlights important guidelines to be established to prevent ethical disagreements with patients and family members. Specifically, the authors suggest that ECMO centers specify (1) guidelines for patient selection, (2) consent process, (3) family engagement and education, (4) protocols for circuit configuration and concomitant care, (5) duration of ECMO therapy, (6) futility, (7) managing impasse, and (8) Quality Assurance [29]. The authors specify that the consent process should include indications for ECMO withdrawal in case of futility and further indicate that venoarterial ECMO of greater than 3 weeks or venovenous ECMO for greater than 3 months should be considered as unusual circumstances.

The management of ECMO therapy in patients without a decannulation strategy is further complicated when the patient is awake and an active participant in their care. A case report by Moon et al. presented a 53-year-old patient on venovenous ECMO for acute respiratory failure [30]. After 4 weeks of ECMO treatment, recovery of native lung function appeared unlikely, and a lung transplant was suggested to the patient. The patient refused transplantation due to cost and unspecified personal concerns, however. After discussion with the center's ethics committee, a written do not resuscitate (DNR) was obtained and the plan to forgo further oxygenator changes was agreed upon. After 95 days of ECMO therapy, however, the patient showed signs of radiographic improvement, and he was successfully weaned off ECMO care after 104 days. Due to the novelty of prolonged ECMO therapy, it remains a challenge for physicians to fully define the futility of treatment, as it is unclear which patients will recover on prolonged ECMO treatment.

In 2013, a physician survey was conducted to examine the nature of authoritative decision-making during venoarterial ECMO care [31]. The purpose of the study was to assess physician attitudes toward the doctor-patient engagement in ECMO therapy versus a medical professional dominated form of decision-making. This survey of 179 physicians concluded that the majority of physicians with experience in administration of venoarterial ECMO are in favor of physicians having authority for decision-making. The majority of the physicians surveyed also

http://dx.doi.org/10.5772/intechopen.76506

felt that authority in decision-making should extend to termination of venoarterial ECMO therapy against the wishes of the patient's surrogate. They credited this finding to the perceived complexity of the technology and the inability to properly inform and educate the patient and patient surrogates. Without suitable patient and patient surrogate understanding of the complex treatment plan, proper joint decision-making in ECMO therapy may be difficult to achieve.

The ethical dilemmas surrounding long-term ECMO therapy highlight the importance of maintaining good rapport with both the patient and their family. The technology surrounding ECMO is complex, and it is important for the physicians to have honest conversations with patients and their families to ensure that the benefits, risks, and limitations of ECMO therapy are well understood. One can envision a future where technological and therapeutic advancements obviate the need for careful navigation of ethical issues, but at present, the onus is on the physician to bridge the gap between patient preferences and realistic outcomes.

7. Future directions

If current trends are indicative of the future, ECMO will continue to be used for long-term respiratory and circulatory support, with the duration of support continuing to increase. Currently, animal studies in ECMO are focusing on high-mobility devices, with the current designs being compact, paracorporeal, and portable. The immediate goal of these devices is to allow the patients to freely ambulate with minimal assistance, with the long-term goal of allowing patients to leave the ICU, and possibly leave the hospital.

Advances in control systems may allow for the development of adaptive ECMO systems, which can automatically modify the blood and sweep gas flows to match the metabolic demands of patients. These devices aim to allow for increased mobility, greater device efficiency (and smaller size), and improved safety. Currently, such devices are in benchtop or animal studies, without incorporation into clinical practice. In one study of six adult pigs placed on venovenous ECMO, a control system was able to maintain automated blood and sweep gas flows over a 6-hour period [32]. Other such reports exist in the literature, and ECMO is ripe for application of advancements in biomedical engineering.

One further area of investigation is the use of novel surface coatings to reduce the need for anticoagulation and improve the biocompatibility of the ECMO circuit. Development in this area will reduce the risk of hemorrhagic and thromboembolic complications associated with ECMO and may prove to reduce immune cell activation and infectious complications as well.

Author details

R. Gregory Conway, Douglas Tran, Bartley P. Griffith and Zhongjun J. Wu*

*Address all correspondence to: zwu@som.umaryland.edu

Department of Surgery, University of Maryland School of Medicine, Baltimore, Maryland, USA

References

[1] Hill JD, O'Brien TG, Murray JJ, et al. Prolonged extracorporeal oxygenation for acute post-traumatic respiratory failure (shock-lung syndrome): Use of the bramson membrane lung. The New England Journal of Medicine. 1972;**286**(12):629-634

[2] Conrad S, Rycus P, Dalton H. Extracorporeal life support registry report 2004. ASAIO Journal. 2005;**51**(1):4-10. http://ovidsp.ovid.com/ovidweb.cgi?T=JS&NEWS=n&CSC=Y&PAGE=fulltext&D=ovft&AN=00002480-200501000-00002. DOI: 10.1097/01.MAT.0000151922.67540.E9

[3] Paden M, Conrad S, Rycus P, Thiagarajan R. Extracorporeal life support organization registry report 2012. ASAIO Journal. 2013;**59**(3):202-210. http://ovidsp.ovid.com/ovidweb.cgi?T=JS&NEWS=n&CSC=Y&PAGE=fulltext&D=ovft&AN=00002480-201305000-00003. DOI: 10.1097/MAT.0b013e3182904a52

[4] Barbaro R, Paden M, Guner Y, et al. Extracorporeal life support organization registry international report 2016. ASAIO Journal. 2017;**63**(4):456-463. DOI: 10.1097/MAT.0000000000000603

[5] Wang C, Chou C, Ko W, Lee Y. Rescue a drowning patient by prolonged extracorporeal membrane oxygenation support for 117 days. The American Journal of Emergency Medicine. 2010;**28**(6):750.e7. http://www.sciencedirect.com/science/article/pii/S0735675709005567. DOI: doi.org/10.1016/j.ajem.2009.11.011

[6] Kon ZN, Wehman PB, Gibber M, et al. Venovenous extracorporeal membrane oxygenation as a bridge to lung transplantation: Successful transplantation after 155 days of support. The Annals of Thoracic Surgery. 2015;**99**(2):704-707. http://www.ncbi.nlm.nih.gov/pubmed/25639416. DOI: 10.1016/j.athoracsur.2014.04.097

[7] Biscotti M, Gannon WD, Agerstrand C, et al. Awake extracorporeal membrane oxygenation as bridge to lung transplantation: A 9-year experience. The Annals of Thoracic Surgery. 2017. DOI: 10.1016/j.athoracsur.2016.11.056

[8] Hoopes CW, Kukreja J, Golden J, Davenport DL, Diaz-Guzman E, Zwischenberger JB. Extracorporeal membrane oxygenation as a bridge to pulmonary transplantation. The Journal of Thoracic and Cardiovascular Surgery. 2013;**145**(3):862-868. http://www.ncbi.nlm.nih.gov/pubmed/23312979. DOI: 10.1016/j.jtcvs.2012.12.022

[9] Camboni D, Philipp A, Lubnow M, et al. Support time-dependent outcome analysis for veno-venous extracorporeal membrane oxygenation. European Journal of Cardio-Thoracic Surgery. 2011;**40**(6):1341-1347. https://www.sciencedirect.com/science/article/pii/S1010794011004969. DOI: 10.1016/j.ejcts.2011.03.062

[10] Kon ZN, Dahi S, Evans CF, et al. Long-term venovenous extracorporeal membrane oxygenation support for acute respiratory distress syndrome. The Annals of Thoracic Surgery. 2015;**100**(6):2059-2063. http://www.ncbi.nlm.nih.gov/pubmed/26296269. DOI: 10.1016/j.athoracsur.2015.05.088

[11] Khorsandi M, Shaikhrezai K, Prasad S, et al. Advanced mechanical circulatory support for post-cardiotomy cardiogenic shock: A 20-year outcome analysis in a non-transplant unit. Journal of Cardiothoracic Surgery. 2016;**11**(29. http://www.ncbi.nlm.nih.gov/pubmed/26892226). DOI: 10.1186/s13019-016-0430-2

[12] Rousse N, Juthier F, Pinçon C, et al. ECMO as a bridge to decision: Recovery, VAD, or heart transplantation? International Journal of Cardiology. 2015;**187**:620-627. http://www.ncbi.nlm.nih.gov/pubmed/25863737. DOI: 10.1016/j.ijcard.2015.03.283

[13] Javidfar J, Brodie D, Costa J, et al. Subclavian artery cannulation for venoarterial extracorporeal membrane oxygenation. ASAIO Journal. 2012;**58**(5):494-498. http://www.ncbi.nlm.nih.gov/pubmed/22929897. DOI: 10.1097/MAT.0b013e318268ea15

[14] Javidfar J, Brodie D, Sonett J, Bacchetta M. Venovenous extracorporeal membrane oxygenation using a single cannula in patients with pulmonary hypertension and atrial septal defects. The Journal of Thoracic and Cardiovascular Surgery. 2012;**143**(4):982-984. https://www.sciencedirect.com/science/article/pii/S0022522311012232. DOI: 10.1016/j.jtcvs.2011.10.061

[15] Camboni D, Akay B, Sassalos P, et al. Use of venovenous extracorporeal membrane oxygenation and an atrial septostomy for pulmonary and right ventricular failure. The Annals of Thoracic Surgery. 2011;**91**(1):144-149. https://www.sciencedirect.com/science/article/pii/S0003497510016474. DOI: 10.1016/j.athoracsur.2010.07.036

[16] Machuca T, de Perrot M. Mechanical support for the failing right ventricle in patients with precapillary pulmonary hypertension. Circulation. 2015;**132**(6):526-536. http://ovidsp.ovid.com/ovidweb.cgi?T=JS&NEWS=n&CSC=Y&PAGE=fulltext&D=ovft&AN=00003017-201508110-00009. doi: 10.1161/CIRCULATIONAHA.114.012593

[17] Extracorporeal Life Support Organization. ELSO guidelines for cardiopulmonary extracorporeal life support. Version 1.4. Ann Arbor, MI, USA; 2017. http://www.elso.org

[18] Cheng R, Hachamovitch R, Kittleson M, et al. Complications of extracorporeal membrane oxygenation for treatment of cardiogenic shock and cardiac arrest: A meta-analysis of 1,866 adult patients. The Annals of Thoracic Surgery. 2014;**97**(2):610. http://www.ncbi.nlm.nih.gov/pubmed/24210621. DOI: 10.1016/j.athoracsur.2013.09.008

[19] Meuwese C, Ramjankhan F, Braithwaite S, et al. Extracorporeal life support in cardiogenic shock: Indications and management in current practice. Netherlands Heart Journal. 2018;**26**(2):58-66. DOI: 10.1007/s12471-018-1073-9

[20] Rupprecht L, Lunz D, Philipp A, Lubnow M, Schmid C. Pitfalls in percutaneous ECMO cannulation. Heart, Lung and Vessels. 2015;**7**(4):320 http://www.ncbi.nlm.nih.gov/pubmed/26811838

[21] Tissot C, Habre W, Soccal P, et al. Successful lung transplant after prolonged extracorporeal membrane oxygenation (ECMO) in a child with pulmonary hypertension: A case report. Research In Cardiovascular Medicine. 2016;**5**(3):e32545

[22] Extracorporeal Life Support Organization. ELSO Guidelines on Anticoagulation. Ann Arbor, MI, USA; 2014. http://www.elso.org

[23] Hanshi A, Masoud SA, Al Othmani F. A case study of harlequin syndrome in VA-ECMO. Qatar Medical Journal. 2017. DOI: http://www.qscience.com/doi/full/10.5339/qmj.2017.swacelso.39, 10.5339/qmj.2017.swacelso.39

[24] Villa G, Katz N, Ronco C. Extracorporeal membrane oxygenation and the kidney. Cardiorenal Medicine. 2015;**6**(1):50-60. https://www.karger.com/Article/Abstract/439444. DOI: 10.1159/000439444

[25] Sun H, Sun C, Ko W, et al. Infections occurring during extracorporeal membrane oxygenation use in adult patients. The Journal of Thoracic and Cardiovascular Surgery. 2010;**140**(5):1132.e2. https://www.sciencedirect.com/science/article/pii/S0022522310007373. DOI: 10.1016/j.jtcvs.2010.07.017

[26] Biffi S, Di Bella S, Scaravilli V, et al. Infections during extracorporeal membrane oxygenation: Epidemiology, risk factors, pathogenesis and prevention. International Journal of Antimicrobial Agents. 2017;**50**(1):9-16. DOI: 10.1016/j.ijantimicag.2017.02.025

[27] Lehr CJ, Zaas DW, Cheifetz IM, Turner DA. Ambulatory extracorporeal membrane oxygenation as a bridge to lung transplantation. Chest. 2015;**147**(5):1213-1218. DOI: 10.1378/chest.14-2188

[28] Turner DA, Cheifetz IM, Rehder KJ, et al. Active rehabilitation and physical therapy during extracorporeal membrane oxygenation while awaiting lung transplantation: A practical approach. Critical Care Medicine. 2011;**39**(12):2593-2598. http://ovidsp.ovid.com/ovidweb.cgi?T=JS&NEWS=n&CSC=Y&PAGE=fulltext&D=ovft&AN=00003246-201112000-00001. DOI: 10.1097/CCM.0b013e3182282bbe

[29] Ramanathan K, Cove ME, Caleb MG, Teoh KLK, Maclaren G. Ethical dilemmas of adult ECMO: Emerging conceptual challenges. Journal of Cardiothoracic and Vascular Anesthesia. 2015;**29**(1):229-233. http://www.ncbi.nlm.nih.gov/pubmed/25440649. DOI: 10.1053/j.jvca.2014.07.015

[30] Moon S, Lee H, Moon J, et al. Prolonged maintenance of VV ECMO for 104 days with native lung recovery in acute respiratory failure. ASAIO Journal. 2016;**62**(2):e17. http://www.ncbi.nlm.nih.gov/pubmed/26461237. DOI: 10.1097/MAT.0000000000000293

[31] Meltzer EC, Ivascu NS, Stark M, et al. A survey of physicians' attitudes toward decision-making authority for initiating and withdrawing VA-ECMO: Results and ethical implications for shared decision making. The Journal Of Clinical Ethics. 2016;**27**(4):281-289

[32] Kopp R, Bensberg R, Stollenwerk A, et al. Automatic control of Veno-venous extracorporeal lung assist. Artificial Organs. 2016;**40**(10):992-998. http://onlinelibrary.wiley.com/doi/10.1111/aor.12664/abstract. DOI: 10.1111/aor.12664

Chapter 15

Ventricular Assist Devices

Faruk Özalp and Stephan Schueler

Additional information is available at the end of the chapter

http://dx.doi.org/10.5772/intechopen.79509

Abstract

Heart failure is a common and debilitating disease with about 40 million affected worldwide. While there has been some improvement in the optimal medical therapy over the last two decades there is a worldwide stagnation in the number of heart transplantations which is only available to a very few selected patients. The emergence and progress in mechanical circulatory support strategies over the same period has provided a real hope for those patients who have otherwise similar life expectancy to terminal cancer patients. Devices like the IABP have been around for longer but it was the advent of extracorporeal pulsatile and especially the so-called second and third generation ventricular assist devices that provided a real progress in the surgical treatment of heart failure. Devices like the HeartMate II and the HeartWare MVAD found widespread application as intracorporeal continues-flow left ventricular assist devices. Initially the licences were for bridge to transplantation but more and more patients are now receiving these devices as destination therapy. There are certain specific complications like device thrombosis, bleeding and driveline infection that are related to these devices and are the focus of current research and development so that over the next decade or so that we can anticipate that newer devices may provide a direct alternative to transplantation with the advantage of its availability off the shelf. The ensuing increased usage of these devices will possibly reduce the cost to more affordable rates for the health care providing institutions worldwide which will make them available to millions of patients who have otherwise a very bleak outcome.

Keywords: heart failure, heart transplantation, mechanical circulatory support, ventricular assist devices, VAD complications

1. Introduction

Heart failure (HF) is a common condition affecting 37.7 million people worldwide. In majority of affected patients it can be debilitating chronically if not immediately lethal in some. The burden on the affected individual as well as the wider society is considerable. Currently the best available treatment for worsening end-stage HF despite optimal medical therapy is considered to be heart transplantation with the caveat that it is available for only very few patients who are deemed eligible to be accepted on the waiting lists and survive long enough without precluding end-organ dysfunction for a suitable organ to become available. For the rest the outcome is very poor with an average survival of 50% at 5 years after diagnosis of HF, rates comparable with the diagnosis of cancer. While early extra-corporeal pulsatile mechanical circulatory support has been around since 1960s, it was the advent of continues flow intra-corporeal ventricular assist devices (VAD) that made this treatment widely available as longer term option to advanced HF patients. Last decade has seen a worldwide surge in the use of long-term left ventricular assist devices (LVAD) that has given a new hope to patients together with new challenges. These challenges are based around chronic driveline infections, right ventricular failure, neurological events and the dilemma between thrombosis and bleeding. Recently the focus of research and development has shifted towards alleviation of these complications and development of comprehensive strategies and pathways for acute and chronic HF patients.

2. Heart failure

Heart failure (HF) is one of the most common causes of death while it affects about 37.7 million people worldwide and was identified as an epidemic in 1997 [1, 2]. In majority of patients it can have a debilitating effect chronically if the initial insult is survived. The burden on the affected individual as well as the wider society is substantial. Poor exercise tolerance, chronic lethargy and depression with constant anxiety of sudden death together with frequent hospitalizations are among those factors limiting patients' quality of life (QOL). The burden to the society is highlighted by 1–4% of all hospital admissions in Europe and US being due to HF with an average stay of 5–10 days and readmission rates of about 25% within 1 month and 50% within 2 months after discharge [3].

Over the last two decades the management of HF has improved with optimal medical therapy including ACE-Inhibitors, β-Blockers, loop-diuretics and Spironolactone together with implantable defibrillators and resynchronisation devices. However the best available therapy for advanced HF is heart transplantation with the caveat that it is available for only very few patients who are deemed eligible to be accepted on the waiting lists and survive long enough for a suitable organ to become available. For the rest the outcome is very poor with an average survival of 50% at 5 years and 10% at 10 years after diagnosis of HF. This rate has not changed in the last 20 years whereas the survival when diagnosed with cancer has doubled in the last 40 years. Therefore there is much potential for alternative treatment options of which the ventricular assist devices present a real hope.

3. Mechanical circulatory support

3.1. Emergence of ventricular assist devices

The relative short history of mechanical circulatory support in clinical use started with the invention of the cardiopulmonary bypass machine early 1950s that allowed safe operations on the open heart. The first device to temporarily support the circulation other than for heart operations was reported in 1962 in the form of intra-aortic balloon pump (IABP) [4, 5]. The research into the development of more substantial mechanical circulatory assist devices that was initiated by the National Institutes of Health (NIH) in the US was responsible for most of the progress that followed from the 1960s onwards. Funded by the NIH we had the first reported clinical use of an intra-corporeal and then extra-corporeal ventricular assist devices in 1963 and 1966 respectively by DeBakey's group [6]. A total artificial heart (TAH) was developed in Baylor College of Medicine and then implanted in 1969 by Cooley. Much progress in the following 30 years has been around sizeable extra-corporeal devices that were driven pneumatically with substantial consoles. These were relatively successful so-called first generation short-term devices with pulsatile flow pattern allowing patients in acute heart failure to bridge to recovery or transplantation but were burdened with high rates of mortality and morbidity. Patients were bed-bound, unable to mobilise and could only be supported for few days to weeks. The lack of long-term durability of these devices was the main factor to restrict the use only as a short-term bridge to transplantation.

The next big step towards more usable devices took shape around the millennium with a new so called second generation devices that were smaller therefor implantable and intra-corporeal. These pumps provided a continues flow (CF) pattern generated by an axial rotor which was suspended mechanically in its casing. The lack of pulse was a shock to the medical community that required some debate and time to get over. These CF VADs also required thinner drivelines that helped to reduce the infections often originating from exit sites of large cannula and drive lines of the first generation devices. To date the most commonly used example of these devices is the HeartMate II which is still used frequently. Other rarely used examples were Jarvik 2000 and Micromed DeBakey VAD.

Another quantum leap happened more recently in the last decade when there was a surge in the number of implanted LVAD's worldwide triggered by both the new licences obtained for destination therapies and particularly with further progress achieved with newer so called third generation devices. These devices introduced substantial progress in further miniaturisation, reliability, durability and noise reduction all of which contributed to the usability and long-term manageability of patients who now tend to envisage living with these devices for the rest of their lives. Primary third generation device example is the HeartWare HVAD with recent addition of HeartMate 3 both of which have a centrifugal pump that is magnetically suspended eliminating wear-out with better durability. Miniaturisation meant that they could be implanted entirely intra-pericardial even on smaller adults and children.

Current research focuses in reducing the much feared morbidities. Driveline infections is one and often cited as the 'Achilles' tendon' of LVADs. Progress in transcutaneous energy transmission systems (TETS) promise to avoid the need for drivelines altogether. Special consideration of the right ventricle (RV) is required as the vast majority of VADs is placed for the support of the left ventricle with early and late post-operative RV failure resulting in significant increase in mortality. Strategies have been developed to predict RV failure, to preventively optimise haemodynamic parameters pre-operatively and to improve management post-operatively. The dilemma between pump thrombosis and bleeding can be very difficult to manage and has to be patient specific. Usual long-term strategy involves a combination of warfarinisation and anti-platelet therapy that allows individual attention to patients' tendency to either "bleed" or "clot". Another fascinating area of research is gastro-intestinal AV-malformations and their relationship with von Willebrand factor and CF pattern of these new devices. Newer materials are sought for better biocompatibility and reduced thrombogenic properties.

Due to the unique nature of patients and their LVADs most of established MCS Programs have now comprehensive long-term management protocols involving patients' families, General Practitioners, local emergency departments and hospitals, ambulance services and local government services.

3.2. Current devices

The vast majority of currently used LVADs are the HeartWare HVAD and HeartMate 3. Both are miniaturised and fully implantable into the pericardial cavity and by the use of a centrifugal pump that is magnetically levitated they avoid mechanical wear-out therefore more durable and less thrombogenic. The HVAD has a centrifugal pump that is magnetically levitated with hydrodynamic bearings avoiding mechanical interface resulting with only one moving part that is the pump which is driven by two motors providing a continuous flows of blood. The HVAD System weighs at 160 g and is small enough to fit intra-pericardial in most patients with dilated cardiomyopathy. There have been reports of two pumps for bi-ventricular support and some paediatric use to ages below 10 years all of which placed fully intra-pericardial [7–9]. Only some restrictive cardiomyopathy and smaller children present a challenge due to lack of intra-pericardial space. The HeartMate 3 is similar in design and function with certain differences. These include full magnetic levitation without hydrodynamic bearings allowing for the rotor to operate in wider RPM ranges which in turn allows flows between 2.5 and 10.0 L/min and larger gaps between the rotor and the casing reducing the haemolysis and sheer stress to the blood. There is also an attempt to address the concerns about CF in regards to its causative effects on AVM's by incorporating a degree of pulsatility to the flow profile. The Abiomed Impella device is a different approach which includes the option of percutaneous insertion and placement across the aortic valve with blood inlet area in the LV cavity and outlet area in the ascending aorta reaching flows up to 5 L/min. An axial rotor is positioned at the outlet area. Common complications include haemolysis, device thrombosis, bleeding, vascular injury and arrhythmia [10, 11]. There are numerous other short- and long-term ventricular assist devices available however these are less frequently used by the majority of centres specialising in MCS.

3.3. Patient selection

Each patient in heart failure requires individualised assessment for suitability for MCS implantation which proposes only one aspect of patient management. Patient and device choice depend on the indication and purpose of the MCS implantation. Statistically over the last decade the majority of patients treated with assist devices fall in to Intermacs classes 1–4. **Table 1** describing severity of heart failure according Intermacs classification (Interagency Registry for Mechanically Assisted Circulatory Support) and expected survival of patients in each category which helps to determine the urgency of the intervention as well as its type.

http://dx.doi.org/10.5772/intechopen.79509

Intermacs level	Short code	Definition	Expected survival: action required
Level 1	"Crash-and-burn"	Critical cardiogenic shock, oliguria/anuria, rising lactate levels and liver function tests	Hours/days: immediate intervention required
Level 2	"Sliding fast"	Progressive decline despite inotropic support	Days/weeks: intervention within days
Level 3	"Hospital bound"	Stable but inotrope dependent	Weeks/months: elective MCS vs. Transplant within weeks
Level 4	"Frequent flyer"	Resting symptoms, frequent hospitalisation with decompensation	Months/year: elective MCS vs. Transplant
Level 5	"House bound"	Comfortable at rest, intolerant to minimal activity of daily living	Year/s: elective MCS vs. transplant depends on other parameters
Level 6	"Walking wounded"	Exertion intolerant, can only manage normal activity of daily living	Year/s: elective MCS vs. transplant depends on other parameters
Level 7	NYHA III	Advanced NYHA III	Years: medical management, MCS or transplant not indicated

Table 1. Intermacs classification with definitions and management strategies.

Level 1: patients in this category usually present with fulminant myocarditis or more commonly after complicated myocardial infarction when primary PCI failed to restore the resulting acute loss of pump function of the heart. If there is sufficient evidence that the individual would be suitable transplant candidate than a longer term MCS could be considered but in reality in this emergency setting this evidence is lacking so that in most cases short-term MCS device is chosen as salvage and bridge to decision. Devices to consider for these patients include intra-aortic-balloon-pump (IABP), extra-corporeal-membrane-oxygenator (ECMO) or more recently the Impella device or TandemHeart. While the application of ECMO usually requires a dedicated centre, the insertion and management of IABP or Impella is less cumbersome but only provide partial support of the circulation. Occasionally the Impella device is also used for right ventricular support either in addition to the left sided support or in isolation. There are reports from highly specialised ECMO centres achieving relatively high survival rates for ECMO application on patients with out-of-hospital-cardiac-arrest (OOHCA) and ongoing CPR [12].

Level 2: these patients are deteriorating despite escalating inotropic support and usually show end-organ dysfunction and not expected to survive more than days or weeks. They are either unfit for transplantation due to end-organ dysfunction or not expected to survive long enough for a suitable donor-heart to become available. Considerations for Level 2 patents include destination therapy or bridge to either decision or candidacy/transplantation. Devices for this category include HVAD or HM3 among other less often used devices as well as even less commonly used total artificial heart systems (TAH). More common than TAH is the temporary support of the right ventricle with extra-corporeal CentriMag in addition to an LVAD. If there is complicating respiratory dysfunction, it is easy to add an oxygenator to the CentriMag circuit and await recovery.

Level 3 and 4: these patients have a very poor quality of life being either hospital bound or admitted frequently. They also often have end-organ dysfunction that precludes them from listing for transplantation. If they are suitable for transplantation and have preferable blood group/typing and body weight and if the geographical donor pool is preferable making heart transplantation likely within few weeks or months then waiting for transplantation may be a good option. However in reality in most centres in the world overcoming all of these postulations and receive a successful heart transplantation is preserved to a very few lucky ones. In vast majority patients at this level of disease progression present considerable disease burden and require MCS in an elective fashion. Left ventricular support with HVAD and HM3 are most commonly used. In patients with concomitant right ventricular dysfunction there are different approaches available. Mostly, pre- and post-operative optimisation and attentive management of the body fluid equilibrium are sufficient to prevent right ventricular failure. Sometimes a temporary RVAD with CentriMag is required to overcome the immediate intra- and post-operative insult to the right ventricle. A right sided Impella is also an option in this setting.

Level 5 and 6: patients at these levels of disease progression are usually stable in the short and medium term period therefore could be placed on heart transplant waiting lists with close follow up to early pick up any sign of deterioration or end-organ dysfunction. Some patients in this category present or develop pulmonary hypertension precluding them from listing for transplantation which can be improved with an LVAD therapy rendering them into a candidacy position. Generally these patients are not considered for MCS as the heart failure burden is comparable with the burden of any type of mechanical support is often accompanied. In the coming years this cohort of patients will become increasingly the focus when we can significantly reduce the frequently observed complications related to MCS.

3.4. Peri-operative management

End-stage heart failure with diminished organ perfusion has a detrimental effect to most of organ systems of the body. Renal dysfunction due to reduced cardiac output, liver dysfunction due to cardiac output as well as congestion, nutritional depletion due to dysfunctional gastrointestinal absorption as well as liver dysfunction causing physical debilitation, respiratory dysfunction due to congestion as well as pulmonary hypertension, upwards regulation of the systemic inflammatory responses, cognitive impairment due to hypoxia and psychological implications due to constant anxiety and burden of the disease all contribute to push the individual into a vicious circle and downwards spiral of end-stage heart failure. Any MCS system aiming to alleviate the underlying cardiac dysfunction is bound to fail if these organ systems are not concomitantly addressed.

Aggressive fluid removal with high dosages of loop-diuretics and/or renal replacement therapy in form of haemofiltration may be required on top of optimal medical therapy which includes β-Blockers, ACE-Inhibitors and Spironolactone. The achievement of the ideal fluid equilibrium sets the right ventricle in a best possible starting position to overcome the strains of the operation and the increased cardiac output that will be provided by the LVAD. The use of infused phosphodiesterase inhibitors and inhaled nitric oxide can support the right ventricle in this immediate post-operative period. Cardiac arrhythmia needs to be treated aggressively for the same purpose.

Intensive input from the dietitian as well as physiotherapist and psychologist represent cornerstones of optimal pre- and post-operative management of patients receiving MCS.

3.5. Surgical techniques

The urgency of the procedure and the type of MCS together with the individual clinicians and units experience determines the technique of implantation. Of course there are different approaches to the implantation technique including bilateral small thoracotomies, avoidance of the CPB, using more distal aortic sites for outflow-graft anastomosis and exit point of the drive-line. We will however only discuss the most common approaches of the techniques related to the implantation of the most commonly used devices.

The simple percutaneous insertion of IABP does not require much attention due to its common use and familiarity. The Impella device is inserted percutaneously through the femoral or subclavian/axillary arteries with the help of Fluoroscopy and cardiac catheterisation techniques. The blood inlet area is at the tip of the device which is positioned across the aortic valve in the left ventricular outflow tract well away above the papillary muscles and the outlet area is positioned well above the aortic valve at the level of the sino-tubular junction. Trans-oesophageal Echocardiographic images help exactly position the inlet and outlet areas.

For the implantation of the HVAD the patient is positioned supine and draped exposing the entire front of the trunk including cranially the jugular notch and medial two thirds of the clavicles for the exposure of the subclavian vessels, laterally along the anterior axillary line down to the anterior superior iliac spinosus and further down the lateral thigh and caudally just above the patella. The groins are kept prepared in case femoral cannulation is required for ECMO or additional RVAD support. Standard median sternotomy and ascending aortic and right atrial cannulation is performed for cardiopulmonary bypass (CPB). Techniques avoiding median sternotomy therefor avoiding the need for re-do sternotomy for eventual heart transplantation includes left anterior thoracotomy at the apex which can be localised with TTE, and right parasternal thoracotomy at 2nd ICS can be used with or without CPB. The LV apex is examined and the dimple identified to centre the sewing ring around just lateral to the distal LAD. We use 16 pledged 4/0 Prolene sutures in a horizontal mattress fashion and a layer of sealant to secure the sewing ring in position. Then while the heart is fibrillated a cross incision with a blade is made and the coring device provided in the implantation pack is used to remove a cylindric piece of myocardium within the sewing ring. The HVAD device is then inserted into the sewing ring and fastened with the screw driver provided. The inflow cannula is oriented directly pointing to the middle of the mitral valve which is confirmed with TOE images. The outflow graft is left open momentarily for de-airing. The outflow graft is then sutured with continues 5/0 Prolene sutures just like any other top-end anastomosis right laterally onto the ascending aorta above the ST junction and above the SVC using a side-biting clamp. The clamp on the graft can again be released momentarily before tying the knot for further de-airing of the LV. The driveline can now be tunnelled across the abdominal wall with three exit points in a Z-shaped or V-shaped course initially sub-fascial then subcutaneous. The final exit point is at the level lateral and below the umbilicus either on the right or the left flank depending on patients' handedness and preference which is usually determined pre-operatively if possible. After the driveline is connected to the driver CPB is discontinued slowly and the HVAD started and RPMs set that allow the inter-ventricular septum to be straight and neither bulged to the left nor to the right. TOE is used to assess the septum as well as right ventricular function and aortic valve opening. Volume load, inotropic support, especially Milrinone, inhaled nitric oxide and setting of the RPMs of the LVAD can help to fine tune the patients' haemodynamic equilibrium and prevent RV failure. This is usually the timing for the decision to add an RVAD is made. The implantation of the HM3 is very similar with that of the HVAD with only little differences owing to the design of the pump.

If there is the need for temporary RVAD then CentriMag is often used as extracorporeal centrifugal VAD using the femoral venous cannulation for inflow and a Gore-Tex vascular graft onto the pulmonary artery and tunnelled through the left second intercostal space parasternally and above the pectoral muscle with any aortic cannula attached as outflow. If a more long-term RVAD is required then another HVAD can be used in intra-pericardial position using inferior RV wall or the RA as inflow access and the PA as outflow. The use of TAH could also be considered however the evidence for long-term TAH is scanty.

3.6. Complications

We will investigate not the common complications related to any heart surgery but only those particular to VADs. These include drive-line infections (DLI), pump thrombosis (PT), GI-bleeding, cerebral vascular incidents, right ventricular failure and aortic valve insufficiency.

3.6.1. Driveline infections

Overall DLI incidence is around 10–20% with higher rates observed with devices requiring a pump-pocket or has larger diameter drivelines [13]. This rate is also dependent on patient and procedure risk factors including hygiene, nutritional status, diabetes, urgency of the procedure and implantation technique. Prolonged subcutaneous course is thought to prevent speedy up-migration of potential DLI towards the pump itself with severe consequences however at the same time it increases the potential infection sites by increasing the number of skin breakages to allow the long course. The use of antibiotic containing products deposited at the exit site may also help reduce the infection rate. The burial of the Dacron part of the DL below the skin allowing only silicone-skin interface as well as perpendicular exit of the DL as supposed to lying on the skin can further help reduce the DLI rates. Treatment includes targeted antimicrobial therapy and surgical exploration with debridement and re-routing of the DL. Long-term suppressive antimicrobial therapy is a not too unfeasible option to control and contain infections that are difficult to eradicate or too close to the pump and carry high risk for operative approach.

3.6.2. Anticoagulation

Patients present with different levels of general coagulability, which is why there are rather non-scientific terms like "*clotter*" and "*bleeder*" in existence and in use in the clinical arena. The general state of the patients nutrition and rates of systemic inflammatory response to heart failure as well as to the operative insult has surely more influence to the coagulation tendencies. The resistance to acetylsalicylic acid (ASA) is another more scientific explanation why some patients do not respond to platelet inhibition with Aspirin therefor more prone to thrombosis. Previous events of thrombi especially in the left ventricular cavity or in the left atrium predispose to pump thrombosis. Device type also seems to influence the rates of thrombosis although not proven to be statistically significant. Increased thrombosis is also seen if for clinical reasons lower pump-flow rates are sought with corresponding low RPMs of the device. Consideration to all of the above together with a thrombophilia workup will allow an individualised anticoagulation regimen that requires close monitoring with the available methods. The usual anticoagulation regimen that can be the basis includes initial heparinisation started after 12–24 h postoperative depending on chest tube drainage. Heparinisation is guided by activated clotting time (ACT) at 160–220 s. On postoperative day one Aspirin at around 150 mg can be introduced and later increased to 300 mg per day in single or divided doses. Aspirin response can be measured and monitored with serum anti-Xa levels with a therapeutic target range of 0.5–1.0. Aspirin can be supplemented or replaced with Clopidogrel for resistance or allergy. Dipyridamol is often added to this anti-platelet regimen. Warfarin is introduced on day three or later depending on chest tube drainage and presence of epicardial pacing leads which require removal. The recommended target INR is between 2.0 and 3.0 for most devices.

Surveillance of anticoagulation is routinely done by INR measurements complemented by platelet count and serum LDH. However some centres advocate more detailed assessments including platelet function tests, anti-Xa levels and thromboelastogram (TEG).

3.6.3. Pump thrombosis

The diagnosis of pump thrombosis is suspected primarily if there is increase in pump power with or without pump flow changes. This is due to the fact that the driver has to spend more power to achieve same speed of the rotor which is impeded by the presence of the thrombus either reducing the blood inflow into the cannula or through the pump or the outflow graft or indeed mechanically impeding the rotation of the rotor inside the pump in areas of the rotor bearings. Further diagnostic test is the serum LDH levels which increase relative to baseline surveillance levels. Clinical signs i.e. haematuria, of or laboratory tests for haemolysis the likes of haptoglobin, plasma-free haemoglobin, bilirubin and fibrinolysis products can aid the diagnosis. If the pump thrombosis is large enough to cause reduction of pump output signs of heart failure can resurface. Cardiac imaging with Echocardiogram and/or CT Thorax for visualisation of the thrombus in the ventricular cavity as well as assessment of ventricular filling together with manipulation of the pump speed can be carried out for further differentiate the diagnosis.

Treatment of device thrombosis depends on the severity of the thrombus and its haemodynamic and device related complications. This would include up-regulation of anticoagulation, intravenous heparinisation, systemic thrombolysis or device exchange if the former interventions are not successful. New approaches with intra-ventricular and/or intra-pump thrombolysis and washout are being assessed for safety and effectiveness.

3.6.4. *Gastro-intestinal bleeding*

Intractable epistaxis is mentioned but not further discussed here as often this can be managed successfully with the input of ENT Surgeons. There are several reports and studies investigating bleeding from the entire gastro-intestinal tract (GIT). Obvious predisposing risk factors include reflux oesophagitis, gastritis or inflammatory diseases like Crohn's or Colitis which may present themselves as contraindication for VAD therapy as they will be very difficult if not impossible to manage with full anticoagulation. More intriguing concept in continues flow (CF) LVAD therapy is the often encountered arteriovenous-malformations (AVM) that seems to be associated with von Willebrand factor (vWF) deficiency. There are theoretical and conceptual suggestions that the continues flow pattern of these devices are at least partially responsible for development of AVM's in the GIT. Simultaneously the accelerated speed of the blood through the rotors of these CF pumps is said to be responsible for high shear forces active on the high molecular weight vWF causing distortions/breakages leading to qualitative changes with subsequent reduction of function in relation to platelet aggregation. This combination of AVM's with vWF deficiency gives rise to intractable bleeding occasionally leading to surgical intervention.

3.6.5. *Cerebral vascular incidents*

Intracerebral events are feared for the reason that they are often fatal. They can be of two sometime overlapping pathophysiology namely embolic or haemorrhagic of nature. Embolic events are more often encountered peri-operatively due to particulate matter or air from the operative field reaching cerebral vasculature causing ischaemia. The particulate emboli can originate from preexisting thrombi from the LV or LA cavity, atherosclerotic debris from the aortic manipulation during cross clamping or graft anastomosis or paradoxical thrombi crossing across an undiagnosed ASD. Therefore great care is taken in pre-operative workup to identify these risk factors. Air emboli can be avoided with appropriate and assiduous de-airing manoeuvres aided by CO_2 insufflation of the operative cavity. Later in the follow up period haemorrhagic intracerebral events predominate in frequency and lethality although often overlapped with embolic events that transform into haemorrhagic lesions.

3.6.6. *Right ventricular failure*

Management of the right ventricle in patients receiving LVADs can present itself like a manoeuvre 'between Scylla and Charybdis'. Bi-ventricular assist device implantation has reportedly high mortality therefore efforts are focused into avoidance of RVAD in addition to LVAD therapy if at all possible [14–17]. Strategies have been developed over the last decade that include optimisation of hydrostatic status of the heart failure patients including oral and intravenous pharmacological as well as renal replacement therapies. This effort aims to set the right ventricular filling pressures into the optimal position on the Frank-Starling Curve with the best possible contractility resulting from the actin-myosin relationship. In practice this means to aim to decrease the central venous pressure down to single figures i.e. below 10 mmHg prior to the procedure if there is sufficient time available. Further fluid can be removed using haemofiltration during cardiopulmonary bypass if used. Other peri-operative measures include off-pump and minimally invasive techniques to minimise systemic inflammatory response to the procedure, TOE guided optimisation of the position of the ventricular septum by manipulation of the LVAD speed and the use of pulmonary arterial pressure attenuating pharmacology including intravenous phosphodiesterase inhibitors and inhaled nitric oxide. Comprehensive heart rhythm management including resynchronisation and anti-arrhythmic strategies are required to avoid the undesirable effects of arrhythmia to RV function. Hybrid approaches of endocardial and epicardial ablation for supra-ventricular or ventricular arrhythmias may represent a feasible option in some centres. Continued effort is necessary in the long-term follow up of these patients focussing on hydrostatic optimisation if the right ventricular function is to be kept under control.

3.6.7. Aortic valve insufficiency

The evidence is mounting that show the adverse effect of the continues flow LVADS to the aortic valve [18–22]. Constant closure of the valve during LVAD support encourages fusion of the leaflets leading to stenosis. More importantly the lack of physiological movements of the leaflets during the cardiac cycle leads to worsening of mild to moderate regurgitation with increased morbidity. Over time an increasing portion of the pump flow returns back to the LV cavity creating a short circuit with resulting peripheral hypo-perfusion and LV filling pressures consequently return of heart failure symptoms. Manipulation of pump speeds to achieve sufficient aortic valve opening is proposed by large MCS Centres. Bioprosthetic aortic valve replacement for more than mild aortic regurgitation at the time of LVAD implantation has been advocated by experts more frequently in recent years.

3.7. Long-term management

The patient population with long-term LVAD therapy has been increasing due to the improved technology and the management strategies of the complications. More patients are now receiving LVADs as de-facto destination therapy as there is no other promising treatment option available for patients who do not belong to the lucky few transplant recipients. This increasing population require close and continued care that is very distinct and individualised. A great number of regional health care services, social services and potentially family and friends need to be involved in the care of these patients. Local emergency services and hospitals need to be familiarised with the specific patient profiles. They need not to panic and commence CPR if there is no pulse. They need to know that some arrhythmia is better tolerated than without an LVAD, that deranged anticoagulation does not always require immediate counter measures, that any infection/sepsis can have amplified detrimental effects on RV function and anticoagulation and that their hydrostatic equilibrium may have a very small margin of safety. Social services and local council authorities have to facilitate emergency measure for power cuts. Relatives and friends or carers need to familiarise themselves with the LVAD driver connections to the drive-line, batteries and power cables and what certain alarms mean and how to contact the appropriate MCS Centre. This close monitoring and cooperation can only be achieved with dedicated VAD coordinators taking on a central role between the patient and their carers, the clinicians and local emergency and social services. Well thought through protocols taking into account the geographic particularities and circumstances are required to accommodate the needs of this distinct group of patients that is certain to grow in numbers in the not so far future.

4. Future developments

The technology around mechanical circulatory support is evolving with an exponential speed which makes any prediction beyond few years futile. We can however look into current work that is focusing in the alleviation of VAD complications and is promising to become clinical practice in foreseeable future. One of these is contactless energy transfer that is combined with subcutaneous implantable batteries allowing transcutaneous energy transfer (TET) and avoid the driveline passing through the skin eliminating the 'Achilles' heel' of MCS Systems [23]. Further work involves strategies aiming for early and more sensitive recognition and treatment of certain complications especially the likes of pump thrombosis. These techniques use remote monitoring systems with in-time assessment and intervention of pump readings and parameters to more finely tune the VAD therapy [24]. Improved biocompatibility of materials used and rotor design will surely be helpful to reduce thrombosis risk as well as to reduce shear forces affecting blood components. Further miniaturisation and less invasive techniques of implantation can be expected to become more common place in the near future and will allow to expand the age spectrum of the recipients. Better understanding and management of right ventricular dysfunction may be coupled with more intuitive bi-ventricular support in order to achieve better and sustainable results. With improved results and better control of complications one can expect to broaden the spectrum of recipients to less sick patients and include Intermacs classes 5 and above to preemptively avoid end-organ dysfunction of heart failure patients.

5. Conclusions

Within a relatively short period of emergence the implantation of left ventricular assist devices have made a huge impact in treatment of end-stage heart failure patients. The development of a new treatment method inevitably brings with it new challenges that limit its spectrum of utilisation. LVAD specific challenges which represent the limiting factors are mainly driveline infections, anticoagulation balances, cerebral incidents and right ventricular dysfunction. We can be optimistic that current research will lead to progress in tackling of these challenges so that we will be able to claim that this therapy method represents a first line management plan for HF patients. Notwithstanding the recent encouraging attempts of widening the donor pool to donation after circulatory death, the number of heart transplantation worldwide has reached a plateau and is only available to very few select types of patients. The prospect of much improved mechanical support methods for the circulation with better manageability represents a real hope for patients in wider age spectrum as well as in earlier phases of disease progression. Sooner or later MCS Systems that are available off the shelf and adaptable to each patients needs have the potential to replace heart transplantation for end-stage heart failure. However we may want to mention here that in parallel there are endeavours in bio-engineering and gene-manipulation which could allow speculations into the 'off-the-shelf' availability of authentic spare organs for each person.

Conflict of interest

The authors have no conflicts of interest to declare.

Author details

Faruk Özalp* and Stephan Schueler

*Address all correspondence to: fozalp@gmail.com

Newcastle Upon Tyne Hospitals, Newcastle Upon Tyne, United Kingdom

References

[1] Ziaeian B, Fonarow GC. Epidemiology and aetiology of heart failure. Nature Reviews. Cardiology. 2016;**13**:368-378

[2] Braunwald E. Shattuck lecture--cardiovascular medicine at the turn of the millennium: Triumphs, concerns, and opportunities. The New England Journal of Medicine. 1997;**337**:1360-1369

[3] O'Connor CM et al. Causes of death and rehospitalization in patients hospitalized with worsening heart failure and reduce left ventricular ejection fraction. American Heart Journal. 2010;**159**(5):841-849

[4] Moulopoulos S, Topaz S, Kolff W. Diastolic balloon pumping (with carbon dioxide) in the aorta—A mechanical assistance to the failing circulation. American Heart Journal. 1962;**63**:669-675

[5] Kantrowitz A, Tjonneland S, Freed PS, Phillips SJ, Butner AN, Sherman JL Jr. Initial clinical experience with intra-aortic balloon pumping in cardiogenic shock. Journal of the American Medical Association. 1968;**203**(2):113-118

[6] Liotta D, Hall CW, Henly WS, Cooley DA, Crawford ES, Debakey ME. Prolonged assisted circulation during and after cardiac or aortic surgery. Prolonged partial left ventricular bypass by means of intracorporeal circulation. The American Journal of Cardiology. 1963;**12**:399-405

[7] Shehab S, Macdonald PS, Keogh AM, Kotlyar E, Jabbour A, Robson D, Newton PJ, Rao S, Wang L, Allida S, et al. Long-term biventricular HeartWare ventricular assist device support-case series of right atrial and right ventricular implantation outcomes. The Journal of Heart and Lung Transplantation. 2016;**35**(4):466-473

[8] Tran HA, Pollema TL, Enciso JS, Greenberg BH, Barnard DD, Adler ED, Pretorius VG. Durable biventricular support using right atrial placement of the HeartWare HVAD. ASAIO Journal. 2018;**64**(3):323-327

[9] Conway J, Miera O, Adachi I, Maeda K, Eghtesady P, Henderson HT, Guleserian K, Fan CS, Kirk R, Pediatric VAD Investigators. World wide experience of a durable centrifugal flow pump in pediatric patients. Seminars in Thoracic and Cardiovascular Surgery. 2018. pii: S1043-0679(18)30083-2

[10] Gaudard P, Mourad M, Eliet J, Zeroual N, Culas G, Rouvière P, Albat B, Colson P. Management and outcome of patients supported with Impella 5.0 for refractory cardiogenic shock. Critical Care. 2015;**19**:363

[11] Lauten A, Engström AE, Jung C, Empen K, Erne P, Cook S, Windecker S, Bergmann MW, Klingenberg R, Lüscher TF, Haude M, Rulands D, Butter C, Ullman B, Hellgren L, Modena MG, Pedrazzini G, Henriques JPS, Figulla HR, Ferrari M. Percutaneous left-ventricular support with the Impella-2.5-assist device in acute cardiogenic shock, results of the Impella–EUROSHOCK-registry. Circulation. Heart Failure. 2013;**6**:23-30

[12] Tan BKK. Extracorporeal membrane oxygenation in cardiac arrest. Singapore Medical Journal. 2017;**58**(7):446-448. DOI: 10.11622/smedj.2017058

[13] Intermacs Web Page for Public Statistical Reports: https://www.uab.edu/medicine/intermacs/reports/public-statistical-reports

[14] Taghavi S, Jayarajan SN, Komaroff E, Mangi AA. Right ventricular assist device results in worse post-transplant survival. The Journal of Heart and Lung Transplantation. 2016;**35**(2):236-241

[15] Oezpeker CCO, Schoenbrodt MMS, Ensminger SSE, Gummert JJG, Morshuis MMM. Temporary RVAD support after LVAD–Longterm outcome. The Journal of Heart and Lung Transplantation. 2013;**32**(4):S285

[16] Fitzpatrick JR 3rd, Frederick JR, Hiesinger W, et al. Early planned institution of biventricular mechanical circulatory support results in improved outcomes compared with delayed conversion of a left ventricular assist device to a biventricular assist device. The Journal of Thoracic and Cardiovascular Surgery. 2009;**137**(4):971-977

[17] Takeda K, Naka Y, Yang JA, et al. Outcome of unplanned right ventricular assist device support for severe right heart failure after implantable left ventricular assist device insertion. The Journal of Heart and Lung Transplantation. 2014;**33**(2):141-148

[18] John R, Mantz K, Eckman P, Rose A, May-Newman K. Aortic valve pathophysiology during left ventricular assist device support. The Journal of Heart and Lung Transplantation. 2010;**29**:1321-1329

[19] Lima B, Chamogeorgakis T, Mountis M, Gonzalez-Stawinski GV. Replacement of the aortic valve with a bioprosthesis at the time of continuous flow ventricular assist device implantation for preexisting aortic valve dysfunction. Proceedings (Baylor University Medical Center). 2015;**28**(4):454-456

[20] Cowger JA, Aaronson KD, Romano MA, Haft J, Pagani FD. Consequences of aortic insufficiency during long-term axial continuous-flow left ventricular assist device support. The Journal of Heart and Lung Transplantation. 2014;**33**:1233-1240

[21] Pak SW, Uriel N, Takayama H, et al. Prevalence of de novo aortic insufficiency during long-term support with left ventricular assist devices. The Journal of Heart and Lung Transplantation. 2010;**29**:1172-1176

[22] Jorde UP, Uriel N, Nahumi N, et al. Prevalence, significance, and management of aortic insufficiency in continuous flow left ventricular assist device recipients. Circulation. Heart Failure. 2014;**7**:310-319

[23] Bocan KN, Sejdić E. Adaptive transcutaneous power transfer to implantable devices: A state of the art review. Sensors (Basel, Switzerland). 2016;**16**(3):393

[24] Lampert BC, Emani S. Remote hemodynamic monitoring for ambulatory left ventricular assist device patients. Journal of Thoracic Disease. 2015;**7**(12):2165-2171